Whole Person Healthcare

WHOLE PERSON HEALTHCARE

Volume 1

Humanizing Healthcare

Ilene A. Serlin, PhD, ADTR, General Editor

Marie A. DiCowden, PhD, Volume Editor

Praeger Perspectives

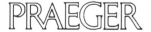

Westport, Connecticut
London

Library of Congress Cataloging-in-Publication Data

Whole person healthcare / Ilene A. Serlin, general editor.
 p. ; cm.
 Includes bibliographical references and index.
 ISBN-13: 978–0–275–99231–6 (set : alk. paper)
 ISBN-13: 978–0–275–99232–3 (v. 1 : alk. paper)
 ISBN-13: 978–0–275–99233–0 (v. 2 : alk. paper)
 ISBN-13: 978–0–275–99234–7 (v. 3 : alk. paper)
 1. Integrative medicine. I. Serlin, Ilene A. [DNLM: 1. Mind-Body and
Relaxation Techniques. 2. Behavioral Medicine—methods. 3. Health Behavior.
4. Holistic Health. WB 880 W628 2007]
 R733.W489 2007
 610—dc22   2007013444

British Library Cataloguing in Publication Data is available.

Library of Congress Catalog Card Number: 2007013444
ISBN-10: 0–275–99231–4 (set)   ISBN-13: 978–0–275–99231–6 (set)
     0–275–99232–2 (vol. 1)   978–0–275–99232–3 (vol. 1)
     0–275–99233–0 (vol. 2)   978–0–275–99233–0 (vol. 2)
     0–275–99234–9 (vol. 3)   978–0–275–99234–7 (vol. 3)

First published in 2007

Praeger Publishers, 88 Post Road West, Westport, CT 06881
An imprint of Greenwood Publishing Group, Inc.
www.praeger.com

Printed in the United States of America

The paper used in this book complies with the
Permanent Paper Standard issued by the National
Information Standards Organization (Z39.48–1984).

10 9 8 7 6 5 4 3 2 1

VOLUME 1: HUMANIZING HEALTHCARE CONTENTS

FOREWORD

When I was a senior resident in internal medicine, I was a little startled to hear one of the most respected senior physicians say to me one day, "You know, Dean, the mind doesn't really affect the body very much. I'm surprised that you believe that it does. And it can't be studied anyway."

This was not *that* long ago—in 1984. And it was at Harvard Medical School's Massachusetts General Hospital, which goes to show how much the field of behavioral medicine has evolved since then.

Because behavioral medicine is a relatively new field, it can be challenging to sort out what is most effective. This three-volume series does a lot of that work for you. It has assembled a group of accomplished experts in the field who can help guide you to understand better what works and what does not, for whom and under what circumstances.

We tend to think of advances in medicine as a new drug, laser, or other high-tech device. It can sometimes be hard for people to believe that relatively simple changes in behaviors, such as diet and lifestyle, can make such a powerful difference in our health and well-being, but they often do.

During the past 30 years, my colleagues and I at the nonprofit Preventive Medicine Research Institute and the School of Medicine, University of California, San Francisco (UCSF), have conducted a series of randomized controlled trials and demonstration projects demonstrating how powerful behavioral medicine approaches can be. We used the latest in high-tech, state-of-the-art diagnostic technology (including quantitative coronary arteriography and cardiac PET scans) to prove the power of low-tech, low-cost, and often ancient interventions.

At the time the conventional wisdom was that the progression of coronary heart disease could only get worse and worse. At best, you might be able to slow the rate at which the disease progressed, but that was about it. We were able to show, for the first time, that the progression of even severe coronary heart disease may begin to reverse using a multifactorial behavioral medicine program of comprehensive lifestyle changes. These included eating a whole-foods, low-fat diet rich in fruits, vegetables, whole grains, legumes, and soy products; getting moderate exercise; practicing stress management techniques, including yoga and meditation; and using support groups to build community and enhance love, intimacy, and healthier communication.

What did we find? Within a month, there was a 91 percent reduction in the frequency of angina, and most patients became essentially pain-free. These patients not only *felt* better, they *were* better; their hearts received more blood flow, and they pumped blood more efficiently. Within a year, we found that even severely blocked coronary arteries became measurably less occluded, and there was even more reversal of their coronary artery disease after five years than after one year. In contrast, coronary artery disease continued to worsen in patients in the usual-care control group. After five years, 99 percent of patients were able to stop or reverse the progression of their heart disease as measured by cardiac PET scans, and there were 2.5 times fewer cardiac events. These findings were published in the *Journal of the American Medical Association.*

Last year, we published the first randomized controlled trial (in collaboration with Dr. Peter Carroll at UCSF and Dr. William Fair at Memorial Sloan-Kettering Cancer Center) showing that the progression of prostate cancer may be affected by a similar behavioral medicine intervention. This study was published in the *Journal of Urology.*

After completing these randomized controlled trials showing how medically effective these behavioral medicine approaches could be, we conducted a series of three demonstration projects showing that these approaches are not only medically effective, but also cost-effective, in people with coronary heart disease. Through our nonprofit institute we began training hospitals throughout the country in our behavioral medicine program that integrates the best of traditional and complementary interventions. Mutual of Omaha found that almost 80 percent of people who went through this program and were eligible for coronary bypass surgery or angioplasty were able to safely avoid it, saving almost $30,000 per patient in the first year. In a second demonstration project, Highmark Blue Cross Blue Shield found that they were able to reduce their costs by 50 percent in the first year and by an additional 20 percent to 30 percent in subsequent years.

On the basis of these findings, Medicare conducted a demonstration project of our approach and another behavioral medicine program based on our work by Dr. Herbert Benson, a pioneer in behavioral medicine who conducted research documenting the power of meditation to elicit what he termed the "relaxation response." Our data were peer reviewed in an all-day hearing at the Centers for Medicare and Medicaid Services by 16 experts, who concluded in a national coverage determination that Medicare should now cover cardiac rehabilitation programs that include behavioral medicine interventions. Since reimbursement is a major determinant of medical practice, this Medicare coverage may help to increase the demand for behavioral medicine practitioners and thus help make the field more sustainable.

Also, medical care costs are reaching a tipping point. Many corporations are beginning to find that their employees' medical care costs are exceeding their entire net profits, which is clearly not sustainable. For example, Starbucks spends more for healthcare for their employees than for coffee beans, and General Motors spends more on healthcare than on steel. As a result, there is a growing receptivity for behavioral medicine programs that have been shown to reduce costs and improve health.

At a time when the power of behavioral medicine approaches is becoming increasingly well documented, the limitations of high-tech medicine are becoming more evident. For example, tens of billions of dollars each year are spent on angioplasty and cardiac stents, even though a recent meta-analysis of all the randomized controlled trials showed that these approaches do not prolong life, or even prevent heart attacks, in stable patients with coronary heart disease. Newer, more expensive technologies, such as coated stents, actually *increased* the risk of having a heart attack. There is a growing realization that it often makes more sense to pay for behavioral medicine interventions than for ones, such as angioplasty, that are dangerous, invasive, expensive, and largely ineffective.

In contrast, the landmark Interheart study examined almost 30,000 people in 52 different countries throughout the world. The investigators found that heart attacks can be prevented in more than 90 percent of people simply by changing nine easily measured risk factors (smoking, lipids, hypertension, diabetes, obesity, diet, physical activity, alcohol consumption, and psychosocial factors), all of which are the focus of behavioral medicine.

Ultimately, behavioral medicine is about transforming our lives, not just our behaviors. Meditation, for example, can be presented as a stress management technique, which it is, but it can be even more powerful if used to help people quiet down their minds and bodies enough to rediscover and experience an inner sense of peace, joy, and well-being.

In our studies, we found that it was not enough to focus on behaviors; we had to work at a deeper level. Many people smoke, overeat, drink too much, abuse other substances, and work too hard as a way of numbing their pain, depression, and loneliness. We found that when we work at that level, people are more likely to make and maintain comprehensive lifestyle changes that are life enhancing rather than self-destructive.

Dean Ornish, MD

Founder and President, Preventive Medicine Research Institute Clinical Professor of Medicine, University of California, San Francisco

PREFACE

Minding the body and embodying the mind are two challenges that face medicine, psychology, and related healthcare disciplines. The better we get—and we are indeed getting better—at treating life-threatening illness, the more we convert previously terminal diseases like cancer and heart disease into chronic illnesses. As life expectancy increases, we expect more from medical care and life itself. The technology that has brought us elegant noninvasive imaging, monoclonal antibodies in the treatment of cancer, statins to lower cholesterol, microsurgery, antidepressant and antipsychotic medication, and microarrays of gene expression, has, oddly enough, created a greater demand than ever for mental methods of controlling and understanding our bodies. It is as though the technological advances in medicine provide not just methods but processes that inspire us to find other ways to manage our bodies better from a psychosocial as well as a biotechnological perspective.

Indeed, the public appetite for integrative approaches to healthcare has grown remarkably. In the past decade the use of integrative services has grown by 1 percent of the population per year (Eisenberg et al., 1993, Eisenberg, Davis, & Ettner, 1997). Americans now spend more money on alternative and complementary medical care than they spend out of pocket on doctors or hospital care. They make more appointments with such practitioners than with primary care doctors. They are clearly seeking something they do not find in modern high-tech medicine. In the past, such contacts were something of a secret—two-thirds of patients did not tell their doctors they were availing themselves of herbal, meditative, or physical treatments such as acupuncture, yoga, and massage. But physicians are increasingly accepting of what is now being called integrative care, and more patients are open about their bimedicality, which is good for both kinds of care.

Another force driving those with medical illnesses to integrative care is the fact that, by and large, integrative services are outside the grasp of health insurers. This means that good old-fashioned market forces drive the development of services. People pay out of pocket for what they want, rather than running the thicket of regulations, approvals, copayments, limitations, and other artificial bureaucracy that plagues healthcare in the United States. People feel more in control of their integrative treatment than of their mainstream medical care. This is a crucial and helpful dimension, since the essence of serious stress is helplessness—the inability to do anything about the stressor. Feeling in charge of a treatment elicits cooperation and a sense of competence. In a classic study of the effect of patient involvement in treatment, Ralph Horwitz and colleagues (Horwitz et al., 1990) examined the effects of beta blockers in reducing risk of death after a heart attack. These widely used drugs, which block arousal of the sympathetic nervous system, are now standard care. Horwitz and colleagues' study demonstrated that these drugs were indeed effective in reducing mortality and that better adherence to the medication regimen was associated with lower mortality. But the surprise in this large randomized trial was that better adherence was also associated with reduced mortality among those receiving *placebo* medication. Apparently, it was their adherence that kept them alive, as much as the medication.

I was asked to see the CEO of a large corporation in the coronary care unit because he was suffering from intractable hiccups. He had suffered a myocardial infarction, and the heart injury may have been irritating his diaphragm. But he had been unresponsive to medication, so they asked me to try hypnosis with him. I saw this man, accustomed to controlling everything around him, flat on his back, wearing little, with tubes going in and out of every orifice. He felt demoralized and helpless. He turned out not to be hypnotizable, but I taught him a relaxation exercise to try to minimize his reactive muscle tension that accompanied the frustration he felt about his illness and annoying symptom. I returned the next day to see how he was doing, and his wife greeted me excitedly, saying he had felt much better after seeing me and was eager to have another visit. Surprised, I asked about his symptom. "Oh, he still has the hiccoughs but just felt so much better after talking to you," she said. When I asked him why, he said, "I have been flat on my back for a week having things done to me. You were the first person who told me there was something I could do for myself." So while objectively I didn't help him with the symptom, finding a way that he could participate in his recovery made a difference to him.

The average doctor spends some 7 minutes with a patient; the average practitioner of integrative medicine 30 minutes per patient. These numbers suggest what is missing in high-tech medical care: attention to the person with the disease. Sir William Osler said that it is more important to know the person who has the disease than the disease the person has. The twentieth century ushered in the era of scientific medicine with the Flexner report, which recommended that medicine be taught in organized curricula emphasizing two years of basic training in the fundamental sciences of medicine, including biochemistry, pathology, anatomy, immunology, and pharmacology. This was a departure from the apprenticeships that had dominated medical training until that time. The Flexner report promoted tremendous advances in healthcare, emphasizing more the science rather than the art of medicine, which was needed, since we were not far from the era of purgatives and blood-letting, which had often inflicted more harm than good. The oldest adage of medicine had been, "to cure rarely, to relieve suffering often, to comfort always." However, in the twentieth century we rewrote that job description to be, "to cure always, relieve suffering if you have the time, and let someone else do the comforting." This was a swing of the medical pendulum too far in the other direction. No matter how good we get at medical treatment, the death rate will always be one per person. Medicine and medical intervention will have to help us live with dying as well as cure diseases.

Whole Person Healthcare addresses this need, presenting in a lively and scholarly way a variety of approaches to helping the person with the disease learn to live better with it. Interventions ranging from essentials of mind-body medicine through psychological and spiritual approaches to art, music, dance, writing, and other applications of creative expression to healthcare are presented by experts in these areas. These experts provide a varied and authoritative review of methods to harness the human in the service of better health. We ignore what is most human in us at our peril. The science and art of psychologically, socially, emotionally, spiritually, and physically expressive intervention in healthcare is growing rapidly and is much needed. These volumes address that need, both for those with medical illnesses and for those who treat them. They are timely and timeless. Enjoy them.

David Spiegel, MD

Willson Professor and Associate Chair of Psychiatry & Behavioral Sciences
Medical Director, Center for Integrative Medicine
Stanford University School of Medicine
Stanford, California

REFERENCES

Eisenberg, D., Davis, R., & Ettner, S. (1997). Trends in alternative medicine use in the United States, 1990–1997. *Journal of the American Medical Association, 280,* 1569–1575.

Eisenberg, D. M., Kessler, R. C., Foster, C., Norlock, F. E., Calkins D. R., & Delbanco, T. L. (1993). Unconventional medicine in the United States. Prevalence, costs, and patterns of use. *New England Journal of Medicine, 328,* 246–252.

Horwitz, R. I., Viscoli, C. M., Berkman, L., Donaldson, R. M., Horwitz, S. M., Murray, C. J., et al. (1990). Treatment adherence and risk of death after a myocardial infarction. *Lancet, 336*(8714), 542–545.

ACKNOWLEDGMENTS

Many people have served as inspiration, believed in this project, and read drafts of various sections. First, our editor at Praeger, Debora Caravalko, has encouraged and supported us through three years of gestation to give birth to these "triplets." Second, I want to thank my family, Florence, Barbara and Erica Serlin, and Jeff Saperstein for putting up with my preoccupation all these years. Friends and mentors, Kirk Schneider, Tobi Zausner, Stan Krippner, and Pat DeLeon were always there with wise advice. Fellow editors, with whom I have collaborated on projects over many years, Marie DiCowden, Kirwan Rockefeller, Stephen S. Brown, Jill Sonke-Henderson, Rusti Brandman, and John Graham-Pole, have been unflagging believers and collaborators in this work. Thanks to Dean Ornish and David Spiegel for supporting the work with their foreword and preface. Finally, all the editors and contributors, whose names appear in each volume, have given generously of themselves and shared their work and expertise.

Ilene A. Serlin, PhD, ADTR

I wish to thank my colleagues who contributed to this volume. In addition to the authors there are many others—clinical and administrative—who work daily to help others heal. I particularly want to acknowledge my mother and father. For years I witnessed their care for myself, our family, and many others in need of healing—physically, emotionally, and spiritually. They set the standard for caring for the whole person.

Marie A. DiCowden, PhD

INTRODUCTION

Mind-body therapies offer an exciting new healthcare frontier. This series introduces the public, healthcare professionals, and students to this future. Mind-body therapies address the complex interaction of mental, physical, and spiritual dimensions of health and illness. Because these therapies deal with the whole person in his or her setting, rather than in terms of isolated disease entities or body parts, this integrative approach is referred to as whole person healthcare. Each volume of this series demonstrates the application of mind-body therapies in a variety of contexts, showing their relevance across a wide range of settings and disciplines. Healthcare practices are expanding from traditional medical settings into new areas such as rehabilitation, wellness programs, and community education—offering practitioners new opportunities and challenges.

These developments are consistent with a variety of recent trends within psychology, such as the "Year of the Whole Person" (Serlin, 2001–2002; Serlin, Levant et al. 2001) and the addition of the word *health* into the mission statement of the American Psychological Association (APA) in 2001. An APA Health Care for the Whole Person Task Force in 2004, under the leadership of APA's president Ron Levant, began to gather evidence of the effectiveness and best practices of integrative collaborative care.

This series presents theory and clinical instruction for bringing a *whole person* perspective to healthcare. Each volume features chapters written by experts in various areas of mind-body healthcare, with case examples and a Tool Kit that lays out basic principles of clinical practice in this area. The afterword for each volume is by a renowned expert in the interface of psychology and healthcare, including the director of the APA Practice Directorate, the director of the APA Education Directorate, a member of the APA Board of Directors, and a former APA president. The preface is written by David Spiegel, Medical Director of the Center for Integrative Medicine at Stanford University Medical Center, and the foreword is by Dean Ornish, Founder and President of the Preventive Medicine Research Institute. This series has been blessed with contributions from some of the most inspired and creative leaders of the psychology and healthcare community.

What is whole person healthcare? Whole person healthcare integrates the best of medical and psychological practices into a biopsychosocialspiritual model. While traditional psychology has celebrated the Decade of Behavior and the Year of Cognition, it is now time for a psychology of the whole person, which integrates behavior, cognition, and consciousness—body, mind, and spirit. It takes into account the impact of life-style on health issues and educates patients to be informed consumers who practice prevention and make changes in their lives toward self-care and health. It relies on experiential as well as theoretical learning and utilizes symbolic and nonverbal as well as linear and verbal modes of expression, data gathering, and verification. Cynthia Belar, APA's Executive Director for Education, called for an integrative psychology:

> I have spent years educating physicians and other health professionals that psychology had a scientific knowledge base and practice relevant to both "mental" and "physical" health . . . the biopsychosocial model cannot be segmented into its component parts without attention to interactive efforts. (Belar, 2000, p. 49)

Russ Newman, Executive Director of the APA Practice Directorate, used the term "strategic resilience" to describe a new collaboration of psychology with healthcare in which lifestyle plays an important aspect of psychological and physical health.

The whole person approach considers the person in the context of his or her world. It seeks to understand the *meaning* of symptoms, as well as their biological and behavioral causes. Adapting a whole person model is becoming critical for healthcare professionals as an increasingly educated public demands integrative approaches. Growing numbers of people are turning to integrative practitioners for the treatment of a broad spectrum of medical conditions, as well as to reduce stress and enhance personal effectiveness through methods such as meditation, yoga, and acupuncture. These techniques are far less effective if applied mechanically and require a new way of thinking about integration. Psychologists and other healthcare practitioners who hold a whole person perspective are showing how to integrate them into the therapeutic process. The enormous popularity of Bill Moyers's television series

"Healing and the Mind" and the revelation in the January 28, 1993, issue of the *New England Journal of Medicine* that over one-third of Americans utilize unconventional medicine, yet do not tell their doctors, signaled a major shift in public attitudes toward healing (Eisenberg et al., 1998). The trend is growing; a rigorous study done in 2004 shows that 80 percent of cancer patients use complementary, alternative, and integrative therapies (Dittman, 2004; Dossey, 1991, 1992). With its emphasis on prevention and education, integrative healthcare is also cost effective (DeLeon, Newman, Serlin, Di Cowden, et al., 1998; Gazella, 2004, p. 83). The National Institutes of Health (NIH) funded a National Center of Complementary and Alternative Medicine to support research into alternative approaches, and the center's budget and prominence have been growing yearly. NIH also issued a "Roadmap" with an emphasis on prevention and education. The Consortium of Academic Medical Centers for Integrative Medicine consists of 23 medical schools with programs in integrative medicine that include education, research, and clinical training.

Mind and body are interrelated (Rossi, 1986). Candace Pert's groundbreaking work on psychoneuroimmunology demonstrated that the processing of emotions often affects physical illnesses and the ability to heal. Research on healthy humans, as well cancer and HIV-positive patients, has shown that significant increases in immune function and positive health outcomes correlate with constructive emotional expression (Pert, 1997). Holistic perspectives on the self can be found in humanistic psychology, humanistic medicine, preventive medicine, health psychology, and wellness practices.

Integrative healthcare addresses a three-fold crisis in our medical systems: (1) the "completely disgruntled health care consumer," (2) the "disenfranchised, disillusioned physician," and (3) the growing perception that our approach to healthcare "is a broken model" (Gazella, 2004, p. 86). Combining whole person psychology with healthcare practices will revive the morale and effectiveness of healthcare practitioners while opening a wide range of opportunities. Since so many Americans already utilize integrative healthcare, but do so with little useful information for quality control or sound decision making, healthcare practitioners can make a large contribution simply by offering a systematic whole person evaluation and providing listings of available resources. This series goes beyond this, building upon state-of-the-art practices and existing literature to describe how a whole person model can be applied in a wide range of settings and areas of practice.

Beyond making sound theoretical sense, an integrative whole person approach is urgent as we face ever-more complex health issues. For example, one-third of California's 2 million teens are very overweight or obese and are at risk for life-threatening illnesses by the time they reach age 30. The highest rates of these at-risk teens are among Latin Americans and African

Americans. In a study carried out by the U.S. Department of Agriculture, over one-half of all American adults are considered overweight or obese, spending about $33 billion each year on diet books, diet pills, and weight loss programs (Squires, 2001). Both losing weight and keeping weight off are psychological issues that require understanding of motivation, stress factors, coping mechanisms, and social support. An encouraging study at the University of California, San Francisco, suggests positive results from an approach to weight loss (PRNewswire, 2000) in which sustained weight loss resulted from training people in two basic internal skills of self-nurturing and limit setting. Psychological interventions give people more conscious control over their lives while improving their self-esteem and sense of meaning (Yalom, 1980). Integrative therapies are also cross-cultural, opening healthcare to diverse, disabled, and marginalized populations.

Psychosocial support groups have proven to be a significant whole person intervention in healthcare. They have increased quality of life and survival time in cancer patients (Fawzy, Fawzy, et al., 1993; Spiegel, Bloom, et al., 1989). Supportive-expressive group therapies are existentially based and aim to help patients live their lives more fully in the face of a life-threatening illness. A wellness model would focus on how to help ordinary individuals cope with such extraordinary circumstances, while support groups address questions of meaning, mortality, and expression.

A NEW INTEGRATIVE PARADIGM

A new healthcare approach must move away from the culture's "scientific materialism"—with its fragmentation of mind, body, and spirit—to a new integrative paradigm. Nobel laureate Roger Sperry described the coming paradigm shift as moving from this scientific materialism to an integrative, holistic, nonmechanistic, bidirectional model. Scientific materialism is based on the Cartesian dualism of mind and body. The new paradigm would provide "a more realistic realm of knowledge and truth, consistent with science and empiric verification" (Sperry, 1991, p. 255), while including the "ultimate moral basis" (Sperry, 1995, p. 9) of environmental and population sustainability. In Sperry's interactionist, nondualistic model of mental and physical states, causation is determined upward from physical states as well as downward from mental states. In this model, the mind affects the body, just as the body affects the mind.

Consciousness, which brings together the physical and mental aspects of experience, comprises the area of meaning, beliefs, and existential choice. An illness such as breast cancer, for example, might involve the symbolic aspects of a woman's body, her attitudes and sensibilities about her life's meaning, and her understanding of the spiritual dimensions of her existence, as well as a confrontation with her mortality. Out of such confrontations can come a renewed will to live, hardiness, and optimism (Maddi & Hightower, 1999).

Stories of death and rebirth descend into sadness and ascend to joy. Disconnection and reconnection are ancient themes reflected in the myths common to all humankind. With the courage to create (May, 1975), new narratives move the self from deconstruction to reconstruction (Feinstein & Krippner, 1988; Gergen, 1991; May, 1989; Sarbin, 1986). These healing narratives are experienced as coherent and meaningful and have been gaining attention in many areas of clinical practice, including family therapy (Epstein, White, & Murray, 1992; Howard, 1991; Omer & Alon, 1997; Polkinghorne, 1988; Rotenberg, 1987). The act of telling stories has always helped humans deal with the threat of nonbeing, and sometimes the expressive act itself has a healing effect (Pennebaker, 1990). Not all expressive acts are verbal, however. Whole person healthcare embraces diversity of technique and approaches that include nonverbal and multimodal modalities such as the expressive therapies and mindfulness meditation (Kabat-Zinn, 1994). The arts are a particularly effective way to bring symbolic expression and coping mechanisms to people who cannot express trauma verbally or cognitively. From a humanistic whole person perspective, the creative act is a courageous affirmation of life in face of the void of death. Art comes from the basic human need to create, communicate, create coherence, and symbolize. The arts are also transcultural, expressing archetypal symbols that are universal throughout history and across cultures. By bringing the body, ritual, and community back into healthcare, diversity is served by countering the dominance of a white, individualistic European male verbal psychological and medical tradition. Whole person healthcare goals include achieving a gender and culture balance of emotional empathy, self-awareness, assertiveness, instrumental problem solving, and expressiveness (Levant, 2001).

The religious and spiritual dimensions of human nature and human fate are ultimate questions that are integrally related to whole person healthcare. Although long banished by Western medicine, spiritual concerns are proving vital in whole person healthcare. One of the three major themes the National Multicultural Conference and Summit sponsored by the APA in 1999, for example, was "spirituality as a basic dimension of the human condition." It recommended that

> psychology must break away from being a unidimensional science, that it must recognize the multifaceted layers of existence, that spirituality and meaning in the life context are important, and that psychology must balance its reductionistic tendencies with the knowledge that the whole is greater than the sum of its parts. Understanding that people are cultural and spiritual beings is a necessary condition for a psychology of human existence. (Sue, Bingham, Porche-Burke, & Vasquez, 1999, p. 1065)

A healthcare system that separates science from spirit is culturally narrow and "may not be shared by three quarters of the world nor by the emerging culturally diverse groups in the United States" (Sue et al., 1999, p. 1065). Spiritually based rituals have been shown to be effective coping strategies for dealing with life stresses (Pargament, 1997) and serious trauma (Frankl, 1959). However, while a national survey showed that 92 percent of all American reported that "my religious faith is the most important influence in my life" (Bergin & Jensen, 1990, p. 5), most healthcare professionals are unprepared to deal with these issues (Shafranske & Malony, 1990). Learning to deal professionally and objectively with these issues is, in fact, an ethical concern (APA, 2003).

STRUCTURE OF THE SERIES

Each volume of this series is designed to guide readers into a different area of whole person healthcare, and each provides a coherent overview of the field. The contributions are transdisciplinary, from practitioners and programs in psychology, medicine, clergy, public policy, and the arts.

- **Volume 1: Humanizing Healthcare,** edited by Marie Di Cowden, lays a foundation of definitions and practices of integrative healthcare for the twenty-first century. It helps practitioners develop protocols and assess efficacy of alternative practices, emphasizes the relevance of integrative healthcare for marginalized populations, and discusses risk prevention, policy, and issues of patient protection.
- **Volume 2: Psychology, Spirituality, and Healthcare,** edited by Kirwan Rockefeller and Stephen S. Brown, focuses on issues of meaning in illness; the role of spirituality; health and mental health; chaplaincy and pastoral care; and research and practice in yoga, meditation, imagery, QiGong, prayer, ritual, and death and dying.
- **Volume 3: The Art of Health,** edited by Jill Sonke-Henderson, Rusti Brandman, Ilene Ava Serlin, and John Graham-Pole, introduces readers to the history and practices of art and healthcare throughout the ages. It presents the history of art and health in ancient healing rituals; shows the relevance of rituals in the growing number of international contemporary art-in-health programs; and discusses applications of art, music, dance, drama, and poetry therapy programs at the bedside, in groups, and in cross-cultural conflict.

SUMMARY

The Year of the Whole Person provides a timely focus for a much-needed collaboration among healthcare professionals. This collaboration can bring together the best practices from psychology and medicine for a comprehensive treatment approach. The current unsustainable U.S. healthcare system urgently needs a more efficient utilization of services; the underserved patients are demanding that their healthcare professionals talk to each other and combine quality traditional and complementary practices—an experience through which healthcare professionals can rediscover their modern yet ancient roles as healers of the mind, body, and spirit.

REFERENCES

American Psychological Association. (2003). Guidelines for multicultural education, training, research, practice and organizational change for psychologists. *American Psychologist, 58*(5), 377–402.

Belar, C. (2000, September). Learning about APA. *APA Monitor, 31*(8), 49.

Bergin, A. E., & Jensen, J. P. (1990) Religiosity of psychotherapists: A national survey. *Psychotherapy, 27*(1), 3–7.

De Leon, P., Newman, R., Serlin, I., Di Cowden, M., et al. (1998, August). *Integrated health care.* Town Hall symposium conducted at the meeting of the American Psychological Association, San Francisco, CA.

Dittman, M. (2004). Alternative health care gains steam. *American Psychological Association Monitor, 35*(6), 42.

Dossey, L. (1991). *Meaning and medicine.* New York: Bantam.

Dossey, L. (1992). Era III medicine: The next frontier. *ReVision: A Journal of Consciousness and Transformation, 14*(3), 128–139.

Eisenberg D., Davis R., Ettner, S., Appel, S., Wilkey S., Van Rompay, M., & Kessler, R. (1998). Trends in alternative medicine use in the United States, 1990–1997; Results of a follow-up national survey. *Journal of the American Medical Association, 280*(18), 1569–1575.

Epstein, D., White, M., & Murray, K. (1992). A proposal for the authoring therapy. In S. McNamee & K. J. Gergen (Eds.), *Therapy as social construction.* London: Sage.

Fawzy, F. I., Fawzy, N. W., et al. (1993). Malignant melanoma: Effects of an early structured psychiatric intervention, coping, and affective state on recurrence and survival 6 years later. *Archives of General Psychiatry, 50*(9): 681–689.

Feinstein, D., & Krippner, S. (1988). *Personal mythology.* Los Angeles: Tarcher.

Frankl, V. (1959). *Man's search for meaning.* New York: Praeger.

Gazella, K. (2004, July/August). Mark Hyman, MD. Practicing medicine for the future. *Alternative Therapies, 10*(4), 83–89.

Gergen, K. (1991) *The saturated self.* New York: Basic Books.

Howard, G. (1991). Culture tales: A narrative approach to thinking, cross-cultural psychology, and psychotherapy. *American Psychologist, 46,* 187–197.

Kabat-Zinn, J. (1994). Foreword. In M. Lerner, *Choices in healing* (pp. xi–xvii). Cambridge, MA: MIT Press.

Levant, R. (2001). *We are not from Mars and Venus!* Paper presented to the American Psychological Association, San Francisco, CA.

Maddi, S., and Hightower, M. (1999). Hardiness and optimism as expressed in coping patterns. *Consulting Psychology Journal: Practice and Research, 51*(2), 95–105.

May, R. (1975). *The courage to create.* New York: Bantam Books.

May, R. (1989). *The art of counseling.* New York: Gardner Press.

Omer, H., & Alon, N. (1997). *Constructing therapeutic narratives.* Northvale, NJ: Aronson.

Pargament, K. I.(1997). *The psychology of religion and coping.* New York: Guilford Press.

Pennebaker, J. W. (1990). *Opening up: The healing power of expressing emotions.* New York: Guilford Press.

Pert, C. B.(1997). *Molecules of emotion.* New York: Scribner.

Polkinghorne, D. E. (1988). *Narrative knowing and the human sciences.* Albany: State University of New York Press.

PRNewswire. (2000, October 18). First obesity treatment to report sustained weight loss-skill training vs. drugs and diets.

Rossi, E. L. (1986). *The psychobiology of mind-body healing.* New York: Norton.

Rotenberg, M. (1987). Re-biographing and deviance: Psychotherapeutic narrativism and the Midrash. New York: Praeger.

Sarbin, T. (Ed.). (1986). *Narrative psychology: The storied nature of human conduct.* New York: Praeger.

Serlin, I. A. (2001–2002). Year of the whole person. *Somatics,* Fall/Winter, 4–7.

Serlin, I., Levant, R., Kaslow, N., Patterson, T., Criswell, E., & Schmitt, R. (2001). *Healthy families: A dialogue between holistic and systemic-contextual approaches.* Paper presented to the American Psychology Association, San Francisco, CA.

Shafranske, E. P., & Maloney, H. N. (1990). Clinical psychologists' religious and spiritual orientations and their practice of psychotherapy. *Psychotherapy, 27,* 72–78.

Sperry, R. W. (1991). Search for beliefs to live by consistent with science. *Zygon, Journal of Religion and Science, 26,* 237–258.

Sperry, R. W. (1995). The riddle of consciousness and the changing scientific worldview. *Journal of Humanistic Psychology, 35*(2), 7–34.

Spiegel, D., Bloom, J. R., et al. (1989). Effect of psychosocial treatment on survival of patients with metastatic breast cancer. *Lancet, 2*(8668): 888–891.

Squires, S. (2001, 10 January). Only high-carb, modest-fat diets work for long. *San Francisco Chronicle,* A2.

Sue, D. W., Bingham, R. P., Porche-Burke, L., &Vasquez, M. (1999). The diversification of psychology: A multicultural revolution. *American Psychologist, 54*(12), 1061–1069.

Yalom, I. D. (1980). *Existential psychotherapy.* New York: Basic Books.

VOLUME EDITOR'S NOTES

Marie A. DiCowden, PhD

Humanizing Healthcare is a collection of chapters that attempts to bring together, in one volume, a larger perspective on the discussions of current problems in the U.S. healthcare system. It is also an attempt to elucidate some
potential solutions to the problems and challenges of healthcare in the twenty-
first century.

While the United States provides the world's most sophisticated, technologically advanced medical care for trauma and acute illness, quality day-to-day
healthcare is sadly lacking. This volume calls for developing an integrated
healthcare system that will embed the best medical care in a framework of
effective healthcare. Promoting health behaviors, managing chronic illness
or disability, and increasing a functional quality of life are the main health
challenges in the United States today. Humanizing Healthcare presents a
case for developing a healthcare system that focuses on treating the health of
the whole person regardless of age, gender, ethnicity, or financial status. This
means viewing healthcare in the opposite way in which the current system
has developed. Instead of focusing on the illness a person has, as medical care
currently does, the healthcare system should focus on the person who has the
illness. Contrary to popular belief, developing such a healthcare system will
not cost more. In fact, it can have the effect of reducing the present costs of
medical care. However, the development of such a healthcare system requires
a shift in thinking. It requires thinking of healthcare much as we do education,
seeing it as a service industry and not merely as a business. A healthcare system that focuses on the person and defines its mission as assisting that person to

function at the highest level possible in all spheres—even when facing illness or trauma—benefits not only the individual but American families and communities as a whole. However, a healthcare system that focuses on illness and has as its primary goal the making of profits rather than the provision of service runs the risk of ignoring health altogether and limiting medical care, when health does deteriorate, in order to maximize the business profits. This not only places American citizens at risk individually but undermines the health and economics of families and communities as a whole. Authors of the chapters in this book base their writings—clinical, administrative, financial, legal and political—on evidence-based approaches that call for new thinking about integrated healthcare and not just medical care. It is not a definitive volume. It does, however, provide, under one cover, a discussion of many of the aspects of healthcare that have surfaced in debates about the current medical care system in this country and points the way to possible solutions.

We are at a tipping point. What happens in the next few years will determine the healthcare and medical care that is provided—or not provided—for us, our children, and our grandchildren. While complete answers have yet to emerge, it is indisputable that leadership to find workable answers is needed. It is needed in all spheres. This means that patients and families, healthcare providers, and educators need to understand evidence-based approaches to integrated health and weigh in with policy makers to embed quality medical care in a sound healthcare system. The chapters in Humanizing Healthcare contribute to this understanding and, hopefully, provide a beginning for such leadership to find workable answers.

Chapter One

HEALTHCARE FOR THE TWENTY-FIRST CENTURY

Marie A. DiCowden, PhD

A DARK PAINTING

A symbolic painting of healthcare in the United States today might envision a long line of hooded, mysterious, yet all too familiar figures emerging on the horizon of the twenty-first century and intoning a litany of mournful chants: the leading industrial country in the world

- has 47 million people uninsured for healthcare
- has 100 million people without healthcare coverage at some point every year
- has a healthcare system that costs 15 percent of its gross national product
- spends $2 trillion yearly on healthcare, with costs that continue to spiral upward
- reports that half of personal bankruptcies filed are due to healthcare costs
- has a separate and unequal healthcare system based on race, ethnicity, gender, and socioeconomic status
- reports that 7 of the 10 leading causes of death are due to poor health behaviors and lack of social support
- ranks 37th in healthcare overall
- ranks ninth in life expectancy
- ranks seventh in infant mortality
- has 65 percent of its population obese or overweight
- reports that 43 percent of all adults suffer from stress
- turns away ambulances from emergency rooms on the average of one per minute.

Such a picture is dark and foreboding (Institute of Medicine, 2006 and 2002). Indeed, it is such an overwhelming specter that the U.S. Congress has refused to deal with healthcare reform in any global manner since the 103rd Congress walked away from the Clinton proposal for healthcare reform over 10 years ago.

Since then, issues have been debated about the need for consumer-driven health savings accounts, revolutionary information technology approaches, and payment for performance. However, these issues are the microcosm of the larger issues that need to be addressed—cost-effectiveness, efficiency and quality, and access to humane care. The challenge is that to fix the entire broken system, all parts and their interactive effects must be retooled at the same time. Given the way in which healthcare delivery has been structured through private insurance policies and private administration of government programs, healthcare debates have primarily centered on reducing the cost of healthcare through rationing benefits and access to services. This makes sense if healthcare is considered only an economic commodity to be sold for profit. However, following that logic, if the focus of healthcare is on profits, then healthcare is not really the issue—profits become the driving force. Therein lies the fallacy. The product of healthcare should be good health. If a person is healthy, that in itself limits the need for healthcare and drives down the cost of healthcare delivery.

WHICH NEW PARADIGM?

Within the community of healthcare providers and consumers, there is an energy driving toward a different conceptualization of healthcare. Patients are beginning to pursue a different set of values, cost notwithstanding. These values include a focus on wellness and prevention of disease, enlarging the understanding of mind-body interactions in dealing with issues of health and illness, and focusing on connections in their social support system (American Psychological Association [APA], 1995, 2006; APA presidential initiative Health Care for the Whole Person, 2005; Berkman, 1995; Cohen, Underwood, & Gottlieb, 2000; Ray, 2004). The American public recognizes that there is a connection between emotional and physical health (APA, 1995). David Eisenberg's landmark study (Wetzel, Eisenberg, Kaptchuk, 1998) and the subsequently updated survey in 1998 (Eisenberg et al., 1998) reported that more people are pursuing psychotherapy to address health issues. These studies also reported that the use of biofeedback to address physical manifestations of emotional and physical illness was on the increase.

While Eisenberg's studies are generally cited as evidence that the American public is using more complementary and alternative medicines (CAM), such as acupuncture, herbals, and massage—which is also true, according to the studies—it is noteworthy that the definition of complementary and alternative healthcare included chiropractic, biofeedback, and psychotherapy for health reasons as well. Clearly the American public has a larger definition of healthcare than strictly that employed by an insurance- and pharmaceutical-dominated healthcare delivery system (Druss, Marcus, Olfson and Tanielian, 2003). And the public is pursuing this larger definition, regardless of cost. In 1993, $13.7 billion a year was spent, out of pocket, on complementary healthcare (Eisenberg et al., 1993). In 1998, this had increased to an out-of-pocket expenditure of $21 billion a year (Eisenberg et al., 1998). A more recent study (Tindle & Eisenberg, 2005) compared the numbers of Americans using complementary and alternative therapies in 2002 with those reporting usage in Eisenberg's 1998 survey. Reported results indicate that there is a stable number of Americans—more than one in three—using one or more forms of CAM. The greatest increases were in the use of over-the-counter herbals, which increased by 50 percent, and the practice of yoga, which increased by 40 percent. Sixty percent to 70 percent of patients still do not communicate with their primary physicians about the use of complementary and alternative practices.

At the same time that patients are seeking new definitions of medicine, practitioners, along with their patients, are also looking for new models of healthcare. There is a growing awareness that the current system of healthcare delivery is different from the clinical reality (deGruy, 1996). In providing healthcare, there are coexisting mind-body problems to be addressed. First is the individual's behaviors and response to stressors in the community. The mind has a reciprocal effect on the body through the psychoneuroimmunological system. Thoughts affect the chemistry of the body and may make the person more susceptible to disease or more resilient. How a person thinks about and copes with stress impacts his health. When a person does become ill, disease also affects the psyche and may further impede a person's recovery (Ray, 2004). Another category of concern includes patients with severe mental illnesses who often have to address comorbid problems of physical health. For example, extreme weight gain, diabetes, and high cholesterol are often associated with some medications prescribed for more serious mental illness. The ability to navigate the healthcare system to follow up on referrals for physical health is a challenge to individuals who do not suffer from mental health disorders; for someone with an acute or chronic mental health challenge, the task is often insurmountable (Marder, Essock, Miller et al 2004). Third, drug disorders are a particular form of chronic illness that bring a cascade of interactive mental and physical health concerns that need to be addressed very specifically for the individual who struggles with these issues (Pincus, 2003).

In general, there is a disconnect in the current healthcare delivery system between the mental/behavioral care and the physical care provided for each of these types of patients. Clinically, several models of healthcare delivery have evolved to attempt to resolve this gap in care: (1) in large settings, for example, through the Veterans Administration or through large health maintenance organizations like Kaiser Permanente, team-based multidisciplinary and interdisciplinary care is generally provided; (2) spurred by insurance models, there is also a focus on provision of most services by a primary care physician, who acts as gatekeeper to other service providers or (3) collaborates with a case manger to integrate mental and physical health services for a patient; and (4) in cases where severe mental illness is the primary issue, provision of on-site primary medical care in such places as state hospitals has also been attempted in some cases (Druss et al., 2004). For a variety of reasons, primarily economic, administrative, and political, none of these models of healthcare delivery has been consistently implemented across the healthcare system. However, the clinical reality that patients do get better when mental and physical healthcare are integrated is well documented (Druss, Rohrbaugh, Levinson, & Rosenheck, 2001). There is a beginning recognition of this mindbody connection through the American Medical Association's adoption of the new health and behavior codes for treatment, which took effect in 2002. These codes can only be used by physicians and psychologists when psychological assessment and interventions are necessary due to a physical health (not a mental health) diagnosis—for example, when relaxation therapy is used to treat pain or cardiovascular disease, or when imagery is used to treat breast cancer and facilitate the effects of chemotherapy. These codes are now reimbursed by all Medicare carriers and many private insurance carriers.

For that reason, there is a clinical move for more and more association, on-site or utilizing a collaborative model, between primary care physicians and mental health providers (Frank, McDaniel, Bray, & Heldring, 2004; James & Folen, 2005). In 2000, and again in 2006, the American Academy of Family Physicians (2006) endorsed the definition of quality healthcare in family medicine as "the achievement of optimal physical and mental health through accessible, safe, cost-effective care that is based on best evidence, responsive to the needs and preferences of patients and populations, and respectful of patients' families, personal values, and beliefs." The development of integrative professional associations, for example, the Collaborative Family Health Association (http://www.cfha.net), and journals, for example, *Families, Systems, and Health*, encourages combined clinical work and research among mental health professionals, family medicine practitioners, and pediatricians. The American Academy of Pediatrics (2006) also endorses care for the whole person by "providing optimal physical, mental and social health and well-being for all infants, children, adolescents and young adults." And the National Academies of Practice (http://www.nap.org), founded in 1981, is also a professional initiative to develop a recognized, distinguished policy forum that promotes quality healthcare through interdisciplinary education, research, and public policy advising.

There are also burgeoning models gaining ground in integrating other CAM practices into mainstream healthcare. The focus in these models is generally on the use of acupuncture and Chinese medicine, chiropractic, massage, clinical nutrition, and herbal therapies (Faas, 2001). There is a large body of evidence, including clinically controlled studies, that reports that these disciplines provide efficacious care (Stux & Hammerschlag, 2001; Thiel, R. 2002; Meeker & Haldeman 2002; Janisse, 2002). The importance of clinical research in these areas is also underscored by the National Institutes of Health (NIH). In 1992, the NIH established the Office of Alternative Medicine, which has evolved into the National Center for Complementary and Alternative Medicine (NCCAM). While still relatively small compared to other government funding, the budget for this office has increased exponentially over the last 14 years. Beginning with a budget of $2 million in 1992, NCCAM reports a budget of $122.7 million for the 2006 fiscal year (National Center for Alternative and Complementary Medicine, http://nccam.nih.gov/about/appropriations/). The Institute of Medicine (2005) also reports that a number of prestigious medical schools have joined the Consortium of Academic Health Centers for Integrative Medicine, which focuses on integrating traditional Western healthcare with CAM practices. These include such medical schools as Duke University, the University of California at San Francisco and Los Angeles, and the George Washington University. Recent studies also report that, while they are generally being taught as elective courses, the number of medical schools teaching CAM courses has risen from 45 of 125 in the 1996–1997 academic year to 98 medical schools in the 2002–2003 academic year (Barzansky & Etzel, 2003).

Unfortunately, there is little crossover at the present time between the models that seek to integrate CAM practices into traditional healthcare and those models that are moving to integrate mental and physical health (Moran 2003). This trend can be traced to several prevailing assumptions: (1) most alternative schools of healthcare, for example, Chinese medicine, embrace a philosophy that they treat both the physical and emotional components of health through various interventions; and (2) while mental health providers may utilize some form of complementary, alternative care, they have been reluctant to embrace other forms of CAM, for example, acupuncture or herbals, due to a perceived lack of evidence-based practice (DiCowden & Scherer, in press). The appointment in 2003 of psychologist Dr. Margaret Chesney as the first deputy director of NCCAM (now acting director) was a move toward fuller integration of a perspective that includes all aspects of the new clinical healthcare initiatives that are emerging.

SPEAKING FOR THE AMERICAN PEOPLE

In 2003 Congress passed Public Law 108-173 to create the Citizens' Health Care Working Group (CHCWG). The mission of the CHCWG was to engage the American people in public forum discussions to determine what the public wanted in healthcare and how to address the current healthcare crisis. Charged to develop recommendations for the president and Congress, this committee presented its report, "Health Care That Works for All Americans," on September 29, 2006 (Citizens' Health Care Working Group, 2006). This report begins by reflecting on the American values that underlie healthcare delivery as expressed in the various town halls. Rather than an economic commodity, healthcare is viewed by the public as a "shared social responsibility," and healthcare is seen as fundamental to the well-being of all Americans, regardless of "health status, working status, age, income or other categorical factors that might otherwise affect health insurance status." It was the general consensus that Americans want a healthcare system "where everyone participates…with benefits that are sufficiently comprehensive to ensure access to appropriate, high-quality care without endangering individual or family financial security" (p. 8). While stewardship of societal resources is considered important, a sense of urgency and a desire for change to be implemented immediately were equally, if not more important.

Recommendations that reflect these values were made for a five-year transition plan to improve the American healthcare system. The overall goal and the first recommendation was to (1) develop a public policy that all Americans have access to affordable and appropriate healthcare services by 2012. Three areas of concern spawned five additional recommendations:

- *Take immediate action to improve security and access.* Recognizing both the financial burden of healthcare and the difficulty in navigating the healthcare delivery system to obtain needed services, the CHCWG recommends (2) that there be a guarantee for financial protection against very high healthcare costs and (3) that, at the same time, local innovative, integrated community health networks be developed. "Fix the delivery system first" was a theme that developed throughout the public forums.

- *Define core benefits and services for all Americans.* The CHCWG recommends (4) that a nonpartisan public/private group be established by law to define a core set of health benefits and update these benefits on an ongoing basis. Health is to be defined to include medical, mental, and dental health. Evidence-based science and expert consensus regarding the effectiveness of treatments should guide the services that are provided with an awareness that advances in research and knowledge will impact the treatments covered. Healthcare services should focus on "wellness, prevention, primary care, acute care, prescription drugs, patient education, and the treatment and management of health problems provided across a full range of inpatient and outpatient settings" (p. 18). These services should be available across the life span.

- *Build a better healthcare system.* Reflecting the citizen demand to "fix the broken healthcare system," the CHCWG recommends (5) that federally funded programs provide integrated healthcare clinically and administratively. This recommendation focuses on the clinical provision of evidence-based best practices as well as on the need for integrating health information and electronic record keeping. A better healthcare system is also defined as one that promotes health and disease prevention and emphasizes patient-provider communications and patient-centered care and research.

Additionally, another recommendation for fixing the broken healthcare system would require (6) fundamental restructuring of end-of-life care and financing of such care. Care should be appropriate and culturally sensitive so that clinical realities, community-based care, and needed nonmedical services can provide individuals and families the kind of care that reflects their values for the last days of their lives.

The CHCWG, as does all of America, struggles with how to pay for these recommendations. It stops short of recommending that these policies be financed by a national health insurance policy. However, participants in the public forums favored a national health program by a margin of three to one (Physicians for a National Health Plan, 2006). The CHCWG did recommend that some proposed actions be financed by reallocating existing state and federal funds. It also recognized that long-term savings could result from implementation of these recommendations, although immediate actions could result in a financial shortfall to retool and integrate the healthcare system. Throughout the public discussions, the CHCWG indicates that a majority of the American people believe that there are sufficient resources in the system to provide the type of care and access that is recommended. They also indicate that if new revenue sources for healthcare financing are needed, a majority of the public is "willing to pay more to ensure that all Americans are covered" (Citizens' Health Care Working Group, 2006, p. 30). National polls have also confirmed this opinion. The most frequent option presented to raise new revenues is consideration of some form of sliding scale income or payroll tax that is specifically budgeted for universal healthcare.

Financial reorientation of the current healthcare system has been a concern with regard to the disrupting effects on the economy if private insurance is replaced with universal healthcare. This has been a highly significant debate in California, where legislation for universal coverage in that state was recently proposed. However, the economic toll of *not* making changes is also inevitable, in addition to the human toll that the current healthcare system now exacts. In light of the values expressed by the American people that healthcare is not an economic commodity, but a shared social responsibility, the financial allocation of current health funds by private payers from services to administration must be noted. A landmark study of the California healthcare system indicates that overall billing- and insurance-related administrative costs account for 21 percent of privately insured spending in that state (Kahn, Kronick, Kreger, & Gans, 2004). A substantial savings may be achieved by integrating the fractured payment system into a single-payer system. Extrapolating from this California study, the estimated amount the United States would save each year on paperwork if it adopted single-payer healthcare administration would be $161 trillion (Harper's, 2006).

PUTTING WORDS INTO ACTION

One model that addresses a majority of the CHCWG recommendations already exists. It has been in existence for close to 20 years (DiCowden, 2003). This program is called a HealthCare Community (HCC) and has a particular meaning that attaches to such a model. The model addresses the issues, in almost all cases, that the CHCWG identified as most important:

- *Immediate access and continuity of treatment is provided.* Because of the heavy financial burden of healthcare and the difficulty in navigating the healthcare delivery system to obtain needed services, the HCC model provides clinically managed services based on integrated funding, and in many cases, services are provided for a fraction of cost or for free. Patients are not terminated from critically needed treatment if funding runs out. Responding to the need to "fix the delivery system first," the HCC model operates on a local basis, integrating physical, emotional, and evidence-based complementary care under one roof. At the same time it provides a hub for integrating a community network of specialists and other health professionals.

- *A HCC provides core benefits and services for all.* Health is defined to include medical and mental health. Evidence-based science and expert consensus are the guiding philosophies for all clinicians when evaluating an individual's healthcare needs. Healthcare services focus on wellness, prevention, primary care, acute care, patient education, and the treatment and management of health problems provided across the life span. All records are electronically kept and integrated. But beyond technical communication, the emphasis is on patient-provider communications and patient-centered care and research.

- *A better healthcare system results.* Fixing the broken system at a HCC means, as the CHCWG recommended, that integrated healthcare, clinically and administratively, is provided. Both administrators and clinicians are trained and focused on appropriate and culturally sensitive care so that needed medical and nonmedical services can assist individuals and families to function with the highest quality of life.

THE BISCAYNE HEALTHCARE COMMUNITY MODEL

Although there are various models that can be considered, because a prototype HCC exists—and has put a majority of the CHCWG recommendations into action for almost 20 years, despite the healthcare funding crisis—a closer look at this model is warranted.

Defined

The Biscayne Institutes of Health and Living, Inc. (http://www.biscayne institutes.org) prototype working program is based on the HCC model of clinical, administrative, and financial integration. The clinical definition of integrative care includes an on-site team that provides traditional Western physical and emotional care combined with alternative services (herbs, acupuncture, and homeopathy). Spiritual practices are supported or not—as the patient wishes—but the individual's belief system is honored as a part of the healing process. Clinical services are available for a continuum of patient needs from primary care through rehabilitation and wellness and prevention. Administratively, the program is governed by a central on-site office that works closely with clinicians. It is financed through patchwork funding, combining dollars from Medicare, Medicaid, and Medicaid waiver programs, state specialty funding for brain and spinal cord injury, state educational funds for special needs children, private insurance, self-pay, and grants. Integrated funding streams are clinically managed to provide some free care (given as scholarships) to those who cannot afford it.

Philosophy

The HCC model is a frontline, community-based program that stands midway on the healthcare delivery continuum between hospitals and individual practitioners. It is designed to follow a patient within the context of the family and community. Programs are available for adults, children, and elders that span the continuum of care from wellness through primary care to rehabilitation. The focus is on health, not illness. However, in times of illness and/or injury, the goal is to provide a seamless flow of services and information to expedite the patient's healing. Following patients closely in a community context, HCC practitioners can provide integrated care or quickly triage a patient to a specialist or hospital, if needed. The HCC also serves as a central community-based care program that coordinates and receives updated information from hospitals and specialists regarding the patient's care needs and helps to monitor services so that they are not duplicated or in conflict. The underlying philosophy is to be humanly responsive to the individual who is undergoing a health challenge in the context of their larger identity within the family and community—and to be a system designed to meet human needs on a human scale.

A highly important aspect of this model is that its focus is on health and quality of daily living—which includes an emphasis on beauty and the healing power of place. The physical structure in which the Biscayne HCC is housed emphasizes wellness and attractive surroundings. It provides a marked departure from traditional medical office, hospital, rehabilitation, and clinic settings. There are numerous group and community rooms, which look like rooms in a home, in addition to a gym, treatment rooms, and practitioner offices. There is an emphasis on soft colors, beautiful furniture, and lighting throughout. Natural light from floor-to-ceiling windows, clerestory windows, and skylights is used extensively. Incandescent and halogen lighting is also used whenever possible. Carefully selected music, which can be individually controlled in local targeted treatment areas, is also integral to healing within the HCC space. Outside landscaping provides blooming plants at alternating times of the year; a meditation garden and fountains, with the calming sound of running water; and visibility of the outdoors in many places within the building.

An important element for staff and patients in this particular model for healthcare delivery is a large, round room known as the meditation room. This room is 1.5 stories high and 120 feet in circumference. While tables and chairs are brought in as needed for various group programs and activities, the room is normally left vacant. It is a place of community gatherings for the patients and for staff meetings and an auditorium for community outreach programs. The room is used for yoga, Tai Chi, and body work in wellness and prevention workshop programs. This room also serves as the circle for meditation that is held at noon, free of charge, for patients, staff, and the community at large. It is in this space that people of all ages can gather in wheelchairs, regular chairs, and on the floor cross-legged to join in silence and to honor the unity of mind, body, and spirit. It is in this space that the integrated philosophy of supporting the individual within the context of family and the community at large is underscored.

Administration

Integrated clinical and administrative services are essential to the mission of providing humane care. There is a constant emphasis on maintaining a flow of information, both verbal and written, among clinicians and administrators. All records are electronic, and patient records are kept in a central chart, regardless of service provided. Review of records by a designated clinical administrator is required before any information is transmitted from the agency to another facility. This ensures compliance with appropriate confidentiality requirements. There is a strong emphasis on cross training of clinicians and administrators where responsibility for communication overlaps. Clinicians are given in-services on, and are required to maintain a responsibility for, clinical documentation and coding. They are also generally educated on the vagaries of billing within the patchwork funding orientation of the current healthcare system. This allows them to be "on the same team" with administrators. By the same token, administrators are given in-services on how to deal with patients with varying issues. Patients are seen as people to be helped—people who may be laboring under physical and emotional stresses—not claim numbers.

Consultation in therapeutic interventions is given to administrative staff as needed to assist them in accomplishing their part of the agency's healing mission.

Administration of services is also integrated among professional disciplines. A core clinical team with a set of basic skill competencies provides services across program lines. This includes Western medicine, psychology, social work, and Chinese medicine. Specialty team members are added as required by a particular program, for example, physical, occupational, and speech therapies; art therapy; teachers; and so on. Team chart rounds are a weekly occurrence on all service programs and are the glue that holds the clinical integration of care together. Patients are discussed and a care plan with specific timelines is reviewed to keep the team focused on the main goals of clinical care for a particular patient. This allows for true integration of services, rather than having each discipline working independently on their own goals and delivering services in a separate silo of care. The weekly team meetings are essential to breaking open the more limited conceptualizations that can occur in the silos of care. They can provide a fertile ground for discussion that will grow new conceptualizations and can contribute to better integrated caring for a patient by all team members.

The Model

The Biscayne HCC model (Figure 1) provides a full continuum of integrative healthcare services under one roof. By the creation of a community within the community at large, it combines individual treatments and privacy with group and social supports. Core and specialty teams may come into contact with the patient in multiple ways in the HCC milieu. This facilitates both patient and practitioner in seeing each other as more human. It allows for more efficiency in clinical care by a quicker identification of the patient's functioning and any relevant symptomatology both within and across disciplines. It also provides a crucial element in healing that many people lack today—a connectedness to a caring social support network. People—patients and staff—feel that they are not in this alone.

In reviewing the wheel of caring that is the HCC model, three core service areas can be seen: integrative primary care, rehabilitation, and wellness and health promotion. Within each of these service areas, there are multiple programs available. These will be discussed in more detail later. The core service areas are supported by ancillary programs. While the term *ancillary* is used, it in no way implies that the support programs are less extensive. In some cases, for example, the Academy (an integrated rehabilitation and education program for children ages 6 through 21), the program is a major thrust of the HCC. However, the term *ancillary program* denotes an expanded definition

Figure 1
The HealthCare Community model

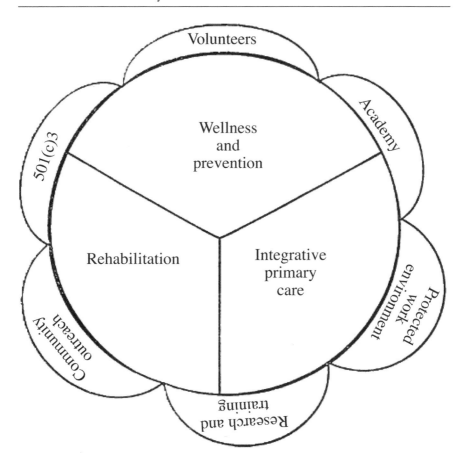

of healthcare. The term *ancillary* is used because the service integrates, in a healthcare setting, a program that is essential to the daily functioning and quality of a person's health that is normally not seen as falling within the purview of the current healthcare system.

Rehabilitation

Within the American healthcare system today, integration of services exists to some degree within the field of rehabilitation. This is good news as integration is not a complete stranger to some practitioners, and this may make it easier to introduce to some healthcare practitioners. Because integration and team care in rehabilitation has been around for over 50 years, it makes sense to begin our exploration of the HCC model in the core service area of rehabilitation.

The HCC has both adult and pediatric rehabilitation programs. The adult program has five specialty areas. Pediatric rehabilitation has two. All areas carry both state and national rehabilitation accreditations. The amount of time a person stays at the HCC facility varies. Patients may spend multiple days a week or only several hours a day. The amount of time depends on the patient's specific assigned services and his choice of involvement in community events that take place through the Wellness and Health Promotion service area on a regular basis, for example, meditation.

Adult Traumatic Brain Injury (TBI) and Neurology Service

Biscayne has a premier, nationally and state-accredited program for reha-bilitation of traumatic brain injury (TBI). Patients are seen for postacute reha-bilitation and followed long-term in the community. Services are provided in both individual and group formats. Cognitive retraining to stimulate brain recovery in an organized, sequential manner is provided through a specified series of activities that can be individualized as needed. Biofeedback, physi-cal, occupational, and speech therapies are provided. Services often work in a transdisciplinary manner so that services can be administered simultane-ously. In Florida, where Biscayne Institutes is located, Chinese medicine practitioners are licensed as primary care providers. Consequently, acupunc-ture and herbals to facilitate the healing process are easily available to patients on this team. Individual therapy and behavioral medicine interventions are also provided along with family and group therapy. Group work is essential to addressing coping and social skills along with the more traditional concerns of depression and anxiety.

Patients with other neurological disorders receive individual and/or group rehabilitation from the same disciplines as TBI patients. A wide variety of people with differing diagnoses are seen, for example, stroke, Arnold Chi-ari syndrome, multiple sclerosis, brain tumors, and so on. In each case, an evaluation is performed, an interdisciplinary care plan is developed with the patient and/or family as appropriate, and weekly team rounds are held both to address progress and set new goals.

Adult Outpatient Medical Rehabilitation

Patients seen in the adult outpatient medical rehabilitation services strug-gle with a wide variety of health challenges. These include such diagnoses as amputation, chronic pain, neuropathy, orthopedic injuries, secondary effects of diabetes, spinal cord injury, and so on. All patients receive the traditional Western services of physical, occupational, and speech therapy as needed. However, they can also avail themselves of biofeedback, acupuncture, and herbs integrated with their allopathic physicians' treatments. Individual and family therapies are provided to address issues of change and adjustment as well as pain management and more emotional concerns related to depression and anxiety. As needed, specialty groups are formed to provide patient support. These groups are organized around specific diagnostic categories, for example, pain management, spinal cord injury, and so on. The groups provide coping and emotional support as well as educational information.

Elders Program

With the growing need to address issues of elders in the community, particularly with regard to issues of aging and cognitive and physical capacities, patients with dementia and Alzheimer's are seen in a separate program. This program is geared to two levels of functioning: (1) those individuals who are at some level of independent functioning within the community and (2) those individuals who are in later stages and, even with nursing assistance, have problems with initiation of mental or social activities. Both groups are provided with sensory stimulation and cognitive retraining appropriate to their level and lifestyle. But the goals are different. For elders in level 1, the goal is to prevent deterioration and promote function. For elders in level 2, the focus is on transcending from past functioning into acceptance of a new way of being, functioning independently as much as possible within a structure. Group therapy is also provided to address issues of loneliness and isolation as well as frustration with the changes associated with aging. Traditional physical, occupational, and speech therapies also are provided to maintain physical functioning, and in some cases, elders choose to participate in Chinese medicine. Therapeutic massage is helpful to this group of people, who often suffer from lack of human tactile contact in their daily lives, increasing their sense of isolation. Therapeutic use of the arts, both visual and musical, provides additional symbolism and a means of communication and stimulation for elders.

Adult Developmental Disabilities Program

The Centers for Disease Control (2006) define developmental disabilities as "a diverse group of severe chronic conditions that are due to mental and/or physical impairments." People with developmental disabilities may have wide-ranging problems in functioning. These problems may include language, mobility, learning, and independent functioning and living. Developmental disabilities are diagnosed during the development years up to 22 years of age. The disabilities are usually pervasive and persist throughout the person's lifetime. Helping these individuals function as independently as possible in the community is important to their quality of life and also the functioning of the overall systems that support them, be these systems privately or publicly funded.

The rehabilitation program for adult individuals with developmental disabilities provides a three-day-a-week program of cognitive retraining and problem solving designed specifically to address independent functioning in the community. Group therapy to provide support and assist in developing coping and social skills is also provided. This consistent structure allows the person to develop to the highest level possible and takes a prevention-oriented approach to maintaining healthy and adaptive functioning physically, mentally, and emotionally. Individual and family therapy is also provided as needed and as requested. The traditional and nontraditional therapies, for example, physical therapy, occupational therapy, speech, and Chinese medicine, are utilized as needed as components of the individual's program to increase function.

Adult Dual Diagnosis Rehabilitation

Individuals with alcohol and drug addictions often have dual diagnoses that involve brain injury, spinal cord injury, or severe orthopedic injuries. The Biscayne HCC admissions criteria does provide for patients to enter the community who are actively using. But patients with an alcohol or drug addiction issue that also need rehabilitation for a variety of problems can be seen providing that they are medically cleared and are actively living in a halfway house that addresses addiction problems or that they are actively participating in an addiction program, for example, Alcoholics Anonymous (http://www. alcoholics-anonymous.org) or Narcotics Anonymous (http://www.na.org).

In addition to the specific services provided for brain injury and neurological and/or outpatient medical rehabilitation, patients are provided a protocol that includes individual therapy and group therapy with others struggling with addictions. Acupuncture protocols specifically developed to address addictions are also provided. Permission for the Biscayne team to coordinate with community-at-large supports, for example, family and/or halfway house staff, is often helpful to the patient and, in some cases, may be considered mandatory for treatment.

PEDIATRIC TBI SERVICE

Children and adolescents up to age 21 with TBI are provided a state- and nationally accredited program that has been termed by reviewers as "the way pediatric rehabilitation should be provided across the country." The developmental stage of the child cognitively, emotionally, and physically is endemic to the type of rehabilitation program that is provided. Children are seen for postacute rehabilitation. They are followed long term to assist in stimulating the brain through immediate recovery and to provide support so that the child may attain the highest level of functioning possible as later age–stage developmental tasks emerge.

Individualized programs of cognitive retraining, group programs to address stage-appropriate coping and social skills, and family therapy for education and support are critical services that are provided. Special education support and physical, occupational, and speech therapies are also integrated. Services are provided as the family desires either after school, if the child returns to a public school, or in the context of the Biscayne Academy. The Biscayne Academy is an ancillary program that provides significant special education services integrated into the healthcare program. Rather than being a school that is added on to services provided, staff are trained to provide educational programs as well as to serve in the role of behavioral assistants. This will be discussed further in the section describing ancillary programs. Because this program is so integrally intricate to the provision of healthcare, a separate chapter on this model is also presented later in this volume.

The Biscayne HCC also provides a unique summer rehabilitation program that services postacute brain injury patients and long-term follow-up for children with brain injury as well as varying disabilities. The program is presented as a summer camp and is organized around a particular theme. All services utilize this theme as the frame for interventions, including cognitive, emotional, and physical care. Themes are always pertinent to current childhood culture, for example, Superheroes, Back to the Future, etc., and are seen as fun rather than rehabilitation.

In addition, the multiple presentations of material via all the different disciplines allow the child to have repetitive stimulation through various modalities of learning.

PEDIATRIC OUTPATIENT MEDICAL REHABILITATION

Children and adolescents through age 21 are also seen for a wide variety of problems in a nationally accredited program. Diagnoses include autism, cerebral palsy, learning disorders, hyperactivity, visual and/or hearing impairments, and mental retardation. No diagnosis excludes a child. Evaluation for admission is done on a case-by-case basis to determine if the child or adolescent can be helped within the community model, even if the child/adolescent may require one-on-one attendance throughout treatment by an aide in addition to the service provider. Pediatric patients that are ventilator-dependent, medically unstable, or determined to have severe behavioral problems that are excessively disruptive to the ongoing mission of the agency, for example, violent, florid psychosis, are referred to more specialized care programs.

Individual, family, and group therapies are integrated with special education, physical, occupational, and speech services. The child may be seen in an after-school program if he attends public school. However, if the child is placed in the Academy program, he is provided treatments integrated with his special education. When the child goes home at 3:00 P.M., his schooling and rehabilitation services are completed. He does not have to be bussed or taken by parents for additional services. This allows the child a more normalized experience and conserves family energy and time.

ACCREDITATION

Although Biscayne rehabilitation programs are provided in an expanded concept of healthcare delivery, the rehabilitation services maintain all standards and accreditations for the highest recognition offered to rehabilitation facilities. Biscayne Rehabilitation is a federally designated Comprehensive Outpatient Rehabilitation Facility. It holds accreditation by the Commission on Accreditation of Rehabilitation Facilities as both an Adult and Pediatric Brain Injury Program and an Adult and Pediatric Outpatient Medical Rehabilitation program. In Florida, where Medicaid services are administered through the state, Biscayne Institute's HCC model holds a Medicaid waiver as a private facility to provide needed healthcare to an underprivileged population. Biscayne Institutes is also a state-designated provider by Florida's Brain and Spinal Cord Injury Council, meeting the accreditation standards for both adults and children.

INTEGRATIVE PRIMARY CARE

The newest service area to complete the continuum of care in the Biscayne HCC model is integrative primary care. Services are provided by two allopathic internists, one of whom is also board certified as a cardiologist; a licensed Chinese medicine practitioner, who also holds a degree in naturopathy; and a psychologist with a specialty in behavioral medicine and rehabilitation.

Patients are referred and treated in the context of three programs: (1) integrative primary care that supplements rehabilitation programs; (2) traditional allopathic patients that are identified as in need of other services and follow-up; and (3) integrative health evaluations and follow-up that provide overall assessment to maintain health or assist patients with complex issues in developing an overall concept of their health issues and making decisions regarding treatment.

Integrative primary care that supplements rehabilitation programs adds great benefit to patients who are undergoing rehabilitation at the Biscayne Institutes. Many rehabilitation patients have complex medical problems with symptomatology and medication changes that are often unreported to the rehabilitation specialist programs. On-site coordination of primary care allows early detection and communication of health concerns that may destabilize the patient medically and interfere with their rehabilitation. Communication among both primary care and rehabilitation providers makes for a more seamless and coordinated view of patient care in a more timely manner that can often avert medical complications and deterioration.

Conversely, many rehabilitation patients with complex issues, for example, spinal cord injury, often have difficulty finding primary care practitioners who understand the complexity and fragility of their rehabilitation issues. Having primary care on-site with rehabilitation that is coordinated in team meetings provides a greater sense of confidence in addressing medical issues for both the patient and the medical provider.

Allopathic physicians at the Biscayne Institutes maintain an ongoing traditional primary care practice for patients with a wide variety of problems. Given their integrative orientation, however, they are focused on addressing issues beyond the physical. Rather than making referrals for emotional or complementary alternative services, physicians have the capability for an on-call integrative team to meet the patient at the time of the patient's regular office visit. This makes for a less anxious and smoother transition for a patient to receive other needed services. It also increases the likelihood of a patient's following up on referrals for future care.

Integrative health evaluations and follow-up are provided to the community with the same protocol but two different goals. One goal is to provide a comprehensive health evaluation for checkup, early identification of any health problems, and recommendations of health maintenance behaviors and services, if needed. The other goal is to assist patients who have complex medical symptomatology and need assistance in developing an overall concept of their health issues and making decisions regarding treatment.

Patients are seen for an interdisciplinary intake that coordinates all medical, emotional, and social history. Information is gleaned about the patient's role in the family, community, and supports and concerning his spiritual or non-spiritual beliefs. This interdisciplinary history is then provided to each of the team members, who do an independent interview to explore specific details, if needed, and a physical. At the end of the interdisciplinary evaluation, the team meets to coordinate findings and produce an integrative report with recommendations for follow-up as needed; these recommendations are placed in order of importance, as agreed on by the team. The patient is then seen to review the report; he has an opportunity to ask questions and is provided with a copy of the comprehensive written evaluation. If the patient needs referrals to specialists, these are made at the time of feedback. If the patient wishes to receive follow-up services at the HCC to address illness/injury or maintain health, these appointments are also made at this time.

Providing such a service allows a patient to view personal health and any health problems in a more global manner. It allows an integrated understanding of the self physically, emotionally, socially, and spiritually. This personal knowledge, and an awareness of available options to maintain health, empowers a patient to become an active participant in his own healthcare—making informed choices about how to proceed, if medical treatments are necessary. It helps a patient navigate the complicated and fragmented health delivery system that, currently, often treats the part that is ill and loses sight of the whole person.

WELLNESS, PREVENTION, AND HEALTH PROMOTION

The wellness, prevention, and health promotion service area is made up of both clinical and educational programs. Clinical programs are an extension to the wellness continuum of services provided in the other two major service areas—rehabilitation and integrative primary care. As noted previously, integrative primary care patients can pursue an evaluation and recommendations to maintain and boost their health. This may entail such diverse involvement and active engagement in health promotion as a patient seeking stress management counseling, acupuncture for wellness, biofeedback, and/or massage therapy for relaxation, for example. Rehabilitation patients who achieve the highest level of functioning possible in the community are also seen to maintain and promote health. Two program examples are the pursuit of wellness through supervised exercise programs after formal rehabilitation has ended and/or ongoing support groups for social engagement.

Education programs are provided through classes and workshops. Various types of yoga classes are held on a weekly basis. They vary from beginner to more advanced practices. Tai Chi and meditation classes are also provided. Workshops are sponsored that run the gamut of wellness promotion and health education. Sample programs include combined presentations with university hospitals, for example, dealing with traditional and complementary approaches to cancer, or programs on stress management, weight loss, nutrition, smoking cessation, or mindfulness approaches to health. The primary goal is to expand the public's understanding of health and how to be an active participant in creating a healthy quality of life.

One particular program is the sponsorship of the Florida Council on Spirituality, Medicine, and Healing. The council is made up of physicians and other healthcare professionals as well as local leaders of varied spiritual traditions. The council holds public information programs that examine different questions relating to overlapping boundaries among varied spiritual belief systems and the process of healing. Some topics have included the role of love in healing and near-death experiences. Each public forum is followed by questions from the audience and closes with a different spiritual group providing an interfaith meditation or spiritual ritual. These have ranged from Buddhist sand mandala constructions to candlelight meditations held on Christmas and Hanukah. The concept is always to honor the spiritual belief system of each person and the innate factors that produce healing.

Based on the concept that the focus of healthcare should be on building health, HCC wellness, prevention, and health promotion programs focus on an individual's beliefs and behavioral factors that contribute to health and/or illness. The interaction between the individual's mind and body and pathogens in the environment are seen as the key elements in whether or not an individual becomes sick. The belief system of the patient is acknowledged as critically important. The emphasis is on education and how the patient can be encouraged to become an active collaborator in treatment and the healing process should the person become ill. This approach echoes the healthcare model of the future (Chiong, 2001; Pincus, 2003; Ray, 2004).

Research is beginning to focus on nonmedical factors that influence a person in resisting illness and living longer (Ray, 2004). Four interactive information systems in the human being have been cited as responsible for health as governed by the psychoneuroimmunological system: the brain, the endocrine system, the nervous system, and the immune system (Maier, Watkins, & Fleshner, 1994). Oakely Ray defines the brain as the first line of defense against illness and sees the mind as the emergent functioning of the brain. Because the body reacts to the mind's beliefs as a product of the brain, it is irrelevant if the belief is true or not. The belief system sets a series of physiological responses into play. In that sense, "belief becomes biology" (Cousins, 1990). Ray (2004) goes on to point out that as stress—defined as an experience when an individual's coping skills are inadequate to meet environmental demands—occurs, it is the coping skills that the person *believes* they have to bring to bear on the situation that are most important. He also cites inner resources that include unconscious assumptions and predictions, social support, and spiritual beliefs as the prime factors in dealing with stress and impacting a person's ability to maintain a healthy state. It is in providing educational and experiential opportunities to address beliefs and develop a social support system through wellness promotion workshops that the HCC, in addition to providing clinical services for prevention of illness, makes one of its greatest contributions to a changed healthcare paradigm.

ANCILLARY PROGRAMS

Figure 1 provides a listing of the ancillary programs that contribute to the basic service areas of the HCC. Issues involved in the first three ancillary programs addressed—the academy, research, and training—are discussed in more detail in later chapters. The Biscayne Academy provides support for pediatric rehabilitation programs by providing special education on-site and integrated with pediatric healthcare delivery. Services are provided for children aged 6–21 with varying disabilities. Data indicate that children that receive services provided in the context of an expanded definition of healthcare, where daily learning opportunities are integrated into health services delivery, achieve better results in all areas—physical, cognitive, emotional, behavioral, and social.

Research and training is provided both for specific disciplines and for integrative and transdisciplinary programs. In addition to utilizing more traditional methods of field research, the primary research focus of the HCC is to implement the International Classification of Functioning, for adults and children, in assessing the efficacy of clinical programs. This reflects the emphasis on increased functioning as the most important aspect in healthcare as opposed to diagnosis. Training for multiple disciplines is achieved through contracts for clinical training with different universities and medical schools. Each professional student in training receives supervision from a qualified, licensed clinician in the field. In addition, they engage in didactic and experiential training programs with multiple disciplines on a once a week basis.

Volunteers from the community at large and rehabilitation patients who have completed their programs yet are unable to return to work in the community are engaged in both the volunteer program and protected work sessions. Peer mentoring; assistance with daily activities in the center, for example, helping the physical therapy department, working in the pet therapy program, and so on; and production of items to sell that convey the meaning of an expanded definition of health are all part of both the volunteer and protected work environment programs. This enables a greater interface with the larger community while allowing patients who have completed programs to give back to the HCC.

A community outreach program also enables the HCC model to plant ideas about the changing model of healthcare by sending teams of clinicians into the community. Examples are teams from the elders program that have set up expanded mind-body programs in nursing homes and assisted living centers. Community outreach has also been fostered through providing wellness teams to local businesses and schools on a time-limited basis to initiate stress management and changes in curriculum. In addition, the HCC is a place that welcomes certain groups to utilize the facility to create a greater connection to the expanded definition of health. The local Kiwanis Club, a service organization that emphasizes "children as priority one," meets at the facility and regularly engages in fundraising activities to support special programs. One such program led to a grant from Kiwanis International for Kiwanis Kids, a service for the early identification of problem areas in development for parents of young children aged birth to six years old.

A 501(c)3, a nonprofit public sector program, known as the Biscayne Foundation also raises monies for research, education, and services needed by those who cannot afford care under the current U.S. healthcare system. Among other activities, the Biscayne Foundation has been able to engage in cutting-edge research that looks at the impact of the arts in healing; provide integrative summer camps for children with disabilities; and develop therapeutic programs for children from underserved immigrant families.

GROWING HEALTHCARE COMMUNITIES

The Biscayne HCC model is a working model that has developed over the last two decades and reflects many of the current recommendations of the CHCWG. It provides efficacious healthcare on a broad continuum of services from rehabilitation through primary care to wellness and prevention services to the local community. Core services emphasize health and wellness and include physical and mental healthcare as well as CAM integrated into the existing system. These services are provided to patients with a widely varying ability to pay and, in some cases, for free. Electronic records integrate all information of the HCC, and the coordinated clinical programs serve as the basis of a local network to quickly refer patients to specialists or hospitals as needed. The HCC also stands as the integrated receiving agent for the patient and patient information when specialty or hospital care is given.

The question arises, How exportable is this model to other locations in the United States, and can it be replicated? Given that the larger definitions of health and basic service areas in the HCC model are universal in addressing human needs, the answer lies in the fact that, currently, this model continues to exist—and to grow year after year—despite the current climate of fragmented funding sources that require a patchwork approach to budget management. As it continues to grow, it is responsive to the needs of the local community.

Utilizing the basic definition of service areas, the HCC can be adapted to other locales. The CHCWG advocates that federally qualified health centers (FQHC) and community mental health centers (CMHC) be examined for feasibility of integrating and expanding local health networks. This is one framework to consider that can include the possibility for change. However, it assumes that the FQHCs and CMHCs are reworked on the HCC prototype to include a combined emphasis on health and ancillary programs that expand the definition of health.

Another method of growing HCCs is for the federal government to contract demonstration projects in several major metropolitan areas as well as in a number of rural areas. Funding through prospective payment, as has been done with elder care in assistive living or with inpatient rehabilitation, would provide a funding mechanism with accountability, while the focus on demonstration projects can be gathering data on efficiency and effectiveness. A third mechanism for growing HCCs can be for the government to provide personal financial incentives for healthcare professionals and administrators to create and maintain nonprofit integrative programs that can demonstrate efficacy across a continuum of care. Another possibility is for nongovernmental organizations to stimulate development of HCCs through grant funds to local providers and agencies.

In expanding and exporting the HCC model, it is critical that local HCCs integrate basic service programs with specific local community needs. Doherty and Mendenhall (2006) indicate the importance of the involvement of local citizens if a sustainable community health initiative is to succeed: "Local communities must retrieve their own historical, cultural, and religious traditions of health and healing and bring these into dialogue with contemporary medical systems" (p. 255).

This initiative must be collaborative, not hierarchical. Individuals and families must experience the relevance of the HCC to their lives and see themselves as active coproducers of their own health.

One such endeavor under discussion is the engagement and integration of the Tribal Doctor program in Alaska into a multicultural health community to eliminate the fragmentation of health service delivery to native peoples. The Inupiat of northwestern Alaska are actively considering how to improve healthcare coordination, decrease costs, and increase efficiency of care. The goal is to provide a spectrum of healing opportunities, recognizing that "individual health resides in the context of that person's life within a family and with a community structure" (Hild, 2006, p. 6). A HCC model would provide such a forum to achieve the basic needs and honor the traditional values of the Inupiat people. Creating a means to be locally responsive, to eliminate health disparities and cost-effectively promote function and quality of life in populations as diverse as the community in Miami and the Maniilaq community in Alaska, is the overarching aim and requires a robust model. The HCC contains the elements for such a vibrant mechanism.

VISION FOR A NEW HEALTH

There is a move toward a new medicine (http://thenewmedicine.org)—a new medicine that treats the whole person, not just parts, when a person is ill. This new medicine looks beyond drugs and surgery to focus on prevention and encourages people to be active participants in their own healthcare.

The doctor-patient relationship in the new medicine is different, too, and emphasizes listening, comforting, and collaborating. But beyond new medicine, we need to move toward a vision of new health. If no man was an island in John Donne's world of the sixteenth century, we are even more intricately interwoven in our connection to one another through the global village we live in some 500 years later. And yet isolation and loneliness abound in daily life and in the delivery of our healthcare services. According to Ornish (1998), people who report feeling alone and isolated have three to five times the rate of premature death and disease as compared to people who have a sense of connection and community. We are creatures of community. If we intend to heal ourselves and our untenable healthcare system in the United States, we need to see our health in the bigger picture of family and community and as a shared social responsibility—a value enunciated by the American people to the CHCWG. Instead of a dark painting, we can then view the brightness of a new health dawning on the horizon of the twenty-first century.

If we intend to change our health system and truly meet the needs of ourselves, our families, and our friends, if we intend to honor the integration of body, mind, and spirit in a quality and cost-effective way, we can. In *The Life We Are Given,* Leonard and Murphy (1995) write, "Ultimately human intentionality is the most powerful evolutionary force on this planet" (p. 61). Where we choose to place our conscious intention has the potential to make major changes in the national policies that affect healthcare in this country. It has the potential to change how we meet the needs of those who seek and those who provide healthcare. It ultimately has the potential to make major changes in the lives of our patients, our friends, our families, and ourselves.

TOOL KIT FOR CHANGE

Role and Perspective of the Healthcare Professional

1. Integrative healthcare means active, regular communication among traditional medical providers, CAM practitioners, and mental/behavioral health professionals.
2. The HCC is one model that provides integrated, frontline health services under one roof in a humane and cost-effective manner.
3. A practitioner of healing arts values both the science and the art of health and living.

Role and Perspective of the Patient/Participant

1. A patient must take an active part in his own healthcare, seeking coordinated care and giving active input into the treatment plan.
2. A patient must be willing to participate as both a giver and a receiver in the community for both his own health and the health of others.
3. A patient must advocate for a coordinated system of healthcare.

Interconnection: The Global Perspective

1. Integrative healthcare is more than simply adding on other services to supplement traditional medical care.
2. Integrative healthcare addresses both the quality of health and the quality of life of the patient in day-to-day functioning.
3. The Citizens' Health Care Working Group report represents what the American people value and want in the healthcare system. It provides a starting point to truly integrate health and medical services.

REFERENCES

American Academy of Family Physicians. (2006). *Family medicine.* Retrieved December 10, 2006 from http://www.aafp.org/online/en/home/policy/policies/f/family medicine.html

American Academy of Pediatrics. (2006). Scope of health care benefits for children from birth through age 21. Retrieved December 10, 2006 from http://aappolicy. aappublications.org/cgi/content/abstract/pediatrics; 117/3/979.

American Psychological Association. (1995). *Public perceptions of the value of psychological services.* Washington, DC: Author.

American Psychological Association. (2006). *Health and behavior codes.* Retrieved December 13, 2006, from http://www.apa.org/practice/cpt_2002.html.

Barzansky, B., & Etzel, S. (2003). Educational programs in US medical schools 2002–2003. *Journal of the American Medical Association, 290,* 1190–1196.

Berkman, L. F. (1995). The role of social relations in health promotion. *Psychosomatic Medicine, 47,* 245–254.

Centers for Disease Control. (2006). *Developmental disabilities: Topic home.* Retrieved December 13, 2006, from http://www.cdc.gov/ncbddd/dd/default.htm

Chiong, W. (2001). Diagnosing and Defining Disease. *Journal of American Medical Association. 285,* 89–90.

Citizens' Health Care Working Group. (2006, September 29). *Final recommendations.* Retrieved November 26, 2006, from http://www.citizenshealthcare.gov/ recommendations/finalrecommendations_print.pdf

Cohen, S., Underwood, L. G., & Gottlieb, B. H. (Eds.). (2000). *Social support measurement and intervention: A guide for health and social scientists.* New York: Oxford University Press.

Cousins, N. (1990). *Head first: The biology of hope and the healing power of the human spirit.* New York: Penguin Non-Classics.

deGruy, F. (1996). Mental health in the primary care setting. M. S. Donaldson, K. D. Yordy, K. N. Lohr, and N. A. Vanselow, Editors. *Primary care and America's health in a new era* (pp. 285–311). Washington, DC: Institute of Medicine, National Academy Press.

DiCowden, M. A. (2003). The call of the wild woman: Models of healing. *Women and Therapy, 26,* 297–310.

DiCowden, M., & Scherer, M. (in press). Division 22 survey of members—2006. *Division 22 Newsletter.*

Doherty, W., & Mendenhall, T. (2006). Citizen health care: A model of engaging patients, families and communities as coproducers of health. *Families, Systems, and Health, 24,* 251–263.

Druss, G., Marcus, S., Olfson, M., Tanielian, T., & Pincus, H. (2003). Trends in care by nonphysician clinicians in the United States. *The New England Journal of Medicine, 338,* 130–137.

Druss, G., Rohrbaugh, R., Levinson, C., & Rosenheck, R. (2001). Integrated medical care for patients with serious psychiatric illness: A randomized trial. *Archives of General Psychiatry, 58,* 861–868.

Eisenberg, D. M., Davis, R. B., Ettner, S. L., Appel, S., Wilkey, S., Van Rompay, M., et al. (1998). Trends in alternative medicine use in the United States, 1990–1997: Results of a follow-up national survey. *Journal of the American Medical Association, 18,* 1569–1575.

Faas, N. (2001). *Integrating complementary medicine into health systems.* Gaithersburg, MD: Aspen.

Frank, R., McDaniel, S., Bray, J., & Heldring, M. (Eds.). (2004). *Primary care psychology.* Washington, DC: American Psychological Association.

Harper's. (2006). *Harper's index for February 2006.* Retrieved November 26, 2006, from http://harpers.org/HarpersIndex2006–02.html

Hild, C. M. (2006). *Multi-cultural health and well-being: A holistic approach to care* (Rep. No. R24 MD 000499). Anchorage: University of Alaska, Institute for Circumpolar Health Studies.

Institute of Medicine. (2002, May 21). *Care without coverage: Too little, too late.* Retrieved February 2, 2005, from http://www.iom.edu/CMS/3809/4660/4333.aspx.

Institute of Medicine. (2005, January 12). *Complementary and alternative medicine in the United States.* Committee on the use of complementary and alternative medicine by the american public. Board on health promotion and disease prevention. Washington, D.C.: The National Academies Press.

Institute of Medicine (2006).Examining the health disparities research plan of the national institutes of health: Unfinished business. Retrieved December 7, 2006, from http://www.iom.edu/CMS/3740/22356/33275.aspx.

James, L. C., & Folen, R. A. (Eds.). (2005). *The primary care consultant.* Washington, DC: American Psychological Association.

Janisse, T. (2002). National institutes of health "Oregon center for complementary and alternative medicine": Value to permanente medical groups and to kaiser foundation health plans and hospitals. *The Permanente Journal.* Fall 2002, Vol 6, 2–5.

Kahn, J., Kronick, R., Kreger, M., & Gans, D. (2004). The cost of health insurance administration in California: Estimates for insurers, physicians, and hospitals. *Health Affairs, 24,* 1629–1639.

Leonard, G., & Murphy, M. (1995). *The life we are given.* New York: Jeremy P. Archer / Putnam.

Maier S. F., Watkins L. R., Fleshner M. (1994). Psychoneuroimmunology. The interface between behavior, brain, and immunity. *American Psychologist, 49,* 1004–1017.

Marder, S. R., Essock, S. M., Miller, A. L., Buchanan, R. W., Casey, D. E., Davis, J. M., et al. (2004). Physical health monitoring of patients with schizophrenia. *American Journal of Pscyhiatry, 161,* 1334–1349.

Meeker, W. C. & Haldeman, S. (2002). Chiropractic: A profession at the crossroads of mainstream and alternative medicine. *Annals of Internal Medicine. 136,* 216–227.

Moran, M. (2003). More patients treated by multiple clinicians. *Psychiatric News, 38,* 14.

National Center for Complementary and Alternative Medicine. (2006). *NCCAM funding: appropriations history.* Retrieved December 12, 2006, from http://nccam.nih.gov/about/appropriations/.

Ornish, D. (1998). *Love and survival: The scientific basis for the healing power of intimacy.* New York: Harper Collins.

Physicians for a National Health Plan. (2006). Our mission: Single-payer national health insurance. Retrieved November 12, 2006, from http://www.pnhp.org

Pincus, H. (2003). The future of behavioral health and primary care: Drowning in the mainstream or left on the bank? *Psychosomatics, 44,* 1–11.

Ray, O. (2004). How the mind hurts and heals the body. *American Psychologist, 59,* 29–40.

Stux, G. & Hammerschlag, R. (Eds.). (2001). *Clinical acupuncture: Scientific basis.* Berlin: Springer Verlag.

Theil, R. J. (2002) Growth effects of the warner protocol for children with down syndrome. *Journal of Orthomolecular Medicine, 17,* 42–48.

Tindle, H., & Eisenberg, D. (2005). *One-third of US adults use alternative and complementary medicine.* Retrieved December 11, 2006, from http://www.researchmatters.harvard.edu/story.php?article_id=801

Wetzel, M., Eisenberg, D., & Kaptchuk, T. (1998). Courses involving alternative and complementary medicine in US medical schools. *Journal of the American Medical Association, 280,* 784–787.

Chapter Two

DEFINING INTEGRATIVE HEALTHCARE: PARADIGM SHIFTING WITHOUT A CLUTCH

William Benda, MD, FACEP, FAAEM and Jeannette Gallagher, ND

IN SEARCH OF THE ELUSIVE NEW MEDICINE

These past two decades, from the mid-1980s to the present, have witnessed a revolution of sorts in the field of healthcare—perhaps even the beginnings of a true paradigm shift. This so-called new medicine has been given a multitude of names: holistic, humanistic, alternative, unconventional, traditional, complementary, integrative, integral, integrated, and more. For the purposes of this volume we will use the term *integrated* as our generic default, but essential to our conversation is the understanding that any true shift in medical philosophy and clinical practice is likely to be in its undeveloped infancy, making names and titles of less consequence at the moment than the inherent meaning behind the words. The most important concept, whether patient or practitioner, is that we must awaken to the reality that health and healing optimally occur when all pertinent factors are addressed, be they physical, emotional, social, or spiritual, and only then may we truly speak of holistic medicine; to quote Sir William Osler (1849–1919), "It is more important to know what sort of patient has a disease than what sort of disease a patient has."

AN INCOMPLETE HISTORY OF MEDICINE

Healthcare, whether orthodox or unorthodox, is not a product of relatively recent times—its historical roots are deeply embedded in both world history and world culture. It was an accepted dictum of ancient civilizations that healers and priests channeled treatment directives straight from the gods, and in return the gods demanded worship for their power to heal. The sire of healthcare was religion, primarily prayer and cleansing, combined with a basic knowledge of illness, wounds, and surgical repair. Today's forensic historian may wish to consult the *Secret Book of the Physician*, which assigned cures based on knowledge from the gods that only the priest could access and interpret (Finger, 2000).

Healing as seen by the ancient Greeks was a family tradition; Aesculapius, the god of healing and medicine, was son of Apollo, senior god of healing. Aesculapius's daughter Panacea was goddess of healing and cures; a second daughter (through Panacea), Hygeia, was goddess of health, cleanliness, and sanitation; son Telesphoros represented recovery from illness; and Aesculapius's wife, Epione, nurturing those suffering from illness and pain, may have been written history's first nurse (Sigarist, 1929). Indeed, the original Hippocratic Oath begins with the invocation "I swear by Apollo the physician and by Aesculapius, and by Hygeia, and Panacea, and all the gods and goddesses...."

A long and gradual evolution in cultural acceptance of healing gratis the gods to healing courtesy of Mother Nature ensued over two millennia, represented by the very logo of our allopathic medical profession—the staff and the snake of Aesculapius. The serpent was thought to be a "holy animal graced with the secret healing powers of the earth...because as it sheds its skin and then appears rejuvenated, it was revered as a symbol of eternal life" (Frazer, 1975, p. xx). Hippocrates himself helped bring an end to this first god-playing-doctor era by decreeing that disease was created and cured not by heavenly influence, but in fact by nature herself—the Greek origin of the word *physician* is *physis*, or "nature" (Shipley, 1945). Life originated from and death returned to an eternal unknown, and disease was a deviation from health, not to be heroically battled, but instead encouraged to find its way back into balance. Thus was born a new therapeutic philosophy and approach to illness—the treatment of collectively shared illnesses, rather than heavenly interventions for individual patients.

Nature as healer held sway over the ensuing centuries and on into the mid-eighteenth to mid-nineteenth-century United States. Not only was her power to heal the dominant cultural paradigm, but the power to call on her for such effort was endowed to one particular entity by virtue of his medical degree—the physician. But who and what exactly was a physician? Nineteenth-century America claimed no established medical orthodoxy—various and sundry practitioners applied their trade without the need for licensure or bureaucratic oversight. Professions are by nature political, and a deep rift soon developed between self-anointed *regulars* (licensed physicians) and designated *irregulars* (unlicensed physicians). To the regular practitioners, the irregulars were the foe, potentially injurious both to the patient and the savings account.

Claiming quackery to be on the rise and a serious threat to modern healthcare, regulars united in their demands for reform via state intervention, requesting legislative definition of medical qualifications, a register of qualified doctors, a medical council representing the profession as a whole, and, most politically potent, a unification of the chaotic state of medical education and examinations (Loudon, 1986). Quality of medical education and thus quality of care, it was said, were hampered by the multiplicity of medical institutions awarding licenses, diplomas, and degrees. Through the creation of a system of formal study, examination, and licensing, it was believed the public would be able to tell the true healer from the false, and irregulars would either abandon practice or face legal consequences.

Communal efforts by the regular medical profession in advancing the quality and standards of its educational endeavors convinced legislators to enact such licensure requirements. Between 1875 and 1900, licensing statutes were instituted by virtually every state in the union, nourished by dramatic advances in medical science and practice (particularly surgery) that sprouted from recognition of the germ theory of disease. By the end of the nineteenth and the beginning of the twentieth centuries, new technologies began to deliver the kind of scientific evidence that would give those faithful to reductionistic philosophies clinical, political, and economic authority; indeed, in 1855, the code of the American Medical Association (AMA) excluded all irregular practitioners from membership (Wolpe, 1999).

In 1910, the Carnegie Foundation, assisted by the AMA, published the Flexner report titled *Medical Education in the United States and Canada* (Beck, 2004). Flexnor's testimony assigned the highest value to those medical schools that had a full-time teaching faculty and that taught a pathological and physiochemical approach to the human body. As a result, only graduates of those schools that received a high rating were allowed to sit for state medical licensing examinations, effectively marginalizing graduates of nonallopathic educational institutions.

Requirements for licensure did not, however, drive all the irregulars from the field, and by the last quarter of the nineteenth century, two unorthodox groups, homeopathy and eclecticism, were considered too well established and attracted too many (voting) patients to be legislated out of business, although numbers of their schools declined dramatically. But extension of licensing to these irregulars did not apply to newer medical professions still struggling for credibility. As osteopathy, chiropractic, naturopathy, and other unconventional professions arrived on the scene, students and practitioners found themselves in the same position as homeopaths and eclectics a century past—charged with practicing medicine without a license. The struggles for validity and recognition by such groups continue to this day and are a topic for another discourse.

Medical necessity does occasionally trump political inequity, however, and soon healthcare began to emerge from under the dominating wing of conventional medicine. Along with the growth of twentieth-century technology came a simultaneous rise in chronic, degenerative illnesses resistant to conventional treatments and increasingly costly to society. Leading causes of morbidity in the nineteenth century, such as trauma and infectious disease, were overtaken by the scourge of cardiovascular disease, autoimmune illness, and cancer. Emotional maladies accompanied such persistent illnesses, and the necessity of psychological as well as physical treatment became both recognized and researched as the twentieth century progressed. The advent of technology also tended to take medicine away from a humanistic focus. With the invention of the telescope by Laennec, the holy grail of medicine became precision. The goal was to gain information about smaller and smaller units and perceive the sources of disease in more microscopic terms. Occasionally, a voice in the wilderness called for development of a new, multidimensional model of healthcare that would attend to all issues influencing health and illness, whether environmental, social, physical, emotional, or spiritual. But such articulations were lost in the winds of conventional ideology until the last decade of the century.

Orthodoxy, whether religious, political, or medical, eventually inspires revolution. Public skepticism of the allopathic medical model began at the end of World War II and grew stronger during the 1960s' decade of dissent. Critics charged that medical institutionalism had placed its own welfare above that of the society it served, ignoring specifically the obligation of self-critique and self-regulation. The response from medicine's political voice, the AMA, was at first dismissive, until the voters began to join the fray. Unregulated fees for service, reimbursement through managed care, and costly defensive medicine had created a perfect storm in healthcare, and the old structures began to crumble (Benda & Weil, 2001). A second tempest arrived in the form of increasing public demand for complementary and alternative medicine, accelerating the erosion of orthodox medicine's hold on the patient. The national debate focusing on repair of the incumbent system began to shift to consideration of a complete reevaluation of priorities and a redesign of healthcare itself.

DEFINE WE MUST

health: A complete state of physical, mental and social well-being, not merely an absence of disease or infirmity.

World Health Organization (1948)

integration: Bringing together of various parts or functions so that they function as a harmonious whole.

Tabor's Medical Dictionary

An entire manuscript could, and likely has, been written delineating nuances large and small inherent to the plethora of names assigned to this so-called new medicine. In our desire for simplicity and our cognizance that definitions change, we will discuss only three: conventional medicine, complementary and alternative medicine (CAM), and integrative medicine. *Conventional medicine* will represent the allopathic model dominant in our Western culture, *CAM* (the mnemonic accepted by the National Institutes of Health and therefore the federal government) will embrace the current abundance of unconventional systems (traditional Chinese medicine, naturopathic medicine, homeopathy, Ayurvedic medicine, and on), and *integrative medicine* will refer to the judicious collaboration of the first two in search of an ideal therapeutic approach. Such collaboration also includes the incorporation of psychological practice steeped in both conventional and unconventional approaches, as health dysfunctions by definition require attention to each individual's mental, physical, spiritual, social, and cultural influences.

Conventional Medicine

Today's cultural icon of conventional medicine is the medical specialist, trained at a traditional institution and employing pharmaceutical drugs, medical devices, and surgery to diagnose and treat disease states. This is in contrast to the late 1800s and early 1900s, when the traditional practitioner was the family physician, caring as best he could for everyone and everything that managed to walk through the front door. As time and technology marched forward, new discoveries and educational advances surpassed the capability of any single individual to absorb the vast amount of information available, deeding the bulk of healthcare delivery to the specialist. Unfortunately, such a shift in medical practice fueled a concurrent shift in medical philosophy as well, and the model of the patient as a collection of individual body parts emboldened science's growing infatuation with reductionistic rather than holistic healthcare. The "ear in room one" or the "laceration in the trauma suite" became standard nomenclature in our educational and clinical institutions, and Osler's admonitions to embrace the patient and not the disease drifted further into our collective historical memory.

Complementary and Alternative Medicine

Since the late 1980s, the public (followed closely by capitalism, Congress, and academic medicine) began to embrace so-called holistic medicine as a potential answer to the chronic illnesses plaguing the twentieth century. Surveys revealed that almost half of the U.S. population had explored such modalities, with numbers increasing annually (although one must accept quite broad inclusion criteria for holistic medicine to interpret such data; Eisenberg et al., 1998).

Although studies showing that CAM use tends be higher for diseases (e.g., cancer, depression, arthritis) often inadequately addressed by conventional means, which may imply an inherent dissatisfaction with Western medicine, surveys show that the public is actually turning to CAM because its doctrines parallel their own personal values and belief systems (Astin, 1998). This is not surprising—although CAM therapies are quite diverse, ranging from well-established cultural traditions (e.g., Chinese medicine) to those yet untested by scientific protocol (e.g., chelation therapy), most all share common underlying philosophies and principles. These include, but are not limited to, recognition of the innate healing capacity of the human body, reliance on the least invasive and least toxic of therapeutic options when appropriate, emphasis of the importance of the relationship between practitioner and patient, and autonomy of the patient, who is informed of all possible options and given control over healthcare choices (Benda, 2002a, 200b, 2002c, 2004).

Integrative Medicine

Integrative medicine was born in the late twentieth century, conceived from the union of conventional and alternative medical theory and practice, just as conventional and alternative therapies evolved in an earlier time from a primal stew of pharmacology, homeopathy, surgery, naturopathy, and countless other established disciplines (Benda & Grant, 2003).

Because conventional medicine had progressively encouraged separation of mind from body, mental health was typically delegated to the field of psychology or psychiatry. Consequently, psychological contributions to the integrative model have, for the most part, been ignored in the development of this new paradigm. While mental health was considered an important component of the mind-body-spirit triad, it was often added on rather than truly integrated. Alternative CAM practitioners, on the other hand, often included mental health as a core aspect of both philosophy and treatment. However, CAM practice has generally failed to incorporate the abundant literature and qualitative and quantitative research of psychology in the promotion of integrative care. Anxiety and depression, most familiar to the integrative (usually MD) practitioner, have received the majority of attention and therapy. But it has became apparent that, although modalities such as acupuncture, massage, energy medicine, and lifestyle changes, including nutrition and physical activity (with the occasional St. John's wort and Valerian), could generally provide benefit, a well thought out, comprehensive therapeutic approach to emotional issues has not yet been developed. This is surprising, given research findings demonstrating neurotransmitter changes secondary to psychological interventions.

With conventional medicine as its dominant sire, integrative medicine seeks scientific proof as the gold standard of efficacy whenever feasible. However, it does recognize the limitations of our current scientific method for investigation of such complex systems as traditional Chinese medicine, homeopathy, and energy medicine. Integrative medicine also inherits many qualities from its more yin CAM parent as well, selecting the least invasive, least toxic, and least costly interventions appropriate to any situation, allowing the body's innate repair mechanism to cure the body, if possible, encouraging strong practitioner-patient relations, and assigning accountability along with autonomy to the one thus afflicted.

From a more philosophical perspective, integrative medicine echoes those early wilderness voices calling for restoration of the focus of medicine on health and healing rather than on disease and treatment. It asks both doctors and patients to pay attention to all relevant influences of life and lifestyle, including diet, exercise, quality of sleep and rest, stress management, nature of relationships to others and to work, and on.

There are, of course, labor pains inherent to the birth of any new paradigm, and the appearance of alternative therapies caused intrinsic discomfort. A hungry public was suddenly offered a multitude of therapeutic choices, but of "unproven" efficacy and safety (not only did centuries-old modalities not lend themselves easily to scientific study, but many of their practitioners feared attempts of validation via research could potentially erode long-held philosophical cornerstones). There was no standardization of training in integrative medicine as there were less than a handful of medical institutions willing to take the political heat of such an endeavor (although as of this writing, 32 conventional medical colleges offer electives in CAM). Finally, and perhaps most importantly, some of the deepest foundational tenets of this new medicine, such as profound and thoughtful self-examination by practitioner as well as patient, often disappeared under the weight of financial and academic priorities.

Such growing pains soon began to exhibit political symptomalogy. As is inevitable in any opinionated discourse, conflicts arose between ideologues on both sides. Academia became partisan. Traditional medical journals published reports of adverse effects from botanical medicines while rejecting studies demonstrating positive clinical outcomes. Alternative medical journals cried foul, pointing to the pharmaceutical industry's influence on editorial decision making. Chiropractic, acupuncture, and naturopathic training institutions sought increased legislative clout and state licensure. Voters and their money entered the fray, and so politicians took note; Congress passed the Dietary Supplement Health and Education Act in 1994, President Clinton created the White House Committee on Complementary and Alternative Medicine in 2000, and the National Institutes of Health established the National Center for

Complementary and Alternative Medicine. This latter development dictated that research funding for unconventional therapies reside under conventional medicine's sphere of influence, spawning further debate as to whether orthodox methodology, flawed as it is in investigating its own paradigm, is an appropriate tool to validate unorthodox systems of health and disease.

Meanwhile, traditional physicians feared losing patients to alternative practitioners, and alternative practitioners feared being co-opted by the orthodox system. Although the integration of alternative and conventional medicine was a step in the right direction, it had not yet given us the necessary redesign of our systems of health and healing, and this proved disappointing to those voices who were no longer crying from the wilderness but had now become culturally mainstream.

WHERE DO WE GO FROM HERE?

Given a steady diet of time, education, knowledge, and technology, conventional medicine has become an amazing, complicated, life-saving, expensive, and mechanistic answer to our healthcare needs. What was once healing has now become science, with science providing the tools with which to heal. But is science truly reflective of a clinical scenario? A patient visits the physician, and the examination and laboratory tests are all within the standard values chosen as normal. At the next visit, the blood glucose (or blood pressure) is near the high end of the acceptable range, still not a real problem, but on the third visit it is several points over the norm. For the conventional practitioner this has become a disease, and he must do something, but what? The usual response is to medicate, and with a modicum of time, both concerns and numbers drift back within normal range. But has the patient regained health? Could not the body still be out of balance, undetectable by blood work or radiographic imagery? And what of collateral damage in the name of healing? According to the Institute of Medicine, in-hospital medication errors injure over 1.5 million Americans each year (one-quarter of them preventable) and may be one of the top 10 causes of hospital deaths in the country (Bates, D. W., Cullen, D. J., Laird, N., Petersen, L. A., Small, S. D., and Servi, D., et al. 1995; Institute of Medicine, 2006).

We have assumed proven efficacy of conventional therapies, convinced that they hold moral and scientific authority over unproven, unorthodox approaches. But a 1978 study by the Office of Technology Assessment of the U.S. Congress (1978) estimated that "only 10–20% of all procedures currently used in medical practices have been shown to be efficacious by controlled trial" a supposition more recently confirmed by other investigators (Imrie & Ramey, 2000). Although great controversy surrounds a multitude of research studies, editorials, and countereditorials delineating the efficacy and safety of both conventional and CAM therapies, the reality must be faced that no one approach can claim any moral or clinical high ground as the one true source of healing.

Perhaps we should return to the philosophies of our distant ancestral healers and consider the possibility that our physical, mental, and emotional health may originate from supernatural (outside the known forces of nature) sources after all. Some of us have sworn by Hippocrates's oath, but have we upheld his beliefs: to pray, meditate, and heal each other? Are our current medical therapies truly healing the patient? What, in fact, is the definition of healing? The absence of disease? Or a state of disease-free lab values? Both disease and health may simply be different extremes of a natural spectrum, complementary underpinnings of life, concepts we cannot really test or define, secrets of the universe. Stephen Hawking states, "We have no idea how the world really is. All we do is build up models which seem to prove our theories (Boslough, 1985)." Perhaps our medical models are just that—small and somewhat crude representations of an elusive masterpiece created by a much greater talent than we.

Healthcare was never meant to end the suffering of the world or the pain and trials of human existence, but to assist in learning to balance life in face of such tribulations. So what is the humanization of healthcare? Alternative medicine as we define it today? Integrative medicine? Integrated? Perhaps it is simply a belief system that continues to develop as long as time progresses, nudging us to let go of that which does not work and accept that which does, not to try to rescue or save the patient from the life they are living or a death they cannot escape.

CONCLUSION

No one can deny the existence of an escalating crisis in the delivery and financing of healthcare in the United States today. A troublesome triad of unregulated fees for service, reimbursement through managed care, and costly defensive medicine has complicated, rather than alleviated, the burden of escalating chronic illness in an aging population. Until recently, our national debate has focused on repair of this system, rather than the creation of a new design. This chapter has been an attempt to encourage consideration to think in different categories.

All new paradigms, past, present, and future, follow a course of initiation, growth, plateau, and decline, followed by the next initiatory phase. Because the underlying impulse is evolutional, such repetitive cycles do not close back on themselves, but move upward as in a spiral—an endless reincarnation toward the direction of theoretical perfection. The paradigm shift we define as integrated healthcare requires such an evolution, away from the simplistic model of body, mind, and spirit and into the more inclusive social, political, economic, metaphysical, ecological, and cosmological dimensions influencing healthcare.

An integrated approach to public health would redefine the ideology of the system rather than attempting to repair the current model. It would seek equitable and universal access, focusing on disease prevention as well as treatment and cure (which may not always be possible). Decisions regarding the provision of healthcare would not simply originate within the medical and reimbursement sectors, but become social contracts among individuals, providers, hospitals, academic institutions, corporations, communities, and governmental agencies. Individuals, accordingly, would become accountable for the impact their behavioral choices have on the community as well as their own personal well-being. Healthcare providers and hospitals would work to prevent illness as well as treat it, placing accountability to the individual and the community above financial profit. Academic institutions would develop programs that promote synergistic training of students of medicine, nursing, pharmacy, CAM, and others involved in patient care. Corporations would recognize the overall value of healthy employees and invest in individual and organizational wellness programs. Communities would acknowledge that health is not only the result of good medical care, but also of adequate housing, sanitation, and education. Finally, government would serve as a safety net, ensuring access to medical care when all other resources fail as well as enacting and enforcing legislation designed to protect both the individual and the healthcare system. Thus the concept of integrated medicine encompasses not only the health of the individual, but of society as a whole (Benda & Weil, 2001).

There is great cause for optimism at this particular moment in our medical and social evolution. After years of eroded confidence, the public is once again seeking a trusting relationship, once again asking their healthcare professionals to take charge of the delivery of service and creation of policy (Kultgen, 1988). The professional also desires to regain the authority and power that was foolishly abdicated to those with conflicting priorities and opposing principles. For the first time in decades, the public and the healing professions are in agreement. Should such synergy continue to grow and develop, no corporate or legislative institution could withstand its mandate. Patient and professional alike are returning, literally and figuratively, to a time when the practitioner sits at the bedside to hold the patient's hand, and the patient looks back with trust and faith.

TOOL KIT FOR CHANGE

Role and Perspective of the Healthcare Professional

1. Medicine is not a known entity, with treatment protocols standard for every patient. It is a field evolving over time, where commonly accepted therapies may be proven

useless and fringe approaches shown beneficial. The healthcare professional must develop and maintain an open mind to maintain balance.

2. One cannot claim to be a true healer without the intention and effort at self-reflection and desire for personal, social, and environmental health.

3. The hierarchy of medical authority and accountability applies to licensing and standards of care only. There is no differentiation among practitioners with regard to moral authority, societal class, or equality of respect.

Role and Perspective of the Patient/Participant

1. The patient has ultimate accountability for his physical, psychological, and emotional health.

2. We will all grow older, lose our beauty, and eventually die. Get over it, and focus on creating and maintaining health in the moment.

3. The future of healthcare cannot be abdicated to the government, managed care industry, or even the practitioner. Only the patient has the moral authority to demand quality of care.

Interconnection: The Global Perspective

1. Healthcare is in the midst of a transition, perhaps even a paradigm shift. The eventual outcome is not known at this moment in time.

2. Both conventional and unconventional medical therapies hold the power to create significant benefit or significant harm. They must be used judiciously and in balance with each other.

3. We are in this life and on this planet to help each other, which in turn ensures our own personal survival and happiness.

REFERENCES

Astin, J. A. (1998). Why patients use alternative medicine: Results of a national study. *Journal of the American Medical Association, 279,* 1548–1553.

Bates, D. W., Cullen, D. J., Laird, N., Petersen, L. A., Small, S. D., and Servi, D., et al. (2005). Incidence and preventability of adverse drug events and potential adverse drug events. *Journal of the American Medical Association, 274,* 29–34.

Beck, Andrew. (2004). The flexner report and the standardization of american medical education. *Journal of the American Medical Association. 291,* 2139–2140.

Benda, W. (2002a). Effects of group psychosocial support in breast cancer patients. *Practical Reviews in Complementary and Alternative Medicine, 4.*

Benda, W. (2002b). Hypnotherapy for the treatment of irritable bowel syndrome. *Practical Reviews in Complementary and Alternative Medicine, 6.*

Benda, W. (2002c). Hypnotic induction eliminates increased sympathetic activity after PTCA. *Practical Reviews in Complementary and Alternative Medicine, 7.*

Benda, W. (2004). From integrative to integral medicine: A leap of faith. In M. Schlitz (Ed.), *Consciousness and healing* (pp. 32–38). St. Louis, MO: Elsevier / Churchill Livingstone.

Benda, W., & Grant, K. L. (2003). The integrative approach to cancer. In D. Rakel (Ed.), *Integrative medicine.* St. Louis, MO: W. B. Saunders.

Benda, W., & Weil, A. (2001). Integrative medicine. In L. Breslow (Ed.), *The encyclopedia of public health.* New York: Macmillan Reference.

Boslough, J. (1985). Stephen Hawking. New York: Universe Avon.

Eisenberg, D. M., Davis, R. B., Ettner, S. L., Appel, S., Wilkey, S., Van Rompay, M., et al. (1998). Trends in alternative medicine use in the United States, 1990–1997: Results of a follow-up national survey. *Journal of the American Medical Association, 18,* 1569–1575.

Finger, S. (2000). *Minds behind the brain: A history of the pioneers and their discoveries.* New York: Oxford University Press.

Frazer, J. G. (1975). *Folklore in the Old Testament.* New York: Hart.

Imrie, R., & Ramey, D. W. (2000). The evidence for evidence-based medicine. *Complementary Therapies in Medicine, 8,* 123–126.

Institute of Medicine, Board of Healthcare Session, Committee on Identifying and Preventing Medication Errors. (2006). Identifying and preventing medication errors. Retrieved July 20, 2006, from http://www.iom.edu/?id=35942.

Kultgen, J. (1988). *Ethics and professionalism.* Philadelphia: University of Pennsylvania Press.

Loudon, I. (1986). *Medical care and the general practitioner.* Oxford, UK: Clarendon Press.

Shipley, J. T. (1945). *Dictionary of word origins* (2nd ed.). New York: Philosophical Library.

Sigerist, H. E. (1929). *History of medicine: Early Greek, Hindu, and Persian medicine* (Vol. 2). New York: W. B. Saunders.

U.S. Congress, Office of Technology Assessments. (1978). *Assessing the efficacy and safety of medical technologies.* Washington, DC: U.S. Government Printing Office.

Wolpe, P. R. (1999). *From quackery to "integrated care": Power, politics, and alternative medicine* (Vol. 8). Philadelphia, PA: Center for Frontier Sciences.

Chapter Three

INTEGRATIVE HEALTH AND LOVING CARE: THE PROMISE AND THE LIMITS

Marc Pilisuk, PhD

INTRODUCTION

When I was a young boy growing up during the great depression, both my parents taught me, by their example, a lesson I was only later able to appreciate. They were concerned deeply with the well-being of others in the human family who had even less than we had. I did not know at the time how important that would be for my own well-being.

My mother also gave me her advice about illness. If I was a little bit out of sorts, she told me to go out and play with my friends. Anything more serious, stay home and let me take care of you, read you stories and feed you chicken soup. Not all parental advice is right, and some things my mother suggested might even have been dangerous. But in this case, an overwhelming body of evidence suggests that Mom was right. Social support is critical to health.

Before examining this evidence, it is useful to reflect on why the importance of social ties should come as a revelation, or even require scientific study. We are evolved as part of an intricately designed planetary system, in which all parts, living and mineral, are interconnected and dependent on one another. Other members of our species form a particularly important part of these connections. Through most of human history, individuals survived within groups of between 15 and 150 people linked by kinship, but also economically, socially, and spiritually and within a particular geographic niche within which they found sustenance. As a late arrival in evolution, conscious thought might be expected to take note of this interdependence, and in many indigenous cultures these connections present a paradigm of thought that frames the meanings of life in daily actions. However, the gift of thought has come with a great deal of flexibility in what we choose to include in the conscious worlds that we construct.

For most of Western medicine and psychology, the assumption is now made that the person is a distinct and separable object of study. Our efforts to understand the human being and to predict human behavior have focused largely on attributes considered to be parts of the individual psyche. This has been true despite powerful evidence to show how interdependent we are with our ecology (Bronfenbrenner, 1977), our attachments (Ainsworth, 1982; Bowlby, 1982), and our relationships (Belenky, Clinchy, Goldberger, & Tarule, 1986).

The ways that love and caring get transmitted are complex. Humans deal in symbols, and much of what we exchange are images of caring and of familiar others with affirming ties to the self. But studies of other animals show the importance of the contact that occurs on a more sensory level. Classic studies by Harry Harlow of the rhesus monkey provided with either a lactating wire mother or a soft cloth mother showed the dramatic positive effects of touch on the baby's development (Harlow & Harlow, 1962). Similarly, classic works on mother-separated infants by Renee Spitz (1974) and again by Bowlby (1982) affirm the critical need for bonding and attachment to a mother figure. The value of physical touch, as in massage, has been demonstrated in a number of studies (Targ, 1997), and the suggestion of four hugs a day is perhaps a worthwhile goal. More controversial are the effects of noncontact therapeutic touch, in which it is hypothesized that energy flows go from the healer to the person being healed. There is some promising evidence to suggest that healing though such practice does occur.

Some of the ways that caring is transmitted are revealed in stories in which the wisdom of our bodies merges with the wisdom of our relationships. That wisdom is central to the healing traditions of several non-Western cultures. But two books provide excellent examples of the wisdom in such stories in our own culture: Bernie Siegel's (1986) *Love, Medicine, and Miracles: Lessons Learned about Self-Healing from a Surgeon's Experience with Exceptional Patients* and Rachel Naomi Remen's (1996) *Kitchen Table Wisdom: Stories That Heal.*

The dominant, person-centered approach fails to take cognizance of the degree to which people are in fact interdependent and that the boundaries of the person are actually quite fluid. A full understanding of the individual depends on an appreciation of the nature, and of the degree, of a person's connections with a broader sustaining ecology and, particularly, with contacts with other people. When an individual's health breaks down, there is often a rift in the ties that sustain the person. One cannot view health holistically while ignoring the major factors that tear people from their social network. We understand health rather poorly without knowing the particular place and the people that give meaning to human lives.

When an individual suffers discomforting symptoms, it is possible to examine the source of the internal infection, the bodily organ working defectively, or the deeply embedded anxieties all to be found within the person. This approach is extremely important for establishing a diagnosis and for prescribing a specific treatment. But if we follow the oft-cited admonition of Dr. William Osler, it may be more important to ask what kind of patient has the illness rather than what kind of illness has the patient (cited in Cassell, 1976). When we do, we find some remarkable similarities among patients experiencing the widest variety of physical and behavioral pathologies. Those who show any one or more of a great variety of maladies, or who die prematurely, are more likely to have weaknesses in the web of supportive ties that represents their network. Those who might otherwise not be considered lacking in network ties typically move into the group with a high risk of breakdown, in some form, following a loss or disruption of their networks (Achterberg, 1998; Pilisuk & Parks, 1986; Sagan, 1988; Seeman, 1996). The form of the breakdown may vary from auto accidents, to depression or suicide attempts, to hypertension or cardiovascular disease, to digestive or respiratory problems, and the timing of the breakdown may be immediate or longer term, as in posttraumatic stress disorder (Pilisuk, Boylan, & Acredelo, 1987).

The importance of integration into a social network was noted in Durkheim's (1897/1951) classic study showing that suicide rates were higher among persons who were not married and who were not linked well to a church or community. The relevance of social ties to mental health was subsequently noted (Ware, 1956). Tolsdorf (1976) documented the weak and fragmented networks of psychotic patients. Now many studies confirm that people better integrated into a social network live longer (Berkman, 1995; Sagan, 1988) and are less susceptible to infectious diseases (Cohen, Doyle, Skoner, Rabin, & Gwaltney, 1997). They are more likely to survive a heart attack (Seeman & Berkman, 1988) and to avoid a recurrence of cancer (Helgeson, Cohen, & Fritz, 1998). These effects appear even when controlling for risks associated with smoking, blood pressure, and obesity (House, Landis, & Umberson, 1988) and therefore highlight the importance of understanding and assessing social networks. The health-promoting or illness-preventing effects of special ties have been documented in work with monkeys, goats, mice, and chickens (Pilisuk & Parks, 1986). Gradually, research in psychoneuroimmunology has provided evidence from controlled studies linking social support to health by documentation of the particular changes within the immune system to be found when individuals are subjected to high stress without the buffering support of a strong support network (Keicolt-Glaser et al., 1984). This research is now quite extensive (Glaser & Kiecolt-Glaser, 1994) and has been related to a theory of what some have described as the fundamental power of love in the healing process (Green & Shellenberger, 1996; Lewis, Amini, & Lannon, 2000).

There is, however, a competing view for which some evidence has accumulated. It states that, while support may be helpful to mitigate the effects of stress, individuals become most vulnerable to some form of breakdown when they no longer have a sense of control over the challenges that they must meet through life (Syme, 1989). This thesis appears, at first glance, to take us back to the individual as the object of study; that is, disempowered individuals are more likely to break down under the stressors confronting them. But under closer scrutiny we see that empowerment is a social process and not a personal bootstrap operation. Special healing powers of spiritual healers and caregivers are a form of empowerment (DiCowden, 2003). Within the fields of community organizing and community development, empowerment has referred to two phenomena. First, the term relates to the ability of poor and disenfranchised people to discover that they do have a voice, and second, it shows a process by which people are enabled to use that voice collectively to address their conditions. The latter is particularly important since it reminds us that power is a concept that takes its meaning in relation to how it is distributed. Those who lack power do so because some other people or forces have more power. Where power is gained by one party, it is lost somewhere else.

In one study, three of the commonly used predictors of health status, that is, social support, locus of control, and life stress, were used with a sample of older adults. All variables showed association with the reported presence of actual symptoms of illness. But for the men in the sample, an increased sense of control and a larger network of friends distinguished males who were able to see themselves as healthy despite the presence of symptoms (Pilisuk, Montgomery, Parks, & Acredelo, 1993). American males are more intensively socialized to obtain mastery. When their control and their networks are in place, they are more likely to discount the importance of their symptoms (helping to explain lower rates of medical care utilization among men). But for those who cannot sustain an image of control and support (e.g., those whose lives have been marked by chronic unemployment), the low sense of control is internalized as failure and contributes to a decline in one's image of healthfulness. This decline is even more rapid than the identifiable physical disorders and symptoms that ensue. The communities we label as at risk are filled with adults who see few options for giving in meaningful ways to a network they will need for their well-being. They oblige young people to seek their support from others who, like themselves, have been cut off from the supportive connections of a broader community. It is perhaps only a small jump from such studies to the conclusion that health promotion is not only about the provision of treatment services or even preventive services. Health is promoted when communities use their voice to make known their health concerns and to act on them (Minkler and Wallerstein, 2005; Pilisuk & Minkler, 1985; Wallack, 2005).

If we are to conceive of the professional task as one directed in a fundamental way toward reweaving the web of relationships, three considerations should prove useful.

1. Networks, including both their strengths and the rifts and gaps within them, can be assessed and diagnosed.
2. The client for services can be redefined to include the context of a healing network.
3. The relationship of the professional is to a client who is no longer an ailing individual but an imperfectly functioning set of relationships and resources.

ASSESSING NETWORK HEALTH

The plotting of the web of exchange tunes us to look at individuals both as recipients of activities generated by others and as generators of activity as well. Precise networks of who is connected to whom can be plotted. The overall plot has a distinctive size and structure—densely or loosely interconnected, hierarchical or equally assessable to all, closed to specific groups or open to outsiders. The linkages can be described according to what flows between people—material help, companionship, or emotional sharing.

Functional or *interactional* qualities describe the relationships of pairs of individuals in a network. In this we are looking not at the form of the web, but at the qualities of the links. We examine such qualities as frequency of contact and friendship duration. In addition, the *mode of contact* describes the ways individuals communicate, such as directly face-to-face or via telephone or e-mail. *Intimacy* refers to how an individual describes the closeness of a relationship. *Multiplexity* refers to the number of different exchanges (emotional support, physical help, social contact, or money) that can occur between two individuals. *Symmetry* (see Barnes, 1969) refers to the degree of mutuality or reciprocity in any relationship. *Functional stability* describes changes in the way in which the network is used over time. Surely ties may be strong or weak, intimate or formal, and reciprocal or unilateral. They may reflect single or multiple role relationships and may be hierarchically ordered in accord with power relationships. The links may be a source of companionship, emotional support, or instrumental assistance (Pilisuk & Parks, 1986). Various scales and measures select aspects of the network of greatest interest to particular assessments. Some of the most important aspects of a network for health include elements of multiplex relationships (many types of exchange) and opportunities for reciprocation (Pilisuk & Wong, 2002). These are more often found in close or intimate networks and are considered critical in mitigating the trauma and subsequent breakdowns in health that are associated with grief or loss. However, the strength of weak ties emerges when clients need to network to find new resources to move on to a new job, a new living situation, or a new primary relationship (Granovetter, 1973). The more extended network can help the professional in the tasks of rebuilding family networks, locating and strengthening the work of natural helpers, resolving disputes, building coalitions, humanizing places of work, and linking people facing similar challenges to one another.

These concepts may be viewed as central to the tasks of counseling and psychotherapy. Feminist theory places relationships at the center of human development and examines how disconnections occur and how therapy may be seen as an effort to deepen relationships. Miller and Stiver (1997) apply the principles to the cultivation of healing relationships in families and in therapy. But just as individual family members cannot be fully helped without attention to their dysfunctional families, families cannot be adequately helped without attention to the pathology of their communities, and communities suffer from the pressures of a global economy, which must also be addressed (Weissbourd & Kagan, 1989). While professionals have an obligation to address larger policy issues, they also have a major role in facilitating the actions of local communities. Many of the practical interventions are grouped under the concept of capacity mapping and capacity building (Gutierrez & Lewis, 2005; McKnight & Kreitzman, 2005).

One question frequently raised is whether people who have been challenged deeply by years of isolation and alcoholism, by serious psychoses, or by the learned helplessness of life in the ghetto or in a refugee camp can truly be full partners in the restoration of their social networks, their neighborhoods, or their communities. A number of studies note that schizophrenics treated in the developed nations as flawed individuals requiring pharmacological interventions show remarkably high rates of reintegration into normal roles in less developed countries where they receive no drugs but are expected to return to normal roles within a caring community (Irwin, 2004; Vedantam, 2005). One project addressed another unlikely candidate of transformative efforts: the health of elderly people living in single-room-occupancy hotels in San Francisco's Tenderloin district. The population includes a large percentage of old people displaced by the closing of mental hospitals. Many are socially isolated, afraid of being mugged if they leave their rooms, and afraid of asking their landlords to deal with broken appliances and toilets, infested cabinets, and unsafe and unclean stairwells. They share their surroundings with mentally and physically disabled younger people, recent immigrants, and the homeless in a section with high crime rates and 300 times greater population density than the rest of the city. The Tenderloin Senior Outreach Project began modestly with one-on-one conversations to address the serious isolation of aged and ill residents of one deteriorated single-room-occupancy hotel. It evolved into a coalition of tenants' organizations in 20 hotels. Twelve years later, they were able to claim safer and better housing, merchant safe houses for protection against muggers, better nutrition, active social involvement, shopping chaperones, political activity on behalf of local immigrant (Cambodian and Vietnamese) groups, access to the press and to the mayor's office, and regular training for and participation in political advocacy on issues from the local to the global (Minkler, 2005; Pilisuk & Minkler, 1980).

REDEFINING THE CLIENT

Viewing the embedding connections of people, we are able to shed the image of a client as an ailing person. Instead, we find a web of exchanges that punish some people, isolate others, and fail to provide sustenance to meet the physical and emotional needs of many. The client is no longer an abused or unfortunate victim but part of a threadbare social fabric that must be rewoven (Sarason, Sarason, & Pierce, 1990).

How does the healthcare professional infuse love and social connection? Love, or embeddedness into a network of caring and reciprocal expectations, may be nurtured. It cannot be prescribed as if it were a particular pill or an added activity to be included on a checklist. The healthcare professional can, however, apply a knowledge of its importance in several ways. At the client level this involves a great deal of active search for the existing familial or community network and a willingness to work outside of the comfort zones of office or agency (Cohen, Underwood, & Gottlieb, 2000). To the extent that the health problems were created and sustained by social dislocation, the remedies must include social reintegration. For the professional to make full use of the beneficial aspects of reciprocity and of multiplex or complex relationships, he needs to sensitively be aware of what networks are already in place and also what the clients have to give.

At the professional level the context of helping may be critical. The remedies dispensed now add yoga, meditation, behavioral training exercises, and herbal remedies to the drugs and surgeries heretofore dispensed. But an important aspect of the individual-focused medical model persists. The professional as a lone practitioner, overworked and disconnected from other practitioners, presents a poor role model for the client. It is a model of work that places the healer at increased risk of breakdown.

The cost to the natural helper may be even greater. Natural helpers play a large and often unseen role. As the population ages and life expectancy increases, the number of caregivers needed grows dramatically, and most care for the frail elderly is provided by family members. An example of the *burden* of caregiving is provided by the typical primary caregiver. She (women far outnumber men in this role) spends an average of six hours and 28 minutes per day assisting with medication, personal hygiene, household chores, transportation, and shopping. The amount of instrumental assistance in care provision can be great. Forty-six percent of the caregivers are required to help the disabled person get in and out of bed. This can pose a tremendous problem to many caregivers who are themselves older people and whose physical strength is seriously tapped in providing this instrumental assistance. A very high prevalence among caregivers of certain emotional consequences—notably depression, anger, and chronic fatigue—has been well documented. When a spouse or parent becomes highly dependent, an inevitable change occurs in the lifescape. The questions before the caregiver include, Is my relative in pain? Can I handle this situation physically? Am I doing enough? What does one do about incontinence, or passivity, or asocial behavior? An experience of grief over the loss of ability and of a relationship as it has been known often occurs. This grief differs from loss through death. Death is final and brings with it a closure to a relationship. Loss here is open ended (Parks & Pilisuk, 1991; Pilisuk and Parks, 1988). The point of the caregiver illustration is that natural helpers need the professionals and the society they represent to enable them to reduce the physical and financial burdens to permit families members to do what they do best, that is, provide love and companionship.

The egocentric view of personal health takes society off the hook. It also removes the hook that we professionals sorely need to be effective. Too often, we stand helpless to address the rifts in a fabric torn by people being downsized at work, displaced by development or by long-term illness or disability or caught in the destitution of deprivation. The rift in a supportive network may be from the disruptions of war, removing the soldier from home and family, killing some, permanently disabling others, disrupting family expectations for being a partner or a parent, and creating another generation of people bearing the symptoms of PTSD and unable to fulfill the promise of their attachments. In its wake are the displaced and uprooted refugees, mostly children, left without parents, or shelter, or potable water.

Some poor communities, particularly some communities of color, have literally survived by the strength of their informal ties (Malson, 1983; Stack, 1974). But survival with a high level of suffering is more the norm. Poverty, defined both as a lack of critical resources and as a source of cultural adaptations to lives of struggle, also contributes to rifts in the supportive web that sustains health (Belle, 1983). Those who are poor are believed to be responsible for their lack of success. To be poor is not only to lack material things, but also to experience the scorn of others and the often internalized scorn of oneself. It is to see one's circumstance as an incurable consequence of fate. In Freire's (1970) *Pedagogy of the Oppressed,* the steps are laid out on how to teach by asking questions and listening. As poor and illiterate peasants learn the signs and labels for common items, they gradually come to realize that these symbols are constructions that were created by people. Alternative constructions can be created to fit their own experience and the experience of their family, tribe, or village. Such constructions permit a perceptual world in which caring relationships are more securely in place.

Examples of such efforts appear in projects everywhere. At their best they go beyond the crises faced by a particular person or even a particular community and are linked to larger efforts toward transformative social change. One example is the project Quipunet, a unique virtual community.

It all started from a desire to help our country from afar by combining the ideas of a tiny group of Peruvians living all over the world. They created a virtual village composed of engineers, students, professors, diplomats, and housewives, all bonded by a common goal: to help their very poor country. They joined forces and created Quipunet (http://www.quipunet.org) entirely on the Internet. Overcoming distance and national borders, they learned how to communicate and cooperate over the Internet to plan and execute ideas. They learned how to make virtual seminars, create bridges of help, forge a communication network, and organize and direct tasks from afar, working in cyberspace as if it were a real office. Their desire to help rural areas faced a harsh reality of the digital divide. They found poor or nonexistent infrastructure, expensive connectivity, lack of awareness, and complete indifference to outsiders and to the wonders of the Internet. They were dismayed, but they kept on. Gradually, they empowered villagers by giving them a window and connection to the outside world.

Their mission is to provide education, information, and aid to those places most in need in South America, especially Peru. They have not provided education as we originally envisioned it; instead, they have empowered many people through their projects.

Their work has empowered the women carpenters in Ica, Peru. Instead of buying the benches and desks needed in their kids' school, the project paid for the training of some of the mothers, for the materials, and for the tools. They made all the school's furniture. They helped to empower small farmers by teaching better techniques to make their farms viable.

They helped to empower the street kids in Huancayo, who before had been stealing in the streets, to learn to be shoemakers, and they encouraged high school kids by promoting virtual writing contests.

The small group of volunteers who comprised the virtual village are keenly aware of what it has accomplished without help from big organizations. The way that people in the Andes build hanging bridges serves as a metaphor for the project. Women and children start by gathering simple stalks of dry grass that they twist into thin threads with their callused hands. These threads thus formed get rolled again and again, forming first a thin rope, then a thick one, until they end up as thick coils of rope that later will be tied to form a mighty cable that will be the support for the bridge. Each of the volunteers is but a stalk of grass, yet together, they have woven a strong rope. Their appreciation of their collective efforts serves as a model to the local people who join in the projects. They have formed a for-profit company where profit is not their main concern but rather the ways and means of more widespread caring. From the Andes and from the jungles of Peru, by presenters who have never used the Internet, they are creating new products and new markets and helping once more. They have learned how important they all are to the success of the organization. One example of how this works is a seminar the people of Cusco have produced, a virtual Trip to Cusco: The Land of the Incas. Whether using mountain paths or electronic highways, it is one creative example of trading traditional knowledge for technical knowledge. Much of the work is done at a distance, and its products travel by paths through the forest and by the Internet highway. Quipunet empowered the people, and the people empowered Quipunet.

An offshoot of Quipunet, and a good example of how the empowerment goes on, is E-Connexions (http://www.e-connexions.net). One of the founders, Martha Davies, writes,

> We, the doers that started with just the idea of helping our people, received much more than what we gave, and ended up with a wonderful education! Now, we are involved in e-commerce. We will keep on learning and doing, doing and giving, giving and receiving, while we help create new groups of people empowered to take an active part in the shaping of their own future in this Information Age.

Other projects elsewhere in the world have built community gardens on the rooftops of tenement houses, brought street theater and free clinics to migrant farm workers, or mobilized communities to action against toxic wastes that were contaminating their wells. The best of these have gone on to organize larger constituencies of people more concerned with caring for humans than with expanding corporate markets. The best of these also share a joy, creativity, and sense of closeness to the human community and the political. They will stand up to those whose economic and political power have deprived communities of their health-generating connections and resources. Concepts of love, trust, kindness, caring, sharing, giving, receiving, influencing, teaching, belonging, and relating are important parts of the human condition that can only be studied, nurtured, or appreciated by examining and enhancing individuals' connections to others. My parents were right.

TOOL KIT FOR CHANGE

Role and Perspective of the Healthcare Professional

1. The healthcare professional needs to focus on the patient's health in the context of the patient's support network and assess the rifts and gaps in the patient's social network as well as in the individual himself.

2. The relationship of the professional is to a client who is no longer an ailing individual but an imperfectly functioning set of relationships and resources.
3. The healthcare professional needs a willingness to work outside the comfort zones of office or agency and actively seek out and enlist existing familial or community networks in the healing process.

Role and Perspective of the Patient/Participant

1. The patient must be willing to take personal responsibility for his health and health challenges.
2. The patient must seek coordinated healthcare and be willing to employ healing and health promotion lifestyle changes, for example, yoga, meditation and stress management, or behavioral training exercises and nutritional vigilance, in conjunction with traditional medical and surgical remedies.
3. The patient must be willing to strengthen positive support ties with friends, family, and community.

Interconnection: The Global Perspective

1. Individual health is dependent on the health of the community and, ultimately, on the ecological health of our planet.
2. Healthy communities promote better health for everyone, physically, socially, economically, and spiritually.
3. Caring and concrete sharing of time and resources for family, friends, and neighbors need to occur at times other than those precipitated by natural and other disasters, for example, Hurricane Katrina, earthquakes, or terrorist attacks.

REFERENCES

Achterberg, J. (1998). *The healing web of human relationships.* Paper presented at the Creating Integrated Care Seminar, San Diego, CA.

Ainsworth, M. (1982). Attachment: Retrospect and prospect. In C. Parkes & J. Stephenson-Hinde (Eds.), *The place of attachment in human behavior.* New York: Basic Books.

Barnes, J. A. (1969). Networks and political processes. In J. Clyde Mitchell (Ed.), *Social networks in urban situations: Analyses of personal relationships in Central African towns.* Manchester, UK: Manchester University Press. 51–76.

Belenky, M. F., Clinchy, B. M., Goldberger, N. R., & Tarule, J. M. (1986). *Women's ways of knowing: The development of self, voice, and mind.* New York: Basic Books.

Belle, D. E. (1983). The impact of poverty on social networks and supports. In L. Lein & M. B. Sussman (Eds.), *The ties that bind: Men's and women's social networks* (pp. 89–103). New York: Haworth Press.

Berkman, L. F. (1995). The role of social relations in health promotion. *Psychosomatic Medicine, 47,* 245–254.

Bowlby, J. (1982). Attachment and loss: Retrospect and prospect. *American Journal of Orthopsychiatry, 52,* 664–678.

Bronfenbrenner, U. (1977). Toward an experimental ecology of human development. *American Psychologist, 32,* 513–531.

Cassel, J. (1976). The contribution of social environment to host resistance. *American Journal of Epidemiology, 194,* 197–223.

Cohen, S., Doyle, W. J., Skoner, D. P., Rabin, B. S., & Gwaltney, J. M. (1997). Social ties and susceptibility to the common cold. *Journal of the American Medical Association, 277*, 1940–1944.

Cohen, S., Underwood, L. G., & Gottlieb, B. H. (Eds.). (2000). *Social support measurement and intervention: A guide for health and social scientists.* New York: Oxford University Press.

DiCowden, M. A. (2003). The call of the wild woman: Models of healing. *Women and Therapy, 26*, 297–310.

Durkheim, E. (1951). *Suicide: A study in sociology.* New York: Free Press.

Field, T. (1997). *Memorandum: Touch Research Institute.* Miami, FL: University of Miami School of Medicine.

Freire, P. (1970). *Pedagogy of the oppressed* (D. Tweedie, Trans.). New York: Continuum.

Glaser, R., & Kiecolt-Glaser, J. K. (Eds.). (1994). *Handbook of human stress and immunity.* San Diego, CA: Academic Press.

Granovetter, M. S. (1973). The strength of weak ties. *American Journal of Sociology, 78*, 1360–1372.

Green, J., & Shellenberger, R. (1996). The healing energy of love. *Alternative Therapies, 2*, 46–56.

Gutierrez, L. M., & Lewis, E. A. (2005). Education, participation, capacity building in community organizing with women of color. In M. Minkler (Ed.), *Community organizing and community building for health* (pp. 240–253). New Brunswick, NJ: Rutgers University Press.

Harlow, H., & Harlow, M. (1962). Social deprivation in monkeys. *Scientific American, 207*, 136–143.

Helgeson, V. S., Cohen, S., & Fritz, H. L. (1998). Social ties and the onset and progression of cancer. In J. C. Holland & W. Breitbert (Eds.), *Textbook of psycho-oncology.* New York: Oxford University Press.

House, J. S., Landis, K. R., & Umberson, D. (1988). Social relationships and health. *Science, 241*, 540–545.

Irwin, M. (2004a). Reversal of schizophrenia without neuroleptics. *Ethical Human Psychology and Psychiatry, 6*, 99–110.

Kiecolt-Glaser, J. K., Garner, W., Speicher, C. E., Penn, G. M., Holiday, J., & Glaser, R. (1984). Psychosocial modifiers of immunocompetence in medical students. *Psychosomatic Medicine, 46*, 7–14.

Lewis, T., Amini, F., & Lannon, R. (2000). *A general theory of love.* New York: Random House.

Malson, M. (1983). The social-support systems of black families. In L. Lein & M. B. Sussman (Eds.), *The ties that bind: Men's and women's social networks* (pp. 37–57). New York: Haworth Press.

McKnight, J. L., & Kreitzman, J. P. (2005). Mapping community capacity. In M. Minkler (Ed.), *Community organizing and community building for health* (pp. 158–172). New Brunswick, NJ: Rutgers University Press.

Miller, J. B., & Stiver, I. P. (1997). *The healing connection: How women form relationships in therapy and in life.* Boston: Beacon Press.

Minkler, M. (2005). Community organizing with the elderly poor in San Francisco's Tenderloin district. In M. Minkler (Ed.), *Community organizing and community building for health* (pp. 272–288). New Brunswick, NJ: Rutgers University Press.

Minkler, M. & Wallerstein, N. (2005). Improving health through community organizing and community building: A health education perspective. In M. Minkler (Ed.), *Community organizing and community building for health*. New Brunswick, New Jersey: Rutgers University Press. 26–50.

Parks, S. H., & Pilisuk, M. (1991). Caregiver burden—Gender and the psychological costs of coping. *American Journal of Orthopsychiatry, 61*, 501–509.

Pilisuk, M. (2001). Ecological psychology, caring, and the boundaries of the person. *Journal of Humanistic Psychology, 41*(2), 25–37.

Pilisuk, M., Boylan, R., & Acredelo, C. (1987). Social support, life stress and subsequent medical care utilization. *Health Psychology, 6*, 273–288.

Pilisuk, M., & Minkler, M. (1980). Supportive networks: Life ties for the elderly. *Journal of Social Issues, 36*, 95–116.

Pilisuk, M., & Minkler, M. (1985, Winter). Social support: Economic and political considerations. *Social Policy*, 6–11.

Pilisuk, M., Montgomery, M., Parks, S. H., & Acredelo, C. (1993). Locus of control, social support and stress: Gender differences in the health status of the elderly. *Sex Roles: A Journal of Research, 8*, 1–20.

Pilisuk, M., & Parks, S. H. (1986). *The healing web: Social networks and human survival*. Hanover, NH: University Press of New England.

Pilisuk, M., & Parks, S. H. (1988). Caregiving: Where families need help. *Social Work, 33*, 436–440.

Pilisuk, M., & Wong, A. (2002). Social network assessment. In R. F. Ballesteros (Ed.), *The encyclopedia of psychological assessment* (pp. 901–907). London: Sage.

QuipuNet. (2006). *What is QuipuNet?* Retrieved April 18, 2005, from http://www.quipunet.org/English/About_us/?&item=1

Remen, N. (1996). *Kitchen table wisdom: Stories that heal*. New York: Riverhead Press.

Sagan, L. A. (1988, March/April). Family ties: The real reason people are living longer. *The Science*, 21–28.

Sarason, B. R., Sarason, I. G., & Pierce, G. R. (1990). Traditional views of social support and their impact on assessment. In B. R. Sarason, I. G. Sarason, & G. R. Pierce (Eds.), *Social support: An interactional view* (pp. 9–25). New York: John Wiley.

Seeman, T. E. (1996). Social ties and health: The benefits of social integration. *Annals of Epidemiology, 6*, 442–451.

Seeman, T. E., & Berkman, L. F. (1988). Structural characteristics of social networks and their relationship with social support in the elderly: Who provides support. *Social Science and Medicine, 26*, 737–749.

Siegel, B. S. (1986). *Love, medicine, and miracles: Lessons learned about self-healing from a surgeon's experience with exceptional patients*. New York: Harper and Row.

Spitz, R. (Producer). (1974). *Grief: A peril in infancy* [Motion picture]. (Available from the New York University Film Archive, 1947.)

Stack, C. (1974). *All our kin*. New York: Harper and Row.

Syme, S. L. (1989). Control and health: A personal perspective. In A. Steptoe & A. Appels (Eds.), *Stress, personal control, and health* (pp. 3–18). New York: John Wiley.

Targ, E. (1997). Evaluating distant healing: A research review. *Alternative Therapies, 3*(6), 74–78.

Tolsdorf, C. (1976). Social networks, support, and coping: An exploratory study. *Family Relations, 5*, 407–418.

Vedantam, S. (2005, June 27). Social network's healing power is borne out in poorer nations. *Washington Post*, A1.

Wallack, L. (2005). Media advocacy: A strategy for Empowering people and communities, M. Minkler (Ed.), *Community organizing and community building for health*. New Brunswick, New Jersey: Rutgers University Press. 419–432.

Ware, E. H. (1956). Mental illness and social conditions in Bristol. *Journal of Mental Science, 102*, 349–357.

Weissbourd, B., & Kagan, S. L. (1989). Family support programs: Catalysts for change. *American Journal of Orthopsychiatry, 39*, 20–31.

Chapter Four

HEALING ENVIRONMENTS FOR INTEGRATIVE HEALTHCARE

Susan J. Frey, PhD, ND, RN

INTRODUCTION

Common sense tells us that the physical environment affects our lives. During the last half of the twentieth century and into the twenty-first, scientific research has confirmed it. Environments are like our trace elements playing subtle yet crucial roles in the human body. The renowned architect Christopher Alexander (2002) says that "the impact of the geometry of our environment—its living or not-living structure—has a similar nearly trace-like effect on our emotional, social, spiritual and physical well-being....Its space has the most profound impact possible on human beings" (p. 373).

In this chapter we will explore the environment as a catalyst for health and healing: new ways to perceive it, possible ways to use it, and transformative ways to be served by it, from the practical to the poetic.

SPACE AS THERAPY

The Romans defined space *(spatium)* as that which is characterized by dimensions extending indefinitely in all directions from any given point and within which all material bodies are located. It is also defined as outer, interval, purposeful, and opportunistic. It is expansive, whole, interconnected, and architectural. Its application is environmental.

Therapy has a more specific definition: treatment, activity, and healing. Interestingly, the original Greek word, *theraps*, means "servant," and in its original meaning and context, therapy may be expanded here to serve an environmental purpose through participation.

Theraps involves four meanings or levels: level one corresponds to the mutual dependence of the servant and master; level two involves the practice, intuition, and sensitivity to the personal engagement; the third level centers on education, responsibility, and a holistic expertise in initiating tasks; and level four culminates in a holistic healing, not strictly physical, but a spiritual restoration as well (Franck & Lepori, 2000).

The authors of *Architecture Inside Out* (Franck & Lepori, 2000) devote an entire chapter to space therapy, applying it to the art and practice of architecture and the built environment. However, the possibility for space therapy to move beyond the realms of servant-master and designer-client to patient-practitioner is indeed compelling. The patient-practitioner relationship is a mutual and symbiotic one within any given space: the patient-practitioner relationship depends on knowledge, intuition, and sensibility to each other and to the environmental space, and a curative restoration requires mutual participation that is holistic, purposeful, expansive, and interconnected. In terms of the fourfold meaning of therapy, "the aim of space therapy is to unify the practical aspects of the built environment as service to the more existential ones related to well-being" (Franck & Lepori, 200, p. 83). The awareness that space impacts the healing experience and the fundamental biorhythms of our being challenges readers to perceive the environment, and their role in it, in new ways.

For centuries, great architects and visionaries have used their intuitive understanding of space to create functional and inspired environments—cathedrals, gardens, spas, museums, schools, habitats—space that not only engaged the senses, but often transcended them. In the past few years, scientists and architects have begun to collaborate to extend that intuitive understanding to a research-based one. In the spring of 2004 the new Academy of Neuroscience for Architecture was established in California as a partnership of science and architecture to measure psychophysiologic responses to the environment. Actually, such collaboration was not new at all, just acknowledged. Neuroanatomist Marian Diamond published so-called enriched environment research on rats as early as 1962. The research was subsequently duplicated with several other species, including humans, with similar results. The findings, now conclusive and expanded into multisensory research, showed the direct link between environment and brain function—altering the environment changed the brain (Hutchison, 1986). Areas of the brain responding to such environments include the cerebellum (movement, balance, sensory integration), cerebral cortex (sensory-motor processing), olfactory bulb (smell, memory), and hippocampus (neurogenesis). Functions of the brain responding to environments include emotions, stress management, memory, immunity, and consciousness (Eberhard & Patoine, 2004). Other studies on multisensory research have included areas of imagery, sound, smell, spatial orientation, electromagnetic fields, touch, and movement. Imagery research has expanded from early studies at Texas A&M University and the Johns Hopkins University Hospital, where they measured the stress response and imagery—simply viewing plants and other nature imagery reduced stress hormones within three minutes (Khalsa, 1997)—to the Pablo Picasso Alzheimer's Therapy project at the Museum of Modern Art in New York and Boston's Museum of Fine Arts. Using art viewing as a therapeutic tool to engage minds damaged by dementia, the therapy helps engage parts of the brain involved with procedural memory, which governs routine activities. Temporary but palpable improvements have been noted in the museum tour participants. In addition to improving moods and behaviors up to several days, the experience sparks interpretive and expressive powers, engages cognitive and physical responses, and creates connections (Kennedy, 2005). As Oliver Sacks, MD, notes in his work with memory-impaired patients, it is not just a visual experience, but the retention of an emotional memory. Since the brain is driven by emotion and connected to the immune system, these connections are environmentally driven.

Sound and imagery studies have been documented in many surgical suites. The auditory pathways are not affected by anesthetics, so they continue to transmit sound. Linda Rogers, a composer of children's music, established the Audio Prescriptives Foundation, combining guided imagery and anxiolytic music following a three-year study at the New York Hospital that showed a direct correlation to lowered anxiety levels measured by an increase in finger temperature. Anesthesiologist Ralph Spintge, MD, says, "Physiological parameters like heart rate, arterial blood pressure, salivation, blood levels of ACTH, prolactin, HGH and cortisol show a significant decrease under anxiolytic music compared with pharmacological preoperative medication. EKG studies demonstrate sleep induction through music in the preoperative phase" (Gaynor, 1999, p. 84).

Conversely, sound may act as a stressor. Research in neonatal intensive care units on developmental neurobiology has demonstrated that high levels of light and noise can adversely affect the still highly plastic brain of a premature infant (Eberhard & Patoine, 2004).

Therapeutic sounds, such as toning, water, and bird sounds, Tibetan bowls, quartz crystal bowls, percussion instruments, and Gregorian chanting have played a role in the therapeutic environment. Gaynor (1999) documents his use of sound therapy in his oncology practice, while the authors of *Sound Choices* (Mazer & Smith, 1999) introduced the CARE channel in 1992, a 24-hour environmental channel in hospitals providing nature videos and instrumental music for broadcast over in-house patient television (Mazer & Smith, 1999).

Lighting and color research over the past 50 years has led to innovation in the built environment. The majority of research has centered on fluorescent lighting in schools, although recent studies have measured natural daylighting in schools. The studies, once controversial, demonstrated the deleterious effects of cool-white fluorescent tubes, linking their flicker effect and compromised light spectrum to excessive cortisol levels and excessive blinking. Over the past 20 years, Dr. John Ott (1986) and the Environmental Health and Light Research Institute in Alberta, Canada, have published major studies linking fluorescent lighting to hyperactivity, fatigue, and low performance, while demonstrating improved behavior and academic performance under full-spectrum lighting (artificial or natural). In 1991 Jacob Liberman, OD, PhD, published *Light: Medicine of the Future* as a compilation of light studies and light therapies. The light therapy evolved out of the full-spectrum lighting research in the early 1980s and has become a treatment of choice for seasonal affective disorder. Using light therapy with individual patients, Liberman noted improvements in visual acuity, visual attention, and mood, along with increased socialization, higher academic testing scores, and general well-being.

Full-spectrum light studies contrasting natural daylighting with artificial or fluorescent lighting, commissioned by the Pacific Gas and Electric Company in California, were conducted over a two-year period by a reputable architectural research team. The findings were published in 1999 to the amazement of the architectural community: students in the most natural daylighting conditions progressed 20 percent faster in mathematics and 26 percent faster in reading (Heschong, 1999).

Multisensory research related to environmental influences expanded to more esoteric areas of research, including smells, energy fields, movement, and touch. Historically, touch was not considered an environmental influence; however, when opportunities for touch therapies were integrated as dedicated spaces into the built environment, touch became part of the environmental experience. The Touch Research Institute at the University of Miami School of Medicine became the focus of most of the controlled studies on touch therapies. Many of the early studies were initiated with infant trials, but subsequent work addressed stress and performance levels of the medical students. Physiological responses following sessions of chair massage included lowered resting heart rates, lowered ACTH and cortisol hormones, and increased alertness secondary to brain wave changes. Dr. Tiffany Field's pioneering work in touch therapies on infants and adults moved into areas of autism, bulimia, and posttraumatic stress disorder. Patients in these categories of diagnosis benefited by lowered stress hormones, elevated moods, increased relatedness, and improved sleep patterns (Field, 1997). Since the advent of Field's research, many hospitals have recognized the value and benefits of therapies for both staff and patients for pain management, stress management, and healing. A recent survey published by the American Hospital Association in May 2006 found that 82 percent of the 1,007 hospitals responding included massage therapy among care options, with 70 percent using it for pain management. In addition, the Hospital Based Massage Network was organized to support massage and touch therapies pursuant to the integration of complementary care and allopathic medicine in healthcare.

Smell may be the new frontier of neuroscience, according to Jim Bower (Lanier, 2006), a computational neuroscientist at the University of Texas at San Antonio and the leading expert on olfaction. Bower and his colleagues are out to solve the olfactory mystery since the sense of smell has no parallels to our other senses. Quoted in the May 2006 issue of *Discover* magazine, Bower's research has led to a new understanding of language—that the cerebral cortex, the largest part of the brain, may have evolved out of the olfactory system through a specific neural circuitry; that is, according to Bower, "the way we think is olfactory" (Lanier, 2006, p. 28).

Research on various types of energy reactions on cellular function has been published by the biophysicist Jan Walleczek. The research reveals that low-frequency electromagnetic fields (ELF) trigger cellular changes, particularly on T-lympocytes: ELF exposure can cause interference with regulating the uptake of blood calcium and either stimulate or inhibit the action of immune cells, depending on the level of exposure. High-technology equipment has been associated with ELF, along with radiation and other environmental contaminants. Valerie Hunt's complementary and groundbreaking research into human energy field chaos patterns has demonstrated profound implications for healing (Hunt, 1995).

Related energy field research on movement, brain wave activity, and immunity conducted at the Beijing College of Traditional Chinese Medicine revealed increases in brain wave coherence and the production of the antioxidant superoxide dismutase (SOD) in test subjects performing Qigong and other martial arts movements (Wildish, 2000). The neuropsychologist James Prescott at the National Institute of Child Health and Human Development has documented that lack of movement leads to physiologic deterioration of brain neurons, while vestibular stimulation leads to gains in dendritic connections (Hannaford, 1995). An interesting observation has been noted around vestibular stimulation: the cerebellum of the brain connects to the vestibular canal in the ear, creating the cerebellar-vestibular system (CVS). Children prone to inner ear infections often demonstrate coordination difficulties, and nursing home patients who frequently use rocking chairs maintain better balance and proprioceptive responses. This finding has been attributed to the act of rocking stimulating the CVS and also to the rocking movement as a mild form of aerobics. Rocking the baby is not only therapeutic for the infant, but for the rocker, too.

Rocking and movement bring us to another complementary area of research— meditation, mindfulness, and intentional breathing as stress management modalities. These modalities are reliant on a *theraps* approach through intentional and dedicated areas that can facilitate meditation practices. Mounting scientific research supports these therapies to improve health, well-being, and longevity.

The data available on mindfulness research can be summarized by key points: effects on brain wave activity increase mental focus and heightened awareness; lower cortisol levels reduce stress; lower blood lactate levels promote relaxation; higher NK cell counts boost immune function; increased levels of superoxide dismutase, catalase, and glutathione stimulate antioxidant activity; decreases in LDL and total cholesterol along with increased HDL; increased levels of hormone prolactin ameliorates depression, according to studies published by the Art of Living Foundation in Germany (Naga, 1998; Sharma, 2003).

The Dalai Lama recently shared insights on benefits of meditation at the meeting of the Society for Neuroscience in Washington, DC (2006), which drew over 30,000 researchers. Richard Davidson presented a study on meditation at the University of Wisconsin that was supported by the Dalai Lama's Mind Life Institute, in which the brain waves of meditating monks were compared with novice meditators. The Dalai Lama's presence was not without controversy, despite his endorsement of science. The controversy sparked was not around the research, but the fact of his status as a religious leader. Some attendees saw his speech as a refreshing attempt to break down intellectual boundaries, while others were offended by his addressing issues of neurobiology. What appeared to be significant was the opportunity to dialogue about science and spirituality within a context of mutual respect. Recently published research at the Massachusetts Institute of Technology on meditation and relaxation have confirmed previous studies showing that people and animals learn best when given "mind" breaks between tasks (Kleeman, 2006).

Gary Zukav (1989), author of *The Seat of the Soul,* served as an inspiration to the exploration of *theraps*. Delving into the science of intuition, Zukav makes a relevant referral to the role of intellect and knowledge: "The intellect is meant to expand perceptions....The experiences of the intellect are experiences of knowledge…and for each level of knowledge, you are held responsible for how you use it" (p. 83). The knowledge and research directly pertain to the third level of *theraps,* which centers on education, responsibility, and holistic expertise in initiating tasks. Understanding the role of the environment opens us to new possibilities for integration, connection, and a humanized healthcare system for minds and spirits.

ELEMENTS OF HEALING ENVIRONMENTS

We return to the architect Christopher Alexander (2002) in a quote about wholeness: "The living character of space is visible as a characteristic of the integrated whole....The vital part played by wholeness as the fundamental substratum that governs the behavior of the world extends far beyond architecture and art....It is the wholeness which is the real thing that lies beneath the surface, and determines everything" (p. 98). The elements of a healing environment work as a whole: the interdependence of patient/practitioner; the sensitivity to the relationship; the responsibility to use knowledge and connections appropriate to healing; and the restorative outcome for both parties. Nothing is passive in this dynamic exchange. It is a matter of physics. What lies beneath the surface, like the trace elements, determines everything.

There may be many and diverse approaches to a healing environment, but all approaches begin with knowledge and the intention for wholeness. The capacity to support life and community all emerge out of wisdom and purposeful intent. For instance, intensive care units, all highly focused, uniformly hardwired for supertechnology and clinical practices, seem very dissimilar to community health centers, where the experience may be more eclectic and chaotic. Yet they share similar sensibilities for wholeness that will affect outcomes for both patients and practitioners. An Alzheimer's residence may share similar environmental considerations with a standard nursing home, yet there are great differences in the participants' experience for wholeness. Following are some examples about differences and similarities of elements in healing environments and the possibilities for achieving wholeness using space as therapy. The first step to understanding cause and effect conditions in any environment begins with an awareness of that environment and the specific intention for its use. Environments are catalysts to healing but often present interesting challenges. Effective solutions invariably surface unconsciously through intuition, and sometimes paradoxically, as the following example of space as therapy demonstrates.

Community Hospital

The space is in the United States. The specific location is a locked psychiatric ward in a small community hospital in the north shore of Massachusetts. The intention for the space was to provide an environment for children, aged 4–15, who required crisis stabilization. The solution for the space came out of Holland (Kirkwood, 2006).

Snoezelen, a Dutch word for sensory integration rooms, originated in the 1980s in response to the rising number of sensory-impaired individuals. It is used as a comfort room for relaxation and sensory integration. Sensory integration rooms are particularly suited to autism-related disorders and oppositional behavioral patterns. It is an exquisite example of using the environment as therapy. The therapeutic models for calming and controlling angry outbursts entail a multisensory approach. On the basis of the stimulation of the five senses through tactile surfaces, music, imagery, colors, lighting, smell, and even taste, the sensory integration rooms offer positive, therapeutic experiences for the staff and patients. The hospital staff who have used the space attest to its therapeutic value. Several selections of equipment can actually lull a person into feeling a detached sense of calm.

The environment acts as a catalyst to access the limbic system of the brain, affecting feelings and memory. Elements, such as the vibrating floor mat and the rotating disco ball, create a soothing, mesmerizing effect and promote relaxation and well-being. The use of color seems practically illogical: deep reds and rose tones on surrounding walls; a black floor mat that lights up with white stars when stepped on; one wall lit by black light, causing stars to glow green; and six-foot colored light tubes that gurgle and glow. The environmental choices seem paradoxical—overstimulating to create calm, yet for this population it works like Ritalin for attention deficit issues.

The intention was clear: to provide a therapeutic experience, without drugs, using the environment as the therapy. The environment is participatory, integrative, and focused. For a population of patients with sensory deficit disorders, it is the perfect solution. Apparently, it is working for a few of the staff, too!

Recent research in the field of sensory integration addresses two similar yet unique concepts. The use of the term *sensualization* originated in the field of brain science in the twentieth century. This form of sensory enhancement was based on studies involving measurements in fluctuation, amplitude, and frequency of brain waves directly affected by the subconscious and by multisensory input. Some of the specific findings included an increased awareness of subtle emotional and physical sensations, a so-called felt shift; an increased capacity for brain synchronization and relaxation; and increased capacities for superlearning, which increases abilities for processing and retrieving information. The sensory integration rooms essentially fall into this category as catalysts of relaxation for a specific population of children who could respond therapeutically (Hutchison, 1986).

A more recognized term, *synesthesia,* dates back to the 1880s when Francis Galton published a paper in *Nature* on the phenomenon of blending of the senses. Until recently, it was merely a curiosity, but neuroscientific research began to uncover brain processes that could help scientists understand how it worked. Scientists acknowledge that synesthesia occurs in the general population and is often inherited. People whose senses, two or more, blend together may see colors in sound, see black numbers in colors, and experience tastes associated with images. They experience the ordinary world in extraordinary ways and are providing valuable clues to understanding the functions of the brain. So far, it is not widely accepted that synesthesia can be created environmentally, but it has not been ruled out.

A common explanation for synesthesia is that affected people are simply recalling childhood associations; another point of view is that they are being metaphorical (Emmite, 2006). But a more intriguing theory is that synesthesia occurs because of cross activation, in which two normally separate areas of the brain elicit mutual activity. After all, we now know that the brain is plastic, adaptive, and meaning-driven and that cross activation occurs in both hemispheres of the brain. By creating conditions for synesthesia in multisensory environments, we may activate memory pathways for certain populations, but not all. For instance, patients suffering with Alzheimer's disease require a different application of neuroscience.

Residential Group Home

The space is in the United States. The specific location is a residential group home for Alzheimer's patients in a suburb of Boston, Massachusetts. The intention was to create a home for a specific population of patients who would not adapt to a typical nursing home facility. The design of the environment reflects an understanding of the cognitive decline of these patients, how the brain changes, how behavior and perceptions are modified during the course of the disease, and most importantly, how wholeness impacts the progression of this disease (Eberhard & Patoine, 2004).

John Zeisel, PhD, a researcher in sociology and architecture, reported his research in the *Gerontologist* in 2003. Zeisel asserts that environmental modifications for Alzheimer's patients are often more effective than drug and behavioral therapies: "Environments conventionally designed for the cognitively able appear to put stress on Alzheimer's patients" (p. 78). The intentions behind the design modifications are to reduce stress, afford the patients more control over their lives, reduce feelings of isolation and helplessness, and create a haven of safety and personal identity. Damage to the hippocampus (the area of the brain capable of neurogenesis) renders the patients incapable of mapping their environment—difficulties discriminating colors, distances, and architectural details cause anxiety and frustration. One of the common symptoms associated with the Alzheimer's population is the problem of wandering and lack of orientation. An understanding of basic quality of life issues offers creative opportunities to provide solutions. In this case, there are no drugs or policing that can be as effective as space therapy.

Informed architectural design dictates specific modifications to the built environment: exiting or egress from corridors to side walls, not corridor ends; color contrasting of corridor doors; purposeful walking paths and defined spaces; objects for orientation at strategic points; and personalized touches that provide a sense of place and identity. One of the most exciting elements in this facility is the therapeutic garden, where patients walk, sit, socialize, breathe fresh air, garden, and witness nature and the changing seasons—the full cycle of wholeness reflected in nature and the patient's environment (Eberhard & Patoine, 2004).

Critical Care Unit

One very specialized hospital environment is the critical care unit (CCU), an environment where opportunities for space therapy are often limited. It was employment in such an environment in the 1970s that offered me my first real awareness of the environment and its impact on patients and my own well-being. I subsequently abandoned healthcare and matriculated to the university to study environmental design.

The environment of a critical care unit is fast-paced, focused, and essentially about technology and function. And yet the critical needs of its population, both patients and staff, center on connection and healing. While technology has its place, and a critical place it is, humanistic and healing elements are often missing. The environment is one way to introduce them, but it takes imagination. Over several decades as a designer I rarely, if ever, experienced any CCU, built or conceptualized, that embraced all levels of space therapy—but one came close. In 1999, at Roger Williams University in Rhode Island, a senior architectural student presented his senior thesis to a group of architectural jurors, including myself as a qualifying member. The assigned thesis project was to design a residential campus and hospital facility located in North Dakota that specialized in eating disorders. One of the areas singled out for innovative approaches was a dedicated CCU as many of these young patients were admitted in critical status. Prior to presenting his model and working drawings for the CCU, he shared a brief narrative about his inspiration for this unusual space. His father had recently passed away in a CCU, having suffered many years with heart disease. His father spent the last three weeks of his life supine, tethered to technology in the very sterile environment of a typical CCU. The young student pondered his father's experience over the semester and visited several local hospitals. He realized that his father's last days were a far cry from any feeling of wholeness or connection. Basically, his father's orientation to the environment was the ceiling—that was his view, an unrelenting view of stained white ceiling tiles and glaring, flickering fluorescent lighting. Out of that empathic perception, the student designed an aquarium in the ceiling of his CCU. A critical care unit seems a far cry from a brain facility, but they share a common goal—space as therapy, one imagined, one fulfilled.

HealthCare Community–Based Program

The space is in the United States. The specific location is a metropolitan outpatient program and school situated in the southern coast of Florida. The nonresidential center offers rehabilitation, health promotion programs, and integrative primary care, education centered on a holistic and integrative wellness model (Biscayne Institutes of Health and Living, 2006; DiCowden, 2003). The environment not only supports the mission, but is integral to it. The architectural focal point is a magnificent, circular-shaped domed meditation space that serves the institute and the greater community. The space is large enough to accommodate movement therapies and performing arts. Scheduled and spontaneous meditation sessions are open to the patients, staff, and community on a regular basis. While the facility does not represent any religious or spiritual bias, it has hosted Tibetan Buddhist monk meditations, sand mandala installations, art making, and multicultural events as part of its integrative healthcare model. In addition, several classrooms have been designed using the principles of multisensory research. Visually connected to the great circular room is a magnificent meditation garden, replete with water fountain, statuary, and cascading bougainvillea, ideal for individual or group meditation or communing with nature. This is an environment inviting participation, a natural response to healing.

Birthing Center

The space is in Europe. The specific location is a birthing center in Ravenna, Italy. The environment reflects the culmination of research and creativity by the designers who studied the physiology, psychology, ergonomics, and biorhythms of the childbearing process (Franck & Lepori, 2000). They observed that birthing in the Western medicine modality encouraged a supine and passive position for the mother, which produced the lowest contraction efficiency, increased maternal discomfort, and more complicated deliveries. Also, the internal rotation of the baby within the pelvic canal became more difficult and painful for the mother in a fixed position. In their research, the designers uncovered advantages for the mother if she moved between a variety of different positions during labor, which resulted in less pain, more efficient contractions, shorter labors, and improved cardiopulmonary functioning for the baby. Moreover, water can facilitate the birthing process by alleviating pain and accelerating dilation. The findings dictated the environment. Instead of a typically centrally located bed where the patient is exposed and passive, the center of this space was left open and a low platform placed to one side, low enough so that the mother could squat, kneel, recline, or sit. Rings mounted on a low wall, moveable birthing stools, and hanging towels from the low ceiling offered opportunities for the mother to stretch, hang, or lean during the labor. A specially designed bath was positioned in the space to allow the mother to float, recline, and even give birth in the water. The choice of positions, movements, and activities placed the mother in an active, participatory role and the staff in a supportive one—a working example of *theraps*, where the healing elements (water, movement, special layout, ergonomics) in the environment supported all parties and encouraged a natural process to be connected to natural biorhythms and sensibilities.

HEALTHY BUILDINGS

Writing about healing environments without addressing air quality issues in buildings would be, at the very least, inconsistent. Prior to the twenty-first century, most of the informed, organic building was happening in western Europe. The Dutch were among the first to recognize health as a design element and that air quality in contemporary buildings was a mounting problem. Breathing is the key function of any organism, and most of us take it at face value. We assume that we are breathing correctly and healthfully. Not so for many of us who are breathing in sick buildings. Breathing confronts us with the environment, and though not considered one of our senses, breathing connects us to each other and to every function of the human experience—our organs, our emotions, our consciousness, and our cosmos. Breathing in healthy environments is fundamental to the healing process, and breathing life into the symbiotic and functional relationship of the participants is space therapy at its best.

The radical Dutch architect Ton Alberts began practicing hatha yoga while searching for a cure for a serious illness many years ago. It was by this path that he developed a way of defining architecture in a more humanistic way (Holdsworth & Sealey, 1992). Over many years his organic buildings have been noted for the lowest energy consumption for office buildings in the world. In a foreword to *Healthy Buildings,* Sealy says, "A building is a third skin. A building has to be as comfortable as our own skin; it lives, it breathes, it surrounds us without oppressing us. A building has to be as healthy as we want our own body to be" (Holdsworth & Sealey, 1992, p. 11).

Architect Bill Holdsworth and climatologist Antony Sealy were one of the first environmental teams to describe the work of healthy building design, including their own methods developed in the 1970s known as Environmentally Controlled Human Operational Enclosed Space. Their work preceded acknowledgments by the World Health Organization, which has estimated that over 30 percent of commercial buildings, including healthcare facilities, suffer from sick building syndrome. Nicholas Tate (1992), author of *The Sick Building Syndrome,* cites studies showing that up to 25 million workers suffer air pollution illnesses, including multiple chemical sensitivity, asthma, bronchial infections, and other major organ systems related to respiratory, gastrointestinal, neurocardiovascular, genitourinary, and skin diseases.

Holdsworth and Sealy (1992) apologize for paying scant attention to the importance of color, art objects, and nonarchitectural elements—their focus was primarily on air quality as the foundation of a healthy building. However, they admit to recognizing and appreciating all elements in the environment as equally important in contributing to our sense of well-being and healing: "It is not that I feel them beyond my ability to present them; it was the knowledge that readers themselves should be able to take part in the creation of a new architectural form of thinking" (p. 3). Fortunately, the new form of thinking has moved along the lines of aquariums in ceilings, clean air, urban gardens, sensory integration rooms, birthing pools, art museums, meditation rooms, sound environments, and researched-based environments. This direction is space therapy in action.

Exploring the elements of healing environments leads us directly to nature. Architect Christopher Alexander (2002) refers to the properties in nature: "these properties must be viewed as fundamental to the existence of the wholeness in the world…and might one day be understood as a single law which underlies the entirety of everything we know as nature" (p. 244). They are not independent. They overlap. They are aspects of the whole. We cannot separate ourselves from our environments or our experience. It is all connected.

SPACE BEYOND SPACE: INTEGRATING INFLUENCES

For thousands of years, nature has been revered as a healing element in many cultures. Early in the twentieth century, the eminent architectural historian Giedion (1941) warned his readers that American architecture was in danger of becoming "style," replete with dangers toward formalism. He prophesied that architecture's future enrichment would evolve organically by contributions from countries on the rim of Western civilization and from the Far East.

The early colonists responded to Native American and South American influences in environmental design during the twentieth century, a response that has been strongest along the California coast and bordering states. Mexican architecture especially draws on a unique and rich culture that mixes the heritage of the Toltecs and Mayans with that of the Spanish and French invaders. Mexicans have a strong sense of their natural biorhythms and use their sensitivity in daring and subtle ways to connect with the environment: "Our reality is a cross between light and shadow, tears and laughter, innocence and wisdom, life and death. Because it is so complex and unsettling Mexican reality must be understood intuitively through the senses" (Colle, 1989, p. 7). Luis Barragan, one of the most famous architects influenced by Mexican culture, notes that his spaces are formed out of the natural living elements and ideals of beauty, silence, mysticism, and animism—it is an emotional architecture, and it is a spiritual one. The climate lends itself to exotic vegetation so that habitats, community centers, and marketplaces are commonly oriented to central courtyards and gardens.

The garden motif is a quintessential element for any healing environment. It is *theraps* on all levels, inviting us to commune in mutual dependence, engage in sensitivity, take responsibility for cultivation, and prepare for transformation. Gardens may be as elaborate as a botanical greenhouse or as simple as potted geraniums. Gardens are active neuroscience. The potted geranium embodies the range of our known sensory capacities: the flower stimulates sight, while the fragrance activates the olfactory system; the petals, stems, and leaves provide various tactile sensations, and the plant moves with each respiration. Geranium petals are edible and make a tasty summer sorbet, and insects respond to the sounds of the plant's vibrational frequencies. Gardens are human connectors, and the experience of one is often transcendent.

One of the most interesting garden designers responding to elements of transcendence is located in San Francisco, California: Delaney (2001) has designed healing gardens for five hospitals to date (2006). Delaney's healing gardens are fun, participatory, and space therapy at its best—they engage a multisensory experience, use many tenets of neuroscience, and initiate profound connections to the self through interaction with the space and nature. In the early stages of her design process, Delaney operates more like a psychologist than an artist. She investigates into early childhood memories that set the stage for inspiration. This process has informed many of her healing gardens, especially the ones for children: "It is my intention to engage the spectator in the rituals of play within the formality of the garden." The Leichtag Family Healing Garden at the Children's Hospital and Health Center in San Francisco is a testimony to play, healing, neuroscience, and nature. Using movement as the modality to engage the children, Delaney designed a 20-foot dinosaur, the "garden's guardian," which children enthusiastically enter and quickly exit to confront an imposing blue-tiled seahorse-shaped fountain inviting them to drink some water. Moveable benches, lush and medicinal planting, vivid colors, bubbling fountains, and undulating pathways create a remarkable healing adventure. Delaney, a breast cancer survivor, has integrated her personal experience as a patient with her role as a designer to inform others of the possibilities for healing.

Gardens offer healing experiences but have also inspired projects far beyond anyone's vision. The Village of Arts and Humanities, originally a rubble-ridden urban African American community in north Philadelphia, was transformed into an oasis of trees, flowers, mosaics, parks, community centers, offices, and housing by the modern-day alchemist Lily Yeh. Yeh, a Chinese landscape painter and intuitive visionary, recognized the power of nature to successfully integrate cultures and to revitalize a blighted area. Initially working with practically nothing but unemployed residents and a few rakes and shovels, she literally started landscaping with a circle in the center of an empty lot. From that center evolved various cultural icons, wall murals, and simple gardens. Witnessing the environmental transformation, collaborations with local officials began to energize the entire community to eventually transform not only the barren lot into a community center, but the people into an integrated neighborhood, ultimately healing the environment and the people from the bottom up (Murray, 2000).

A less common variety of garden sensibility incorporates the labyrinth as the path to emotional and physical healing. The labyrinth has been a universal symbol as a starting point for inner spiritual exploration. Many famous labyrinths, such as the floor of the Chartres Cathedral in France, have served as inspiration for designers to incorporate labyrinths into landscapes using a variety of nature elements. The shape and design of the walking labyrinths evoke nature and the inner landscape of all living structures: the twists, turns, and coiling patterns mirror the surfaces of the human brain, the inner ear, and small intestines, while the shape and spiraling of the labyrinth recalls the natural elements of water rippling, webs, and matrices of plant life. Labyrinths can be designed with just about anything, just about anywhere—stones, canvas, plants, mowed lawns, concrete, lighted candles, or sand are a few examples. The whole point of the walking labyrinth is about exploration of our physical, emotional, and spiritual well-being. There is a fundamental difference between walking the labyrinth and walking the maze. Labyrinths are unicursal, with only one pathway leading directly to the center. The maze is multicursal, with one correct pathway to the center hidden among numerous dead ends and diversions. The distinction is subtle but does affect the experience.

In walking a labyrinth the brain's right hemisphere predominates, engaging us in intuitive and feeling responses because we follow the path without any thinking, just moving forward as the labyrinth directs us. However, mazes encourage left brain activity because logic and concrete decision making become involved in avoiding the dead ends and other junctions. Labyrinth or maze, the healing lies in a solitary experience of exploration for the individual or, as in group participation that incorporates music, movement and bonding (Sands, 2001). An example of labyrinth landscaping used for healing may be experienced at the California Pacific Medical Center in San Francisco. There is another, simple way to use the labyrinth—a tactile experience with handheld enamel or ceramic labyrinths that invite the fingers to trace the imprinted pathway, which, in turn, can promote a relaxation response.

Some of the most profound garden experiences have originated in the East, especially the Zen gardens of Japan. The beauty of these gardens stems from their utter simplicity, usually devoid of flowering species but created with moss, stones, water, and trees. The perfect placement of the elements creates calming and tranquil environments, ideal for contemplation but not necessarily meditation. In fact, the original purpose was not a place for meditation because it was considered too bright and open to distraction—the darkened interior meditation halls functioned as ideal settings for meditation. Originally, it was the act of gardening itself that offered healing and cleansing of the soul. The Saihoji Temple garden in Kyoto, Japan, represents one of the greatest inspirations of Zen sensibility. The designer was an enlightened Zen priest named Muso Soseki. The real soul of this garden experience has been associated with its moss, according to Elizabeth Murray (2000), author of *Cultivating Sacred Space:* "He planted the rocks to grow and followed the Zen ideals for gracefulness and understatement…and after one hundred years or so, the stones did indeed grow and the moss began to come…and the real soul of this garden seemed to arrive with the coming of the moss" (p. 64). Japanese gardens are also intended for purification rituals as you wash your hands with water from the stone vessel, preparing yourself to enter sacred space. The Zen garden can be created using traditional outdoor spaces as well as indoor gardens with a simple tray.

A remarkable example of the blending of cultures, vision, and philosophies in a natural landscape is the Abby Aldrich Rockefeller Garden in Maine, exquisitely documented in *Cultivating Sacred Space.* The garden design, dating back to the early 1920s, was influenced by travels to Korea, China, and the Philippines and by the sensibilities of John and Abby Rockefeller. The site selected was the natural woodlands of mosses, lichen, rivers, lakes, and birch trees perched atop granite bluffs with views to Seal Harbor. The intentions for the garden were to combine the natural elements of the woodlands with sculpture gardens and separate flowering gardens, while integrating the Asian sensibilities for design and placement. The collaboration between the Rockefellers and the garden artist, Gertrude Jekyll, lasted almost 10 years and eventually culminated in this stunning integration of cultures, philosophies, and nature. The visual separation of the different elements was united by a strong axial relationship, spiritual paths, and formal gates. Focal points included sculpture, statuary, a reflecting pond, decorative lanterns, and simple benches for sitting. The original flower garden included over 1,600 perennial and annual plant species but was later pared to about 600 flowering species complemented with ornamental grasses. Murray views this garden as a shining and inspirational example of West meets East—blending their philosophies, elements, and sensibilities to create a sum greater than its parts. It is whole, connected, and healing.

As we observe the influence of other cultures in our daily lives, we learn to appreciate the many positive human elements in our own. The secret in creating any home, office, school, or healthcare environment is not comparing, but appreciating. Moreover, environments can share similar sensibilities while remaining quite specific to function. Westerners are now beginning to see the wisdom in this thinking. Over the last decade, westerners have begun to understand and appreciate the very ancient traditions of Asian and Indian cultures and the great sensibilities to the design of their environments. There are remarkable philosophical similarities in belief systems about health and the influence of environments. Nature connections to healing play a prominent role in primitive and advanced cultures, but differences in details and application account for some interesting outcomes.

In India, Vastu Shastra is the ancient Vedic tradition for architecture and design. The tenets for this tradition are based on the belief that every structure is endowed with a life energy *(prana)* that is influenced by the earth's magnetic polarities, directions, the sun and moon, the planets and stars, and the eight points of the compass. The flow of life energy is regulated directionally and architecturally within the space to promote the happiness, health, and natural biorhythms of the people. Each direction of a given space corresponds to specific aspects of the human condition, such as wealth, health, relationships, and so on, and the placement of elements to specific directions within the environment will eventually effect outcomes of the living experience. The principles of Vastu Shastra can be incorporated in varying degrees in all environments—home, office, or clinic (Art of Living Foundation, 2006).

Another Eastern concept of life energy is the Chinese concept of Ch'i, which emerged from shamanistic traditions of the early philosophers of China's Classical period from the eighth to the third centuries B.C.E. The three most foremost philosophers, Lao Tse, Chuang Tse, and Confucius, contributed to the development of the Tao, which acts in the world through the energy called Ch'i. The Tao, translated "the way," is an abstract concept that ultimately is unknowable, beyond description, eternal, and unmeasurable but has determined a whole way of life for thousands of years. Three essential elements of Taoism are a direct sensory contact with nature, intuitive awareness for decision making, and *wu wei:* "to take no action which is not in harmony with the laws of nature." Out of the empirical foundation of the Tao, arts and sciences adopted principles for living: vitality, health, and spiritual well-being could be actualized only when the mind, body, and spirit were unified and harmonious with nature. Moreover, there was no separation between the experience of living "the way" and the environment in which it was lived. This principle set the stage for a design philosophy called feng shui. The practice of feng shui revealed a deep concern for the individual's relationship to the environment and the inherent rhythms of all living matter. Three basic principles emerged: *Pa Kua*, the governing of the orientation of people and buildings to the environment; the Five Elements in nature—water, fire, earth, wood, and metal—in balance; and the flow of Ch'i. These governing principles relied on the intuitive understanding of the connection of the environment to the natural biorhythms of the people, plants, and animals (Wildish, 2000).

Contemporary feng shui practices mimic the concept of *theraps* as space therapy: the symbiotic relationship of the individuals to the environment, each being served by the other; the awareness and intuition required for the personal engagement in the practices; the knowledge and responsibility in initiating and implementing the principles; and the ultimate connection to harmonious living. The more we explore the world and its cultures, the more we see common themes. Fifty years ago, the ancient practice of feng shui would be dismissed as esoteric, but contemporary research is validating it. The scientific understanding for the existence of Ch'i matters little to those who benefit from their beliefs about it, but believers or nonbelievers will be enriched by the experience of it.

PRACTICAL TO POETIC

The menu of options to consider in designing healthy environments is expansive, but one more overriding and relevant factor is the issue of sustainability. The literal meaning of *sustainable* is to uphold, support, and keep from sinking. Applied to the environment, sustainable has important implications for biodegradable, nontoxic, and ecosupportive products integrated with energy-efficient choices for the physical structure; but applied to "space as therapy," it means much more. Sustainable design for healthcare is rooted in nature and creates symbiotic relationships; sustainable practices require intuitive and sensitive engagement; sustainability relies on education and responsibility to initiate the tasks; and sustainable environments promote holism, interconnection, and well-being for everything, literally supporting the web of life. Fortunately, there are resources to assist in the education and implementation of sustainable choices, whether for homes, office buildings, hospitals, refurbishment, new construction, or neighborhood development. Leadership in Energy and Environmental Design was established to define green building standards, promote integrated whole building design practices, and raise public awareness of green building benefits. Benefits are not only therapeutic, but financial as well (Leadership in Energy and Environmental Design, 2006).

The primary intention for this chapter on creating a healing environment was to explore new ways of perceiving the environment as an integrative factor for healthcare practices through the concept of space as therapy; the second intention was to offer examples of possible and diverse ways of using the environment by introducing the elements of healing environments; and the third intention is to suggest ways to be served by the environment from the practical to the poetic.

The practical and poetic may be two sides of the same coin. The environment can be used as space therapy in a number of ways—some rely on belief systems and others on double-blind controlled studies. Either way, the research supports the practical and the poetic—everyone benefits.

Creating a healing environment begins with a sensitive awareness and a specific intention: to breathe clean air presents options to install a freestanding high-efficiency particulate air filter for improved air quality or to use sustainable building products and cleaning materials; to lower stress hormones and fatigue levels, the options may include replacing fluorescent lighting with full-spectrum light fixtures or incorporating natural daylighting into the space; to stimulate immune systems, antioxidant activity, and performance levels, a regularly scheduled chair massage program might be incorporated into a dedicated space; to stimulate the CVS and dendritic connections for improved balance and functioning for the elderly, rocking chairs could be added to common areas; to lower blood lactate levels and increase alertness, group participation in a 20-minute Qigong class introduces an intentional rest period; to lower stress and create relaxation, the options may include the addition of nature sounds, such as water or birdsong, or a simple garden terrarium at a bedside.

Revisiting the aim of space therapy, it is to unify the practical aspects of the built environment as service to the more existential ones related to well-being. There is no one formula for any environment. Like the human body, each environment is unique to the individual living in it—it is the third skin, and like the skin, it responds in its own way. This is not to dismiss the fundamental principles of healing environments—there are basic rules—but to emphasize one factor over another is not the way; everything is important.

The three most salient points to the creation of a healing environment are the informed awareness of the environment, the informed use of the elements of a healing environment, and the integration of the environment within the community of its participants, ultimately creating a whole, the sum being much greater than its parts.

AWAKENING TO WHOLENESS

Every known life form begins as a sphere. It is the most female form there is, so it makes sense that the female would choose that shape for the ovum. In considering the ovum or a perfectly round egg, it is a perfect sphere. The ovum has a membrane around it, and inside the liquid is another sphere, and inside that are two polar bodies, which in turn are spheres. In ancient architecture the sphere represented the flower of life that is the original geometry for all life forms. It represents the whole.

The architect Christopher Alexander (2002) begins his book *The Nature of Order* with a chapter exploring concepts of wholeness and the theory of centers and carries this theme throughout the nearly 2,000 pages of the four volumes: "The wholeness is the most important thing: the local parts exist chiefly in relation to the whole, and their behavior and character and structure are determined by the larger whole in which they exist and which they create" (p. 80). Of course, Alexander is speaking specifically about the life of a building, but his ideas for wholeness have a more expansive implication for a healthcare environment. The building, or space or room, is a whole as a sum of its elements but is still part of the greater whole, the people and community that it serves and the neighborhood, and the town, and state, and country, and cosmos. All are served by that one single environment.

In exploring the concept of wholes, we are simultaneously addressing the elements of geometry and the elements of nature. Alexander describes the many layers of geometry in building construction and questions why American architecture especially has evolved so rectilinearly or, as a nurse educator emphatically described her hospital environment, as "rectal-linear."

Why are round rooms so dramatic? Just the shape alone is memorable, like the domed space at the healthcare institute in Florida. Round rooms are unusual and are not easily adapted to typical building structure, so most of us are forced to deal with rectilinear space. Where am I going with this? Since we have not addressed the geometry of space as part of the healing elements, it seems appropriate to include it in a discursive on wholeness. Just because we are forced to orient ourselves in a rectilinear world does not mean we cannot think in terms of a spherical world—physically, architecturally, and metaphorically. If we think in terms of centers and wholes, a new world of possibilities unfolds. We are able to define wholeness exactly as a structure in a mathematical context, but we can also define wholeness as a relationship in a therapeutic context, and then we can connect the two.

In the late 1980s there was the trend for circular intensive care units, where the patients formed the rim, and the staff, the hub. It seemed to work for a while, but I expect the novelty of the orientation worked better for staff members whose sensibilities were more attuned to creative geometric forms and space therapy concepts. One of the subtle factors impacting the experience of the new units was a resistance to change rigid and accepted notions about space or the unfamiliar experiences of unusual environments. Most of the units were approached from a strong architectural bias related to form and function, but they were not necessarily designed from a perspective of space as therapy. Nevertheless, for those designers and hospitals willing to push the envelope of form and function for purposes of research, we will all benefit (Academy of Neuroscience for Architecture, 2006).

The major themes of this volume center on connection, integration, and healing in healthcare environments but also embrace responsibilities for educating everyone to the possibilities of applying the knowledge anywhere. Every element considered for a healing environment has relevance to schools, offices, and homes. There are no limits to its applications. Humanizing healthcare is about wholeness—the patient, the practitioner, and the environment; humanizing healthcare is about connections—the environment, nature, the cosmos;

humanizing healthcare is about integration of *theraps*—interdependence, intuition, responsibility, and transformation.

Ultimately, humanizing healthcare is about the integration of the mind, body, and spirit of the individual: "At the base of everything is the individual man. It is he who must be integrated—integrated in his inner nature...so that his emotional and intellectual outlets will no longer be kept apart by an insuperable difference of level. To bring this fact into consciousness and to try to overcome it is closely connected with the outstanding task of our period: to humanize—that is, to reabsorb emotionally—what has been created by the spirit" (Giedion, 1941, p. 880).

TOOL KIT FOR CHANGE

Role and Perspective of the Healthcare Professional

1. To truly aid healing, the healthcare professional needs to pay attention and take some responsibility for the environment in which the patient is seen.
2. Attention to color, lighting, air quality, organization of elements, sounds, movement, touch, and smells is important when treating a patient.
3. Education about the continuum of healing in the outer environment of the world and the inner environment of the office for both the healthcare professional and his patient is important.

Role and Perspective of the Patient/Participant

1. A patient must take responsibility for increasing his awareness of the importance of form, color, lighting, sounds, movement, touch, smell, spirit, and nature in his own health.
2. A patient must take responsibility for living as "green" a life as possible to contribute to his own health and the overall health of the community and planet on which he lives.
3. The patient will benefit in mental and physical health by learning about other cultures and ways to integrate modes of living within the community in which he resides.

Interconnection: The Global Perspective

1. All healing is a mind-spirit-body-environment experience.
2. Space as therapy integrates interdependence, intuition, knowledge, responsibility, and restoration.
3. Elements of healing environments include geometry, lighting, color, air quality, sounds, movement, touch, energy fields, smell, nature, spirit, sustainability, and interpersonal connection.

REFERENCES

Academy of Neuroscience for Architecture. (2006). *Advances in knowledge linking neuroscience to understanding of human response to the built environment.* Retrieved August 18, 2006, from http://www.anfarch.org.

Alexander, C. (2002). *The nature of order, book one.* Berkeley, CA: Center for Environmental Structure.

Colle, M. P. (1989). *Casa Mexicana.* New York: Stewart, Tabori, and Chang.

Delaney, T. (2001). *Ten landscapes.* Gloucester, MA: Rockport Publishers.

DiCowden, M. A. (2003). The call of the wild woman: Models of healing. *Women and Therapy, 26,* 297–310.

Eberhard, J. P., & Patoine, B. (2004). Architecture with the brain in mind. *Cerebrum, The Dana Forum on Brain Science, 6,* 71–84.

Emmite, D. (2006, May). Hearing colors, tasting shapes. *Scientific American Mind,* 17.

Field, T. (1997, March). *Memorandum: Touch Research Institute.* Miami, FL: University of Miami School of Medicine.

Franck, K., & Lepori, R. B. (2000). *Architecture inside out.* Chichester, UK: Wiley-Academy.

Gaynor, M. (1999). *Sounds of healing.* New York: Broadway Books.

Giedion, S. (1941). *Space, time, and architecture.* Cambridge, MA: Harvard University Press.

Hannaford, C. (1995). *Smart moves.* Arlington, VA: Great Ocean.

Heschong, L. (1999). *Heschong-Mahone Group—Architectural research.* Fairfield, CA: Pacific Gas and Electric Company.

Holdsworth, B., & Sealey, A. (1992). *Healthy buildings.* Harlow, Essex, UK: Longman Group.

Hunt, V. (1995). *Infinite mind: The science of human vibrations.* Malibu, CA: Malibu.

Hutchison, M. (1986). *Megabrain.* New York: Ballantine Books.

Kennedy, R. (2005, October 30). The Pablo Picasso Alzheimer's therapy. *New York Times,* 1–5

Khalsa, D. S. (1997). *Brain longevity.* New York: Warner Books.

Kirkwood, J. (2006, January 10). Stimulating rooms calms children with psychiatric disorders. *Gloucester Daily Times,* B1–B2.

Kleeman, E. (2006, May). Relax and think like a rat. *Discover,* 21.

Lanier, J. (2006, May). I smell, therefore I think. *Discover,* 28.

Leadership in Energy and Environmental Design. (2006). *Promotes integrated whole building design and sustainability certification for tax credits.* Retrieved August 18, 2006, from http://www.usgbc

Liberman, J. (1991). *Light: Medicine of the future.* Santa Fe, NM: Bear.

Mazer, S., & Smith, D. (1999). *Sound choices.* Haverford, PA: Hay House.

Murray, E. (2000). *Cultivating sacred space.* San Francisco: Pomegranate.

Naga, V. (1998). P300 amplitude and antidepressant response. *Journal of Affective Disorders, 50,* 8, 45.

Ott, J. (1985). Color and light: Their effects on plants, animals and people. *Journal of Biosocial Research, 7* (1), 78–100.

Sands, H. R. (2001). *The healing labyrinth.* Hauppauge, NY: Barrons.

Sharma, H. (2003). Sudarshan Kriya practitioners exhibit better antioxidant status and lower blood lactate levels. *Biological Psychology, 63,* 281–291.

Tate, N. (1992). *The sick building syndrome* New York: Horizon Press.

Wildish, P. (2000). *The book of Chi.* North Clarendon, VT: Tuttle.

Zukav, G. (1989). *The seat of the soul* New York: Fireside / Simon and Schuster.

Chapter Five

INTEGRATIVE HEALTHCARE IN HOSPITALS

Wayne Ruga, PhD and Annette Ridenour

INTRODUCTION TO INTEGRATED HEALTHCARE IN HOSPITALS

Five thousand years ago, as the hospital was in its early stages of development, all hospital healthcare was integrated and highly humanized (Huelat, 2003). Similarly, prior to about 70 years ago, all farming was organic. In both instances, what has happened in the meantime—the industrialization of healthcare and agriculture—has mechanized both of these natural processes and, in doing so, has removed many of the sensitive values that individuals of a more humanistic persuasion hold as being precious.

In the United States today, a tension is palpable between those individuals who aspire to faster and more efficient progress for its own sake, in contrast to those who actively strive toward progress through the expression of more humanistic values. The signs of this tension are present in almost every community across the country. For example, on one hand, the big-box discounters—such as COSTCO—have become as prevalent as the local post office. On the other hand, the so-called Main Street preservationists are succeeding in preserving and/or restoring the small-scale, localized mom-and-pop shop culture that serves to anchor a place in its history, culture, and values. Frequently, both these polarized artifacts of contemporary cultural values exist within the very same community as graphic evidence of these conflicting local cosmologies. Additionally, it is worth highlighting that not all U.S. hospitals are caught up in this imperative for faster and more efficient progress. In the light of the many that are, there are—and always have been—a value-driven contingent of providers that have remained grounded in their roots of traditionally based practices, such as the Indian Health Service, for example (Huelat, 2003). The role of integrated healthcare in hospitals requires that we examine the core purposes of healthcare and hospitals.

In conducting this examination of core purposes, the proponents of integrated healthcare maintain that healthcare is more effectively provided, and hospitals achieve their purposes better, when the dual aspects of both curing and healing are addressed—or integrated—within the organizational culture, operations, and facilities of a healthcare organization. The integration of these dual aspects does present a challenge in today's world. Nevertheless, there are outstanding exemplars that demonstrate the benefits of accomplishing this integration, as the case studies in this chapter illustrate.

This chapter explores and discusses the tensions that make integrated healthcare challenging to the more mainstream hospital cultures, as these tensions exist and get played out in the everyday, mainstream marketplace of hospital-based healthcare delivery. In exploring these tensions, and the conflicting values that underlie their presence, the discussion and supporting case studies will provide the reader with the background understanding that will enable the reader to (1) clarify his own position relative to the provision of integrated healthcare delivery in hospitals and (2) develop a more critical perspective on the arguments that influence decisions about hospital-based integrated healthcare.

HISTORICAL BACKGROUND

Developing an understanding of the historical background of integrated service delivery within U.S. hospitals requires a longer view into the history of healthcare. Taking this longer view makes it possible to trace the dis-integration that the modern historical period has brought into mainstream practice. Additionally, this longer view enables the ability to highlight and better understand those pioneering healthcare providers that have sought to be proactive in their pursuit of providing integrated healthcare to hospital services.

The classic text that best portrays this historical background is Thompson and Golden's (1975) *The Hospital: A Social and Architectural History.* Interestingly, it should be noted that the primary factors that have had the greatest impact on the nature of hospital service provision are—as Thompson and Golden indicate—both social and architectural. In their text, Thompson and Golden argue for a four-point framework to understand the historical evolution of hospitals by analyzing the forms of their nursing units. The four elements of this framework are "the healthful environment it provides for patients, the amount of privacy it allows patients, the extent to which it exercises supervision and control over patients, and the efficiency with which it can be operated" (p. xxviii).

In contrast to this four-point analytical framework, Verderber and Fine (2000) present a six-point framework for understanding the historical evolution of the hospital. Their model has the benefit of standing on the shoulders of Thompson and Golden's as well as being formulated 25 years later. Verderber and Fine's framework is based on the common themes that exist within a historical era. Consequently, their framework contains the following six elements: (1) the ancient, (2) the Medieval, (3) the Renaissance, (4) the nightingale, (5) the minimalist megahospital, and (6) the virtual healthscape.

The advantage of Verderber and Fine's (2000) framework is that it highlights the evolution of the dis-integration of healthcare delivery. In the first three elements of their framework—the ancient, Medieval, and Renaissance—clearly most, if not all, hospital-based healthcare was integrated. The nightingale era marks the period when the scientificization of medicine began to dominate practice and hence served to cause its dis-integration.

During the next era—the megahospital—this dis-integration expanded still further, and the hospital became seen as an efficient machine for the delivery of healthcare services. The tide only began to turn in the most current era, which Verderber and Fine (2000) describe as the virtual healthscape. In characterizing this post-1990s era, they state that "the information age is profoundly influencing how we define health and how we care for ourselves" (pp. 14–15).

Although it is clearly true that the information age has enabled great strides in supporting progress within healthcare, it is not the panacea that Verderber and Fine (2000) suggest it is. For example, a recent article in *World Hospitals and Health Services* (McConnell, 2006) describes the enormous gulf that exists throughout the underdeveloped world with regard to integrated care for people with disabilities. A key finding of this article is the point that health, social care, and mental health services all experience systemic difficulties in delivering these services in an integrated fashion.

Of course, the situation that this article discusses is not limited exclusively to underdeveloped countries or even to those people who have disabilities. Indeed, in hospital-based care within the United States today, much progress can still be made in delivering an integrated approach to the conventional array of mainstream healthcare services. For example, it is well documented that a common source of medical error is the result of a pharmacist making a substitution of a prescribed medication without first confirming the possible consequences of this judgment with the prescribing physician. In this instance, meaningful progress can be achieved simply with improved communication. As both these examples highlight, the term *integrated healthcare* can take on a variety of distinct meanings, in addition to the meaning that is the primary focus of this book. Nevertheless, all these meanings stem from a common source—the industrialization of medicine.

CURRENT TRENDS TOWARD INTEGRATION IN HOSPITALS

It is exciting to have watched the first Planetree Unit in San Francisco, in 1985, expand its influence beyond the boundaries of this initial site and grow to the degree that, 20 years later, there are almost 100 sites today. However, as a linear progression, this emerging trend will take almost 1,000 years to impact the remaining balance of U.S. hospitals. In the face of this harsh reality that limits the more rapid spread of Planetree's influence, what are the prevailing trends that exert an influence on the integration of healthcare services within hospitals?

A snapshot of the field of hospital-based healthcare as it exists today, in 2006, does not reveal an encouraging picture for the future of dramatically expanding the degree of integrated services. Across this field, a constant pressure is experienced to do more faster, cheaper, and smarter, and although the proponents of integrated healthcare argue that the provision of these services increases effective patient care while reducing costs, their argument has not significantly impacted the mainstream providers. It seems that every step forward that science and technology provides, the healthcare industry's performance outcomes go a step in reverse—or even worse (Nakashian, 2006).

Yet peppered throughout this hospital-based healthcare industry snapshot, it is possible to identify those glimmering brilliant beams of progress, like the Planetree Units, although they do noticeably remain so few and far apart. For reasons that many integrated healthcare advocates and champions find difficult to understand, the fuel that illuminates these beacons does not seem to be easily transferred into the vision, mission, and purpose of many other hospitals.

The very nature of this fuel is well understood by several leading consultants, as it is not unique to the field of hospitals. For example, Pine and Gilmore (1999), in *The Experience Economy*, explain the source of this fuel and discuss how to use it most effectively. For Pine and Gilmore, this fuel is synonymous with developing memorable positive experiences for the patient, visitor, hospital staff, and healthcare practitioners.

However, Heifetz (1994) provides the missing link—which addresses the more systemic issues of providing integrated services within hospitals and their sustainability over the transitions of new administrative and governing influences—by his distinguishing what he calls "adaptive" work. Heifetz argues that a shortfall in organizational progress is a consequence of not understanding the distinction between technical and adaptive work.

Heifetz's (1994) view is that all systemic progress is a leadership challenge. Indeed, if these brilliant beams—such as Planetree—are truly industry exemplars of a more effective means to deliver hospital-based healthcare services, what can Heifetz's position contribute to accelerating the rate of integration? In his distinguishing adaptive work, Heifetz claims that learning is required—for the overall organizational system, for the individual care provider, and for the patient. This adaptive learning that Heifetz advocates is a completely different level of learning than the so-called technical learning that Pine and Gilmore's (1999) scripted performance can accomplish. Considering the sustainable longevity of the case study examples within this chapter, each one seems to lend support to Heifetz's (1994) claim with regard to the presence of adaptive learning that all the relevant stakeholders appear to have accomplished in their lives.

It seems, however, that the difficulty in accelerating the rate of integration within hospital-based healthcare services is that this adaptive learning that is required is not simply a formulaic training, such as reading Pine and Gilmore (1999) and merely operationalizing the understandings they offer. Rather, the kind of learning that Heifetz (1994) advocates is analogous to speaking with an individual who seeks healing over curing, compared to an individual who is not capable of distinguishing between the two.

This analogy, and the tension that it characterizes, seems to be comparable to the tension that exists as a healthcare organization attempts to increase the incidence of integrated services within their delivery protocols. Unfortunately, this snapshot of the hospital field as it exists today does not indicate a trend that is supportive of the type of adaptive learning that Heifetz (1994) argues is required to produce the systemic and sustainable improvements that integrated healthcare services can offer to the practice of hospital-based medicine.

In this regard, it is instructive to note that the Robert Wood Johnson Foundation, one of America's leading foundations that supports innovation in healthcare, publishes an annual journal, *To Improve Health and Health Care*. Volume 9 of this journal contains a list of the contents of the eight previous journals—nowhere can an article about integrative healthcare be found (Isaacs & Knickman, 2006).

THE IMPORTANCE OF INTEGRATED SERVICES IN HOSPITALS

The mission of the Integrative Medicine Alliance (2006) is "to deepen the quality of the human experience of healthcare." This notion, of "deepening the quality of the human experience," seems to strike a resonance across the range of many healthcare–related stakeholders with a more humanistic perspective. Indeed, a review of Planetree's list of core elements, as outlined in the case study example that follows, reveals an intelligent congruence between each of these core elements and a clear intention to "deepen the quality of the human experience."

For example, the very first Planetree (n.d.) core element is "the healing partnership of human interaction." The academic, professional, and lay literature all contain a multitude of personal accounts—both from patients and healthcare practitioners—that lament the poverty in the quality of the human interaction that is commonly found within conventional healthcare practice today. Clearly one very important reason to increase the incidence of integrated services within hospitals is because of the positive impact this will have on the quality of the human experience, which is linked through research studies directly to the tangible benefit of improved medical outcomes (Kleinman, 1988).

Quite specifically, and as one of the many possible examples, the literature provides support for the case of medical noncompliance to be as high as 50 percent (Talking Rx, 2005). A key factor in this measure of poor clinical performance is the very site of the human interaction that is inherent within healthcare service delivery and the degree to which this interaction has an impact on the quality of the healthcare delivery experience of the patient. The research has shown that the perceived quality of the patient's overall healthcare experience has a direct relationship on the patient's rate of compliance (Mishler, 1984).

Consequently, an argument can be made that an additional reason to increase the incidence of integrated services within the hospital is that the medical outcomes are likely to be improved, if, in fact, these integrated services are effective at deepening the quality of the human experience (Isaacs & Knickman, 2006). This argument becomes particularly compelling when it is understood that these means to improve outcomes are not technologically sophisticated, expensive medical devices—rather, on the contrary, the means to accomplish this improvement are the low-tech and inexpensive practices, such as compassionate listening, that are the common sense artifacts of human-centered cultural values, as is evidenced within the examples that the following case studies illustrate.

CASE STUDIES

This section consists of four case studies that examine the sustainable presence of integrated healthcare in a hospital setting. Each case study is divided into four sections to facilitate comparison across all of them. These four sections describe (1) the healthcare organizational context; (2) the individual who served as the champion for the integrated services; (3) the integrated modalities provided; and (4) the relationship between the organizational unit, where the integrated services are provided, and the overall hospital.

The four case studies that follow concern (1) the Vidarkliniken in Jarna, Sweden, (2) Planetree in Derby, Connecticut, (3) Scripps Center for Integrative Medicine in San Diego, California, and (4) North Hawaii Community Hospital in Kamuela.

CASE STUDY 1: THE VIDARKLINIKEN

Organizational Context

The Vidarkliniken is, perhaps, the most widely acclaimed and recognized hospital for integrated care in the world (see Coates & Siepl-Coates, 1988). It is presented as the first case study, although it is not in the United States, because of its acknowledged exemplar status.

The Vidarkliniken is only one component of a large-scale intentional community located approximately 50 miles south of Stockholm, in a village called Jarna. This community was founded, in 1935, initially to provide an anthroposophical curative home for children. Since that time, the community has expanded in its scope, while maintaining its commitment to the anthroposophical principles upon which it was originally founded.

The anthroposophical philosophy was founded by Rudolph Steiner in the late nineteenth and early twentieth centuries. This philosophy is all encompassing, insofar as it is an integrated approach to all of life. An important element of this approach is that of anthroposophical medicine, which serves as the guiding principle for the design and operations of the Vidarkliniken.

Within the village of Jarna today, in addition to the Vidarkliniken, there is a substantial biodynamic farm, a college for teaching these farming principles, several Waldorf schools, numerous curative homes for children and adults, more than 80 dwelling units, a significant performing arts center, and a multitude of additional related buildings. The Jarna-based Rudolph Steiner Seminariat serves as the educational and cultural focus for the entire community.

The Champion

Erik Asmussen moved to Stockholm prior to the outbreak of World War II. As an architect, he designed the first Waldorf school and developed a unique local style of vernacular architecture that is distinctive to the Jarna community. For almost 50 years, Asmussen worked within the community of Jarna, constantly experimenting with architectural expressions that were based within the anthroposophical philosophy.

Erik Asmussen is designated as the champion for the integrated approach to healthcare of the Vidarkliniken because of the variety of

(Continues)

(Continued)

ways that the design of the building supports, facilitates, and reinforces the clinical functions of the hospital. Additionally, because anthroposophical medicine is—by its very nature—an integrated approach to healthcare delivery, Asmussen's designation as the champion is an acknowledgment of his creative interpretation of anthroposophical principles into the design of this facility.

Asmussen's creative interpretation of these principles is apparent immediately on approaching the Vidarkliniken. The shape of the building, the pattern of the window openings, the use of color on the exterior all signal a very distinctive sensitivity. Entering the building serves to heighten the awareness and experience of these sensitivities, as it is reinforced by the spatial composition, the use of thoughtfully crafted local materials, subtle qualities of color, and the intelligent manner in which daylighting is introduced within the building to complement the use of electrical lighting.

The Integrated Modalities Provided

The Vidarkliniken is dedicated to the practice of anthroposophical medicine. It has been created to provide medical and health-related care to the anthroposophical community of Jarna. The Vidarkliniken is a component of the Swedish federal healthcare system, and as such, it provides high-quality socialized care to those individuals who seek its services. It contains a total of 74 inpatient beds.

The Vidarkliniken provides a full range of both inpatient and outpatient care appropriate to a secondary level community hospital with no surgical services. In addition to a range of conventional allopathic healthcare services, the Vidarkliniken provides those services that are unique to anthroposophical medicine. For example, the colors of the inpatient rooms vary to reflect the anthroposophical modality of chromotherapy. Consequently, an inpatient may be moved several times during the course of his stay to be placed in those inpatient rooms that provide the therapeutic colors that are consistent with his treatment plan.

Similarly, curative eurhythmy spaces are designed to encourage richly expressive bodily movements that are intended to harmonize the being of its participants. These eurhythmy spaces provide an ideal means to illustrate the specific contribution that the architectural design makes as a therapeutic modality itself that cannot be taken as separate from the medical practice it is designed to support.

Relationship between the Hospital and the Community

For the purpose of this unique case study, it is not appropriate to isolate a single organizational unit that practices integrated healthcare and discuss its relationship to the hospital, as it is in other case study examples that follow. Rather, in the case of the Vidarkliniken—where the entire hospital is completely integrated in its approach to healthcare—it is more appropriate to consider the relationship between the entire hospital and the overall community within which it is situated.

One of the unique characteristics of Jarna as an intentional anthroposophical community is the seamless integration of all the community's physical components to one another. Part of the reason for this harmonious experience of overall integration is the direct result of the visual cohesion of the community's physical components, which is a consequence of Asmussen's tenure as the resident architect. Notwithstanding, however, this visual cohesion throughout the community reflects the very nature of anthroposophy, which requires that all elements of the approach, irrespective of its scale, are inherently integrated to each other, and all to the whole.

Consequently, there is no separation—functionally or experientially—between the Vidarkliniken and the rest of the community. For example, the Vidarkliniken is not a place that only sick people go to. On the contrary, the hospital is operationally integrated into the daily life patterns of the community residents due to its art and movement programs, meditation garden, café, and gardening activities, to name just a few.

CASE STUDY 2: PLANETREE

Organizational Context

Across the United States, and increasingly in Canada and Europe, Planetree (http://www.planetree.org) has become synonymous with patient-centered healthcare and its unique approach to the provision of integrated healthcare services within a hospital setting. Founded in 1978, Planetree is a practical demonstration of the tangible benefits of consumer-driven healthcare delivery.

(Continues)

(Continued)

In 1985, Planetree opened its first fully operational healthcare unit. This was a single nursing unit within a large medical center in San Francisco. From then until now, Planetree has expanded its direct care, providing operations to more than 95 separate locations, demonstrating both the feasibility and desirability of patient-centered healthcare as an approach to a more consumer-responsive method of healthcare delivery. To this end, Planetree serves as a resource, a facilitator, and a network for those institutions that choose to subscribe to the cultural values that underpin this approach.

The international Planetree headquarters are located in Derby, Connecticut. The headquarters produce the resources that disseminate the Planetree concept, expand its provider base of new sites, and support its expanding network. Each individual Planetree provider—whether it be a small rural hospital or a major medical center, a primary care service provider or a long-term care service organization—is responsible for the operation of its own services within the template that has been developed by Planetree. For the purposes of this case study, the Griffin Hospital, in Derby, has been selected to illustrate Planetree's integrated approach to hospital-based healthcare delivery.

The Champion

Planetree was founded by Angelica Thieriot, who served as its champion during the initial years of developing its first demonstration project and establishing the sustainable basis for the organization. Each one of the subsequent Planetree projects has become possible as the direct result of the advocacy of a local champion. Lynn Werdal, in her capacity as vice president for Patient Care Services, served as the champion to bring Planetree to the Griffin Hospital.

In the late 1980s, Griffin Hospital found itself experiencing difficulties with its ongoing financial viability as a consequence of the other local providers attracting their more lucrative, paying patients away. This flight from Griffin was occasioned by a combination of their aging physical plant as well as the upgraded facilities of the competing providers. In their consideration of alternative strategies to improve their competitive position, Ms. Werdal discovered the Planetree organization and took the role of serving as its local champion.

Ms. Werdal succeeded in developing a major new addition to the hospital that functioned entirely as a Planetree site. However, odd as it may seem, the contiguous older hospital was not initially converted to become part of the Planetree project. The proper functioning of a Planetree site requires extreme attention to staff recruitment, orientation, training, continued training, and the ongoing reinforcement of this training. The success of this Griffin Hospital Planetree project is a tribute to Ms. Werdal's dedication to the ideals of Planetree as well as to her personal commitment to develop a patient-centered organizational culture and the training required to instill and reinforce its values.

The Integrated Modalities Provided

The most significant elements that the Griffin Hospital Planetree addition contained were a new lobby, a maternity unit, and an intensive care unit. The new lobby included a Planetree Resource Library, which is a Planetree hallmark, and a public seating area with a grand piano within a multistorey atrium space.

The Planetree philosophy, although it is patient-centered, is also dedicated to improving the health of patient family members, visitors, hospital staff, and the local community. In this regard, all the physical elements of Planetree are thoughtfully developed to support this whole community approach toward health improvement. For example, the resource library is available to the patients, to their families and visitors, and to the community to access those resources that can be used to learn about illness and treatment options as well as about health. Similarly, the spacious lobby with the grand piano is provided to signal a non-hospital-type of experience that can have more positive associations than the typical visitor experience in a more conventional hospital.

The decision to locate the new maternity and intensive care units in the new addition was a strategic decision to improve the hospital's financial viability by providing world-class patient-centered hospital-based healthcare services that would be responsive to the local market conditions. The operational concept for the new maternity unit was based on the increasingly popular single-room maternity care approach that featured the option of having natural childbirth with a care partner present throughout the entire experience.

The new intensive care unit was designed as a unique doughnut plan configuration. This allowed for a naturally lighted exterior corridor that was dedicated to public circulation for the unit and provided small, private waiting areas adjacent to each patient room. The patient rooms formed the next ring within the unit. This arrangement provided the opportunity for an inner core that was dedicated to staff work, with

(Continues)

(Continued)

a separate staff entrance to each patient room. This unique design concept optimized the quality of experience for each of the user groups and had the added benefit of being able to separate the public circulation from the staff circulation and work areas.

Each individual Planetree site has the autonomy to apply the philosophy in a way that best suits its own unique circumstances. Nevertheless, the core elements of Planetree that were available at the Griffin Hospital included the healing partnership of human interaction; empowering patients through information and education; family, friends, and social support networks; spirituality and inner resources; the importance of human touch; healing arts; complementary therapies; architectural design conducive to health and healing; and the nutritional and nurturing aspects of food (see http://www.planetree.org/about/components.htm).

Relationship between the Unit and the Hospital

As mentioned earlier, the design of the new addition to the hospital was based on the Planetree philosophy, while the contiguous original hospital building was not initially upgraded to be consistent with this approach. The rationale for this apparent separation, as explained by Ms. Werdal, was that the justification for the decision to develop the new addition as a Planetree site was predicated on a strategic business-oriented decision, based on an expectation that the new addition would make a contribution toward the improved financial performance of the hospital—which it did, in fact, do.

However, the difficulty in developing a Planetree unit—where the unit does not encompass the entire hospital, as is often the case with Planetree sites—is that the Planetree site must engage with the rest of the hospital for its services, which has the potential of creating an awkward situation for the Planetree site. At Griffin Hospital, for example, the staff who were employed to work on the new maternity unit would be dedicated to that unit and be trained to deliver the Planetree philosophy within that unit. The Planetree patient-centered model requires that every hospital employee who interacts with the patient deliver the Planetree philosophy.

In contrast, the housekeeping department, for example, is a hospital-wide service, with individuals providing this service who might not be dedicated to any specific area or philosophy. This awkward situation applies across a variety of different modalities and hospital services, including those integrated services that would be unique to the Planetree philosophy. For example, the staff on a Planetree unit are eligible to be given massage for their relaxation. In this instance, while the staff on the maternity unit might be given regular massage therapy, those staff on the medical and surgical units in the original building might not be eligible to receive the same benefit.

CASE STUDY 3: SCRIPPS CENTER FOR INTEGRATIVE MEDICINE

Organizational Context

"The Scripps Center for Integrative Medicine offers the best of conventional and complementary medicine....[They] blend evidence-based complementary and alternative therapies with conventional Western medicine in a 'best of both worlds' approach to treating disease, healing and improving health" (Scripps Center for Integrative Medicine, n.d.).

The center is an outgrowth of Scripps Health, located in San Diego, California. In 1924, Ellen Browning Scripps founded Scripps Memorial Hospital and Scripps Metabolic Clinic in La Jolla. Scripps Mercy Hospital, established in 1890, joined the system in 1995. In 2004, Scripps Memorial (located in Chula Vista, California) and Scripps Mercy joined operations to form Scripps Mercy Hospital Chula Vista. The acute care hospital system also includes Scripps Green Hospital and Scripps Memorial Hospital Encinitas. Since reaffiliating with Scripps Clinic in 2000, the system has about 10,000 employees and 11 clinic locations throughout San Diego County.

The Scripps Center for Integrative Medicine began modestly in the late 1990s by offering alternative services for cardiology patients as part of their lifestyle changes for successful cardiology rehabilitation. Championed by Erminia M. (Mimi) Guarneri, MD, FACC, an interventional cardiologist, and Rauni King, RN, who believes in a healthy vegetarian diet, exercise, and meditation, the first center offered a wide variety of wellness and health education classes and programs in a small space in their Shiley Fitness Center.

Phase one of the Scripps Center for Integrative Medicine was opened in October 2004. Schmidt Scanlon Gordon Architects collaborated with

(Continues)

(Continued)

Jain Malkin, Inc., a company that specializes in interior architecture for healthcare, incorporating into its design work evidence-based research in healing environments. The design of the physical environment is a reflection of the holistic philosophy of care. On the basis of environmental research linking a person's physiological wellness with an innate need for nature, the center's architecture and interior were designed to assist the patient in relaxing and releasing stress.

The golden mean is a natural, geometric proportion that has been used for thousands of years to design sacred spaces around the world. This proportion, which is found in the built environment and in nature, is most notable in the spiral of the chambered nautilus. The designers used the proportion as a template for the design of the center, with the spiral inspiring the curves of the walls, the soffits in the ceilings, and the general layout of the space.

The Champion

Dr. Guarneri is the medical director and founder of the Scripps Center for Integrative Medicine. After earning a master's degree in bioengineering, Dr. Guarneri graduated from medical school first in her class. She served her internship and residency at Cornell Medical Center. In 1995, she joined Scripps Clinic as an attending interventional cardiologist. Her impressive curriculum vitae includes membership in the American College of Cardiology, along with board certification in cardiology, internal medicine, nuclear medicine, and holistic medicine. She is a diplomate of the American Board of Holistic Medicine.

Armed with the most up-to-date research on how diet and exercise can reverse heart disease, she became the spokesperson, lead fundraiser, and designer of the new center. A compelling public speaker, Dr. Guarneri roused the community to look at the value of healthy lifestyle changes to improve health and wellness. Along with her codirector, Rauni King, RN, who has been by her side developing the center from the beginning, she has delivered messages of wellness to the community through lectures and an annual retreat. In this way Guarneri and King assist people in transforming their health and therefore their lives.

Dr. Guarneri was a participant in the writing of the American College of Cardiology Foundation Complementary Medicine Expert Consensus Document, published in 2005. Her book, *The Heart Speaks*, tells the stories of heart patients who have benefited from lifestyle changes brought about by various approaches in integrative medicine.

Her work was featured in a 2006 PBS documentary, *The New Medicine*. Dr. Guarneri has been nationally recognized for her leadership in the field.

> Health is more than the absence of disease. Health is living with purpose, meaning, and passion. Finding our role in the human family is what gives us reason to live. If I had to write a recipe for health it would be: Let go of the past, forgive those who have hurt you, and count your blessings every day. Treat your body like a temple, for it is the only house you have. Your body requires proper nutrition, sleep, and exercise. Stress comes from how we perceive a situation, so take a few deep breaths before you say something you'll regret. Practice 'random acts of kindness' and offer your gifts to the world. Listen to what your heart tells you and let it, not your ego, lead the way. When we realize that we can only change ourselves and not others—that, as Gandhi said, 'We must be the change we want to see'—we will heal ourselves and our planet. (Guarneri & King, 2006)

The Integrated Modalities Provided

As part of their efforts to help patients heal themselves through maintaining a healthy lifestyle, the Scripps Center for Integrative Medicine offers classes ranging from group exercise, Qigong, Tai Chi, and yoga classes to support groups, spirituality and meditation, pain management, mindfulness-based stress reduction, and even a class in healthy vegetarian cooking. Integrative treatments and therapies include acupuncture, biofeedback, healing touch, hypnosis, music therapy, and therapeutic massage, among a host of others.

An unusual component of the center is the high level of diagnostic screening and testing it offers. Full body imaging with a PT scan can be either self-referred by an individual or referred by a physician for advanced diagnostic work and early detection cardiac risk appraisal. Advanced laboratory analysis is also available. The success of the center is attributed to this combination of high tech and high touch.

Consultations are available where specialists design treatment plans for patients that encompass alternative approaches to their medical treatment and help them incorporate nutrition, fitness, and nutritional supplements into their plans for staying healthy.

Relationship between the Unit and the Hospital

The center is a well-integrated model. Patients are referred by a physician, or they choose for themselves to go to the center to deal with an

(Continues)

(Continued)

acute illness, for a preventive evaluation, or for improved wellness and lifestyle change. The staff includes three physicians who are integrated medical specialists and three cardiologists. Clinical nurse managers screen the patients and make appointments with a physician. The physician sees the patient and makes recommendations for complementary programs and a personalized care plan. In all cases a physician supervises each patient, and treatments are recorded in the patient's medical records. The patient then decides the level of classes and therapies in which he is prepared to participate.

Prescribed classes and therapies relate to one another and help the patient progress through the process. Because of this, patients are confident that they are not receiving conflicting information from a variety of practitioners. This creates extraordinary convenience and comfort for patients, who are then able to make long-term commitments to lifestyle change. Patients have been known to participate in the program for many years. Therapies are currently given in an outpatient situation. Though the program has not yet been expanded to include inpatient care, this is the next horizon for the center.

So much publicity has been received that centers and hospitals from around the country are continuously calling to tour and learn more about the center's business model. To accommodate this, the center conducts intensive symposiums twice a year to teach the lessons they have learned during their 10 years of development.

The caregivers as well as community members are extremely proud of the center. However, its growth into a position of influence on the Scripps Health System has not always been easy. In the early development of the center, Dr. Guarneri and Ms. King faced numerous obstacles, the most significant being a lack of finances and credibility. Administrators of the health system felt that the center was a wonderful idea, but they were hesitant to fund it without private support. Today, it is one of the most successful integrated medicine models within a hospital system in the country, evidenced by the long waiting list for new patients to be seen and by a very positive financial picture. The administration considers the center its golden child and actively supports its expansion.

CASE STUDY 4: NORTH HAWAII COMMUNITY HOSPITAL

Organizational Context

It is sometimes the small that become giants in their field. This is the case of North Hawaii Community Hospital in Kamuela. Opening its doors to the public in May 1996 with only 40 acute care, 31 medical/surgical, 5 obstetric, and 4 critical care beds, it was surprising that it made national news. Yet the hospital has been an invited presenter to most healthcare design conferences since it opened, and people from all over the world visit it.

North Hawaii Community Hospital is affiliated with Adventist Health, which is headquartered in Roseville, California, and is the U.S. West Coast arm of an international network of over 160 healthcare facilities. The hospital was in the initial planning stages when Earl Bakken chose to retire on the big island of Hawaii and heard of it. He became a champion and major contributor to the direction that the hospital took.

This may be the only hospital that was designed, from its inception, to provide a careful integration of select complementary healing practices with high-quality medical care. North Hawaii Community Hospital's vision is to "treat the whole individual—mind, body and spirit—through a team approach to patient-centered care, and ultimately to become the most healing hospital in the world….As ohana, we value an environment of aloha which nurtures trust, respect, self expression, open minds and hearts" (North Hawaii Community Hospital, 2006). This guiding principle, which borrows words from the native Hawaiian language, gives special meaning to the hospital's connection to its locale and surrounding community.

The use of native design elements, natural materials, and native art and prayers provides an immediate welcome that echoes the spirit of aloha. The openness of the design keeps patients, visitors, and caregivers always in the beauty of natural surroundings. Refreshing harp music plays on the overhead speaker system. A reflective healing garden near the entrance houses a labyrinth with glorious ceramic tiles. Everything in the facility is designed to continue the effort of healing the body and the whole human being.

Elements important in the design of the facility include natural light, full-spectrum lighting, carpet in the patient areas, and the use of green materials and cleaning products that eliminate the typical hospital smell. Cables are buried extra deep to reduce electromagnetic stress, and

(Continues)

(Continued)

the water is quadruple filtered. The corridors are extra wide, and every patient room is oversized, with homelike finishes and amenities. The environment is perceived as safe, patient-centered, and family-centered. Care is both respectful and responsive to the variety of religious and cultural beliefs present.

The Champion

The hospital would not be what it is or where it is today without the efforts of pioneer Earl Bakken. Fascinated with science and technology, electronics, and robotic devices since his childhood, young Earl became a radar maintenance instructor in the Army Signal Corps. He did graduate work in electrical engineering at the University of Minnesota. His first wife, Connie, was a medical technologist at Northwestern Hospital in Minneapolis, Minnesota. This exposed him to the needs of medical technology. In 1949, Mr. Bakken, along with his brother-in-law, started a medical equipment repair company called Medtronic, Inc. in his garage.

Soon he was developing new devices and training medical personnel on usage. A Dr. Lillehei asked Mr. Bakken to make a better pacemaker for cardiac patients. First tested on a single dog, by 1959 it was being implemented for human beings. Within three months of signing a license agreement with the originators of the first implantable pacemaker, the company had 50 orders at $375 each. Today, Medtronic, Inc. supplies about half of the nearly 700,000 pacemakers in annual worldwide sales. The company reached $1 billion in sales by 1991 and continues to thrive by supplying a host of medical technology devices for a long list of health applications.

Earl Bakken personally observed that Medtronic's high-tech products seemed more effective when prescribed and watched over by certain doctors and nurses. He noted that some professionals "would create in their patients the conviction that the technology was indeed going to make them feel better. By believing in the devices, these physicians and nurses were somehow able to transfer that belief to the patient" (Minnesota Medical Association, 2006). This was the start of another passion for him to somehow link high technology with high-touch medicine, focusing on the patient rather than the hardware and the procedure.

Mr. Bakken retired in 1989 and served on the board of his company until 1994. When he and his present wife, Doris, moved to Hawaii and learned about the local healing traditions, he was instrumental in designing the hospital to integrate truly mind-body modalities into the care practice. Today, he is president emeritus of the hospital's board and is still very involved with the future directions of the hospital.

The Integrated Modalities Provided

Patients admitted to the hospital are offered a variety of complementary therapies, including massage, naturopathy, chiropractic, clinical psychology, acupuncture, and healing touch. People come from all the Hawaiian Islands to give birth at this hospital. It is well known for its homelike, supportive environment and the use of midwives and integrated modalities in birthing.

I recently had the opportunity to experience the birthing center firsthand, when my daughter gave birth there. Her husband and I functioned as birthing coaches. The director of integrative medicine is Dr. Jade McGaff, a doctor of obstetrics and gynecology. My daughter and son-in-law, as many young people are doing, sought a more holistic and natural birth for their daughter. They wanted a center that had midwives and promoted natural birth in a safe and beautiful setting. Since there were some potential minor complications with the delivery, they needed the security of a medical center that could offer the best and most advanced medical solutions if necessary. Although the hospital was an hour and a half from where they lived, they chose to go to the North Hawaii Community Hospital because of the combination of services. The primary attractors were the presence of midwives, a beautiful environment, and a philosophy of integrative practices with labor and delivery.

The birthing rooms are large suites that accommodate the needs of the entire family. In the beginning of labor, the entire family was allowed to be present. We shared a home-cooked meal in the labor room. Since my son-in-law is a massage therapist and an herbalist, he came prepared with special energy drinks for Sarah during labor and oils to massage and relax her, along with her favorite aromatherapy. The midwife and Dr. McGaff embraced the family with all of the accoutrements and jumped right in to assist in facilitating relaxation during labor with encouragement, a warm tub, and healing touch. Even though there were six births going on at the same time, the team was extraordinarily attentive, supportive, and professional.

While Sarah was in labor, I heard beautiful native singing in the corridors. I was pleasantly surprised to find a group of native women in beautiful Hawaiian dress going throughout the hospital offering prayers

(Continues)

(Continued)

and songs for the patients in each bed. One lovely, unique quality of the hospital is "code lavender," which, when sent over the loudspeaker, is a call to prayer for a patient.

The therapies are carried out in the patient room, delivered by a team of trained consultant therapists who work for the hospital on an appointment basis. The practitioners are licensed in the state of Hawaii and have applied for and received medical staff privileges. Some of the services are provided gratis, such as healing touch and heart-math breathing exercises to reduce stress and improve hormone levels. Guided imagery CDs as well as relaxation programs on the hospital's 24-hour free channel are offered.

Billing for services is sent to the patient's insurance provider or directly to the patient, if insurance does not cover the particular therapies. Hospital administrators believe that more people would take advantage of these services if they were covered by insurance.

Relationship between the Unit and the Hospital

In this case, the hospital is fully integrated in its provision of healthcare services. This seamless inclusion of integrated medical services has made North Hawaii Community Hospital a desirable place to work and a destination for people wanting to study integrated healthcare models: "Designed as a 'healing instrument,' [North Hawaii Community Hospital] is fast becoming a prototype for the careful integration of select complementary healing practices with high quality medical care" (North Hawaii Community Hospital, 2006).

In 2004, Earl Bakken made a $10 million gift that has allowed North Hawaii Community Hospital to be affiliated with the prestigious and world-renowned Cleveland Clinic. He donated this money to provide state-of-the-art cardiac and stroke medical services to Hawaiian Islands residents. This gift was in conjunction with a $17 million gift to the Cleveland Clinic to develop a unique institute dedicated to researching the medical interconnections between the heart and the brain. This new relationship between high tech and high touch will bring a new perspective to both institutions.

THE FUTURE OF INTEGRATED HEALTHCARE IN HOSPITALS

Three statements can be made, with a fair degree of certainty, that pertain to the future of integrated healthcare service delivery in hospitals. First, the methods by which healthcare is paid for—and therefore made available to the general population—are likely to evolve over time. This will have a consequential impact on the financial models that are used to determine the viability of providing integrated services in hospitals in assessing the contribution of integrated service modalities on organizational financial performance.

Second, in the face of increased pressure to cap the upper limit of gross domestic product spending on healthcare, the already compelling argument for the financial benefits of providing integrated healthcare services in hospitals will become ever more compelling. In this case, tensions will increase as mainstream healthcare proponents continue to use claims of scientific arguments to discredit the medical and financial efficacy of integrated modalities. The reality of this tension received media headlines recently as Prince Charles advocated the integration of United Kingdom–based hospital services at a World Health Organization meeting in Geneva, Switzerland, as a means to improve financial performance and health outcomes and was scorned by the medical establishment in the United Kingdom for his being incorrect on both of these claims.

Third, the philosophical and cultural principles that support the unquestionable presence of integrated healthcare in hospitals—for example, those of Planetree—are noncontentious within these integrated contexts, across a diverse range of cultural geography, and are of benefit to a full complement of healthcare stakeholders. Therefore acceptance and the desirability of these integrated approaches in the future are likely to increase, as these so-called integrated contexts expand their local influence by tangibly demonstrating the practical benefits of integrated healthcare, while at the same time providing experiential opportunities for the adaptive learning that Heifetz (1998) advocates to occur.

The difficulty, of course, in considering future possibilities—as suggested by the three speculations outlined above—is to make rational arguments when it is well established that human behavior is irrational. A fourth certainty can be offered that overarches the previous three: only time will tell.

CONCLUSION

The organizational decision to provide integrated healthcare services within a hospital is not a casual decision—rather, it requires a champion, a supportive community of consumers, and a team of staff, who, if they are not already engaging in integrative practices, are at least willing to be trained in a manner so as to be able to support the provision of these services.

Accordingly, the decision to provide integrated healthcare in hospitals is a very serious business commitment. Although there are compelling arguments in its favor—financial and otherwise—the lack of rigorous planning and implementation of these services can easily risk perilous results. Furthermore, an organizational champion with personal values that are consistent with integrative practices is critical to initiate the introduction of these services and to manage their success.

There are numerous existing, successful models of integrated healthcare in hospitals that can be drawn on for implementation strategies—such as Planetree—as well as opportunities for creative hybrid approaches to be developed in response to local conditions, such as in the case of the Vidarkliniken. In the end, though, in the United States at least, healthcare delivery is currently governed by business plans. Consequently, although it might be possible to develop a pilot demonstration project that provides integrated healthcare and to rely on grants and philanthropy to provide the initial operational support, a sustainable enterprise must be based on a solid "no margin, no mission" financial foundation.

TOOL KIT FOR CHANGE

Role and Perspective of the Healthcare Professional

1. The healthcare provider is responsible for developing, maintaining, and reinforcing an organizational culture that values quality integrative practices.
2. The healthcare provider actively demonstrates a valuing of quality integrative practices within both the physical and social environments as well as with the behaviors of all provider staff.
3. The healthcare provider provides opportunities to increase access and institutional permeability by the community with a combination of educational resources and community-related activities.

Role and Perspective of the Patient/Participant

1. The patient is an informed healthcare consumer, seeking out and engaging with those resources that correspond with personal cosmologies, values, and practices.
2. The patient supports the development of those resources within his own community that are integrative.

Interconnection: The Global Perspective

1. Local special interest groups that are indigenous to the community are best suited to promote an integrative lifestyle and integrative health resources that are most reflective of particular community needs.
2. Communities function best for the people living in them when opportunities for adaptive learning of the community as a whole are provided.

REFERENCES

Coates, G. J., & Siepl-Coates, S. (1988). New design technologies: Healing architecture: A case design of the Vidarkliniken. *Journal of Healthcare Design*. Retrieved April 27, 2006, from http://www.antroposofi.org/vidar/healthcare.htm

Guarneri, M., & King, R. (2006, June). Rx for heart health. *Spirituality and Health*. Retrieved June 1, 2006. http://www.spiritualityhealth.com/NMagazine/articles.php?id=1488.

Heifetz, R. A. (1994). *Leadership without easy answers*. Cambridge, MA: Harvard University Press.

Huelat, B. J. (2003). *Healing environments*. Alexandria, VA: Medezyn.

Integrative Medicine Alliance. (2006). *The Integrative Medicine Alliance: Deepening the quality of the human experience of healthcare*. Retrieved April 30, 2006, from http://www. IntegrativeMedAlliance.org

Isaacs, S. L., & Knickman, J. R. (Eds.). (2006). *To improve health and health care* (Vol. 4). San Francisco: Jossey-Bass.

Kleinman, A. (1988). *The illness narratives*. New York: Basic Books.

McConnell, H. (2006). Integrated care for people with disabilities: An international perspective, *World Hospitals and Health Services, 42*, 47–48.

Minnesota Medical Association (2006) A Change of Pace Retreived December 5, 2006 from http://www.mmaonline.net/Publications/MNMed2006/November/feature-bakken.htm

Mishler, E. G. (1984). *The discourse of medicine*. Norwood, NJ: Ablex.

Nakashian, M. (2006). Increasing health insurance coverage at the local level: The Communities in Charge Program. In S. L. Isaacs and J. R. Knickman (Eds.) *To improve health and health care*, (Vol. 10). San Francisco: Jossey-Bass.

North Hawaii Community Hospital Welcome page. Retrieved June 1, 2006 from http:// www.northhawaiicommunityhospital.org/index.html.

Pine, B. J., & Gilmore, J. H. (1999). *The experience economy*. Boston: Harvard Business School Press.

Planetree. (n.d.). Our Founder. Retrieved April 30, 2006, from http://www.planetree.org/ about/ourfounder.htm.

Scripps Center for Integrative Medicine. (n.d.). *About us*. Retrieved June 1, 2006, from http://www.scripps.org/services.asp?id=6

Talking Rx. (2005). Talking pill bottles to hit the market. Retrieved June 1, 2006 from http://www.msnbc.msn.com/id/8588632/.

Thompson, J. D., & Golden, G. (1975). *The hospital: A social and architectural history*. New Haven, CT: Yale University Press.

Verderber, S., & Fine, D. J. (2000). *Healthcare architecture in an era of radical transformation*. New Haven, CT: Yale University Press.

Chapter Six

INTEGRATIVE HEALTHCARE IN REHABILITATION

Barry Nierenberg, PhD, Robert L. Glueckauf, PhD, and Scott E. Miller, MA

OVERVIEW

This chapter examines rehabilitation in the context of where it has been, how the field has evolved, and where it is headed. We will demonstrate in this chapter that rehabilitation often provides healthcare for individuals with illness and injury that stretch the limits of traditional health services and technology. Furthermore, we will show that rehabilitation as a discipline has now evolved to the point where it can serve as a model that shows the positive consequences following the integration of other areas of healthcare.

It is hoped that this chapter will assist rehabilitation professionals in remaining knowledgeable about newer developments and in utilizing the more integrative approaches to assist their patients. By discussing these integrative approaches, it is the goal of this chapter to give professionals more tools by which they can establish the sense of trust and caring so central to the healing relationship at the heart of the rehabilitation process.

INTRODUCTION

Rehabilitation can be viewed as both an art and a science that aims to assist persons with physical, mental, or sensory impairments to achieve the maximum possible degree of self-reliance, independence, and equality. As asserted by DeLisa, Currie, and Martin (1998), rehabilitation is a concept that should pervade every part of the healthcare system. In its ideal state, it should include prevention and early recognition programs.

The goal of medical rehabilitation is to enhance the functional abilities of people who have acquired a disabling impairment. These impairments cover a broad scope of conditions, congenital limitations, trauma, acute illness, chronic health conditions, and/or other medical episodes that may limit the ability of affected individuals to function independently. The primary outcome is to enable individuals to reside in the least restrictive and most cost-efficient environment, and to do so at their greatest achievable independence level (DeJong & Sutton, 1995).

At its core, rehabilitation is a holistic and comprehensive approach to medical care, carried out through the collective support of multiple caregivers. Professionals involved may include psychologists, physicians, social workers, nurses, physiatrists (physicians specializing in rehabilitation medicine), physical therapists, occupational therapists, vocational counselors, prosthetists, speech and language therapists, recreational therapists, assistive technologists, and other specialists. A team approach is essential in solving the complex problems connected with various disabilities. The *transdisciplinary* team shares the goal of increased independence and improved quality of life for the patients, along with shorter lengths of stay in hospital or other institutional settings and the most efficient use of the healthcare system resources.

In 1980, the World Health Organization (WHO) published the International Classification of Impairments, Disabilities, and Handicaps. In 2001, the World Health Assembly endorsed its revision, the International Classification of Functioning, Disability, and Health (ICF), which provided "a framework for conceptualizing functioning and disability associated with health conditions" (Peterson, 2005, p. 105). As can be seen by the change in the language, the new classification system provides a new focus on health and the person, not the disease. Since that time, the ICF has been accepted by 191 countries as the standard for the classification of health (Bruyere & Peterson, 2005). This new classification system provides a common language for all disciplines involved in health. Since the ICF represents an assimilation of both the medical and social models of disability within a biopsychosocial perspective, it follows that it offers new definitions and ways of conceptualizing ideas regarding terms such as impairment, disability, and handicap. Within this context, impairment is not necessarily viewed as a disease process but instead "represents a deviation from certain generally accepted population standards of functioning" (World Health Organization [WHO], 2001, p. 12). Thus disability now refers to "the outcome or result of a complex relationship between an individual's health condition and personal factors and of the external factors that represent the circumstances in which the individual lives" (WHO, 2001, p. 17). Likewise, is now seen as a disadvantage for a given individual resulting from an impairment or disability that limits or prevents the fulfillment of a role that is normal (depending on age and social and cultural factors). Overall, an individual's health status is now viewed as an outcome of the complex relationships resulting from an individual's interacting with his environment.

DEVELOPMENT OF MULTI-, INTER-, AND TRANSDISCIPLINARY TEAMS

Rehabilitation medicine is a field where many disciplines meet. The joining of these distinct fields has had innumerable short-term and long-term beneficial effects on a patient's life. Further integration in healthcare can also benefit the disciplines themselves by leading to increased mutual enrichment. Each field (psychology, medicine, physical therapy, occupational therapy, speech and language, etc.) approaches the patient with *discipline*-specific knowledge, that is, with their own individual epistemologies, knowledge, skills, and methods existing within the boundary of that discipline.

Multidisciplinary refers to a process where two or more separate disciplines work in parallel or sequentially. Here they use the discipline-specific knowledge base of their individual fields to address common problems. While they are using the knowledge or understanding of more than one discipline to deliver healthcare, the disciplines are not working together. This framework is reminiscent of the familiar paradigm of the two disciplines operating as separate silos of care.

Interdisciplinary refers to a process using methods and epistemology of one discipline while working in another. It consists of workers working jointly, but still from a discipline-specific basis, to address a common problem. For example, when using the knowledge and applications of physics when dealing with the world of space, a new field, astrophysics, was realized. Mitchell (2005) described an interdisciplinary process as occurring when healthcare professionals work jointly yet remain in discipline-specific roles to address a common problem. Again, thinking of the silos of care idea, an interdisciplinary space would be one where the separate silos overlap.

Transdisciplinary refers to an approach involving multiple disciplines and the spaces between them, with the opportunity of new points of view that stretch and develop beyond the original disciplines.

Transdisciplinary Practice in Psychology

Following is a case highlighting psychology practice to illustrate an example of an effective transdisciplinary approach.

Optimal treatment outcomes were necessary with Tom, a 17-year-old white male diagnosed with infantile cerebral palsy. Tom was being seen by a doctoral-level psychology student as part of her practicum placement at a comprehensive outpatient rehabilitation center. Tom had been diagnosed with posttraumatic stress disorder following his exposure to a category three hurricane. Tom's treatment protocol consisted of creating a hierarchy of upsetting details regarding the hurricane, autogenic relaxation training, systematic desensitization, and thermal biofeedback. During the therapist's treatment, she discovered that Tom had a debilitating and significant fear when transferring in and out of his wheelchair and bed due to recent falls and was refusing further physical therapy. A transdisciplinary approach was used involving the psychology student, the occupational therapist, and the physical therapist. It was jointly decided that while undergoing his physical and occupational therapy, the psychology student would be present to coach Tom throughout the treatment. In particular, Tom would be guided through his physical therapy while engaging in autogenic relaxation. His established relationship with the psychology student allowed Tom to trust the process, and his resistance to physical treatment was eliminated after a short time. At a two-month follow-up, Tom reported that he continued to practice his relaxation techniques and had engaged in relaxation at various times when he felt threatened and scared. Both Tom and his primary caregiver, his mother, reported a decrease in resistance to the transferring procedure and an overall positive increase in their relationship.

Another example involves transdisciplinary collaboration between a speech pathology student from a local university and a psychology staff member from a comprehensive outpatient rehabilitation center. Their collaboration concerned Tina, a 48-year-old white woman who suffered from anoxia at birth, with resulting brain injury and cognitive and emotional sequelae. Tina was born in South Africa and moved to the United States in 1986. She attended specialized private and public schools to assist her in her developmental processes and had undergone speech therapy for the majority of her life. Tina was evaluated and began attending treatment for cognitive retraining of the left and right hemispheres to address her developmental disabilities, specifically her deficits in organizational skills, comprehension, sequencing, visual planning, visual discrimination, safety awareness issues, memory, and initiation. Tina also began speech therapy at the facility to address cognitive issues and intelligibility. The speech and psychology staff collaborated as it became clear that Tina was having difficulty completing her treatment.

In addition to expressive and receptive speech difficulties, Tina was having difficulty with her comprehension and sequencing skills when trying to complete a task that taught her the procedures of the structured group, which was typically taught in a verbal format. The psychology staff member evaluation of Tina revealed strengths in her visual skills, so the psychology staff and speech student collaborated to create new group forms for Tina. A grid was created with the 10 sequences listed vertically. Though visual skills were strengths compared to her verbal skills, Tina still had significant visual-spatial and visual discrimination difficulties. The boxes of the grid were made larger, and only one row of procedure steps was presented on the sheet. Additionally, icons were developed that represented each individual procedural step. Treatment for Tina consisted of both clinicians working independently, then jointly, to improve functioning in the identified areas.

NONTRADITIONAL APPROACHES IN REHABILITATION: AN OVERVIEW

There have been a number of new approaches used in rehabilitation medicine growing out of transdisciplinary collaborations between a variety of fields. One of the most widely studied areas has been the treatment of arthritis, where a number of nontraditional approaches are now used. Rheumatoid arthritis is a disease in which the body's immune system attacks its own healthy tissues. The attacks happen most often in the joints of the feet and hands and cause redness, pain, swelling, and heat around the joint. Arthritic conditions occur commonly and can be progressively disabling. Unpleasant side effects associated with conventional treatments for arthritis have been cited as the reason for the wider use and acceptance of complementary and alternative approaches. For example, recently, electromagnetic fields have begun to be explored as an intervention. Here Hulme et al. (2006) reported that pulsed electric stimulation has enough evidence behind it to be considered a promising approach to osteoarthritis. Similarly, Han et al. (2006), in their review, looked at Tai Chi for an arthritis treatment. Tai Chi, also called "Tai Chi Chuan," combines deep breathing and relaxation with slow and gentle movements. In older people, Tai Chi has been shown to decrease stress; increase muscle strength in the lower body; and improve balance, posture, and the ability to move. They found evidence that Tai Chi "improves the range of motion of the ankle, hip and knee in people with rheumatoid arthritis. And, people felt that they improved when doing Tai Chi and enjoyed it" (Han et al., 2006, p. 1). Likewise, the use of herbal supplements, such as avocado soybean unsaponifiables, were shown to have promising results in two studies; further studies would be desirable to verify efficacy (Little, Parsons, & Logan, 2000).

Little et al. (2000) also examined studies of gamma-linolenic acid in the treatment of arthritis and concluded that this herbal intervention may provide supplementary or alternative treatment to nonsteroidal anti-inflammatory drugs (NSAIDs) for some patients. Ultrasound is another nontraditional approach used as an adjunct therapy for the symptomatic treatment of rheumatoid arthritis. Its mechanical energy seems to have some anti-inflammatory as well as analgesic properties (Casimiro et al., 2002). The review of Casimiro and colleagues (2002) provided evidence that continuous ultrasound applied in water to the dorsal and palmar aspects of the hand significantly increased grip. Ultrasound also produced some "increase in wrist dorsal flexion, decreased morning stiffness, and reduced the number of swollen and painful joints" (p. 1).

OVERVIEW AND KEY ISSUES IN TELEHEALTH PRACTICE AND OUTCOME RESEARCH

One of the most promising and widely used newer developments in rehabilitation today is the growing utilization of telecommunication technologies to provide information, assessment, and treatment to individuals with chronic medical conditions. This new field of healthcare communication, variously known as telehealth, eHealth, or telemedicine, has expanded greatly over the past decade in the United States and Canada, particularly in the public health sector (e.g., U.S. Department of Veterans Affairs, correctional facilities, and child protection services). Given its growth and increasing acceptance, we will go into some detail in this chapter.

According to the Telemedicine Information Exchange (2006), there are now in excess of 200 telehealth programs in the United States and abroad, serving a wide range of healthcare needs and patient populations. Furthermore, 40 percent or more of these programs have been in operation for fewer than five years (Glueckauf, Jeffers, & Sharma, in press; Nickelson, 1998).

The terms *telehealth, eHealth,* and *telemedicine* are often used interchangeably to refer to a wide variety of applications of telecommunication technologies in transmitting and receiving health information and healthcare services. Telehealth has been characterized as the use of telecommunications and information technologies to provide access to health information and services across a geographical distance, including (but not limited to) consultation, assessment, intervention, and follow-up programs to ensure maintenance of treatment effects over time and across community settings (Glueckauf, Pickett, Ketterson, Loomis, & Rozensky, 2003). Similarly, eHealth has been defined as the use of interactive technologies, such as the Internet, personal digital assistants, interactive television, voice response systems, and computer kiosks, to facilitate health improvement and healthcare services (Eysenbach, 2001). The term *telemedicine,* on the other hand, has been used more restrictively, referring to the use of modern information technology, especially two-way interactive audio/video communications, computers, and telemetry, to deliver health services to remote patients and to facilitate information exchange between primary care physicians and specialists at some distance from each other (Bashshur, 1997). Although these definitions overlap considerably, the term *telehealth* will be used in the remainder of this chapter, primarily due to its emphasis on the maintenance of health and rehabilitation outcomes over time and across settings. As Glueckauf (1993) and others (e.g., Scherer, 2002) have noted, one of the defining features of all rehabilitation strategies is the importance of showing generalizability of effects to everyday life.

The communication technologies used to provide telehealth services fall into two broad categories: asynchronous and synchronous. Asynchronous communication refers to information transactions that occur among two or more persons at different points in time. Electronic mail (e-mail) is the most common form of asynchronous communication and has been used in the delivery of a variety of healthcare and rehabilitation services (e.g., Glueckauf, Ketterson, Loomis, & Dages, 2004; Gustafson et al., 1999). Synchronous communication refers to information transactions that occur simultaneously among two or more persons. Synchronous telecommunications include (but are not restricted to) computer synchronous chat systems, telecommunications devices for the deaf (TDD), telephone, and videoconferencing.

Chat systems permit users to communicate instantly with one another through typed messages. Users can "chat" in two different ways: (1) through channels or *chat rooms,* in which several individuals communicate simultaneously, or (2) through a direct connection, in which two persons hold a private conversation. During chat room discussions, each person's contribution is displayed on screen in the order of its receipt and is read by all participants in the room (Glueckauf, Whitton, & Nickelson, 2002).

TDD are instruments that facilitate text-based conversations through standard telephone lines. TDDs typically consist of a touch-typing keyboard; a single-line, moving-LED screen; text buffer; memory; and a signal light. The entire unit is approximately the size of a laptop computer (Scherer, 2002).

The most common form of synchronous communication is the telephone. The major advantage of the telephone is its widespread availability and ease of access. The telephone has become the standard mode of communication in psychological practice for conducting preliminary screening interviews, follow-up sessions, and crisis intervention (Haas, Benedict, & Kobos, 1996). Over the past few years, innovative, low-cost automated telephone technologies have become an increasingly viable option in treating persons with chronic health conditions, such as hypertension (e.g., Friedman et al., 1996; Piette, Weinberger, & McPhee, 2000), and in providing support to their family caregivers (e.g., Glueckauf et al., 2005; Mahoney, Tarlow, & Jones, 2003).

Although the telephone is presently the most accessible form of telecommunications technology, interactive videoconferencing is likely to become the modality of choice for delivering telehealth services in the twenty-first century. Public demand for interactive videoconferencing services is expected to grow exponentially over the next decade. This surge of popularity is fueled by the declining costs of videoconferencing equipment and software, increased penetration of telecommunication services, the broadening appeal of the World

Wide Web, and the anticipation of gigabit-speed Internet 2 (Glueckauf, Pickett, Ketterson, Nickelson, & Loomis, 2006; Mittman & Cain, 1999).

The overall results of telehealth research suggest that telecommunication-mediated interventions show promise as effective and efficient modes of treatment for individuals with chronic illnesses and their family caregivers, particularly telephone- and videoconference-based modalities (see Glueckauf, 2002; Piette, Weinberger, & McPhee, 2000; Piette, Weinberger, McPhee, Mah, et al., 2000; Schopp, Johnstone, & Merrell, 2000). A representative study that highlights the potential benefits of telehealth in improving the psychosocial and physiological functioning of persons with chronic illness was conducted by Piette and colleagues (Piette, Weinberger, & McPhee, 2000; Piette, Weinberger, McPhee, Mah, et al., 2000). Here they evaluated the impact of an integrative program of automated telephone disease management (ATDM) and nurse follow-up on the physiological and psychosocial functioning of adults with diabetes. The investigators randomly assigned 280 primarily low-income, underinsured individuals with diabetes from a multilingual county health clinic to (1) ATDM plus home-based nurse follow-up intervention or (2) usual care. Approximately 50 percent of the study participants were of Hispanic origin. The ATDM intervention had a significant positive impact on both traditional physiological endpoints (Piette, Weinberger, McPhee, Mah, et al., 2000) and psychosocial outcomes (e.g., psychosocial functioning, anxiety, self-efficacy for self-care activities; Piette, Weinberger, & McPhee, 2000). Piette and colleagues found that more than twice the proportion of ATDM participants exhibited HbA_{1c} levels within the normal range compared to those of routine care controls from pretreatment to the one-year follow-up. Furthermore, the ATDM group reported significantly fewer depressive symptoms, higher levels of self-efficacy, and fewer days of reduced activity than did control participants during the same time interval. Although the investigators failed to report the findings of the between-group analysis for ethnic differences in HbA_{1c}, they noted that there were no substantial differences in improvement of anxiety, depression, and self-efficacy between primarily English- and Spanish-speaking ATDM participants from pretreatment to the one-year follow-up.

Overall, recent findings (Glueckauf, Fritz, et al., 2002; Schopp et al., 2000) suggest that telehealth may be a promising alternative method for delivering healthcare services to a variety of rehabilitation populations. Study participants reported moderately high levels of satisfaction and comfort with telecommunication technologies as well as significant improvements in both psychosocial and health outcomes. There was also preliminary evidence of cost savings as compared to traditional itinerant health delivery models. These results were consistent with other studies using similar telehealth technologies and rehabilitation populations (Glueckauf & Ketterson, 2004).

SPIRITUALITY AND PRAYER

Another nontraditional practice being incorporated into rehabilitation settings is the increasing use of spirituality and prayer. More and more patients are asking healthcare providers to incorporate spirituality and prayer into the healing process. In this section we will examine ways in which this has been incorporated into the rehabilitation process.

Americans are a religious people. In fact, the 2000 Gallup poll of the American public found that

- 94 percent believe in God
- 85 percent believe that religion is a "fairly" or "very" important part of their lives
- 76 percent report that prayer is an important part of their daily lives
- 61 percent believe that religion can answer all or most of today's problems.

In Nierenberg and Sheldon's (2001) experience in their role as psychologists working with medically ill children, they would be called on to stand with parents at the bedside of their critically ill child. During these times, parents and children were often observed to take comfort as well as blame and guilt from their religious and spiritual beliefs. For example, recently, a 16-year-old boy came to the pediatric rehabilitation unit at our hospital after surviving a traumatic brain injury following a gang-related shooting. Prior to his injury, he was heavily involved in his gang, had frequent brushes with the police, and had not attended school in some time. Recovery following his shooting was slow, and when he regained the ability to communicate, he told almost everyone who would listen that while he was in a coma, he saw Jesus come to him with his dead brother. They told him he would not die and would get better to "have a second chance at life, to not mess up this time." The patient swore he would not go back to his "old ways" and, at his insistence, went to church during his weekend passes home and avoided contact with his old friends. After discharge, he continued on this path and directly attributed "turning [his] life around" to his religious experience. During his stay in the rehabilitation hospital, staff used his religious approach to help encourage participation in required therapies.

FUTURE ROLE OF SPIRITUALITY IN PSYCHOTHERAPY

The majority of mental health professionals polled responded that an increased awareness and inclusion of spiritual factors in psychotherapy is warranted (Burke et al., 1999). In addition, both psychotherapists and clergy acknowledge a need for collaboration as there is considerable overlap in the issues they address (Weaver, Koenig, & Larson, 1997). But despite these acknowledgments, spiritual and religious concerns are often ignored or not appropriately addressed by care providers (Henley, 1999). There are many areas that could potentially benefit by including assessment of spiritual factors. For instance, home hospice for the dying child is one place in which spiritual issues need to be addressed as it has been shown that spiritual and religious factors can increase family adjustment (Goldman, 1996). Likewise, some cultural groups characterize childhood mental illness in spiritual ways, and being able to diagnose and treat in a culturally sensitive fashion may be more accepted (Barlow & Walkup, 1998). And while there are certain caveats that must be considered when exploring the relationship between spiritual and psychological variables, such as maintaining rigorous testing practices and employing methods of experimental design (Thorsen, 1999), it would be shortsighted not to acknowledge their importance.

The area of spirituality and psychotherapy is currently under much investigation. Many questions beg to be answered. Under what conditions does spirituality play a positive role in negative life events for people? Under what conditions does it play a negative one?

For example, we have dealt with a number of children who are nonadherent to their medical regimens, some to the extent where it is life threatening. When asked, some of these children have stated a belief that their illness is "a punishment from God" and that it is not up to them to prematurely "end the punishment with medicine." Unfortunately, these children sometimes persist in this belief in spite of continued therapy and intervention from church clergy.

If, as psychologists, we are supposed to effect change in the attitudes, attributions, and behavior of those people seeking our help, how can we not understand more about their spiritual lives and how it develops?

Clinical Examples

All the theories presented in this chapter are helpful but skirt the issue of how they can be used in a clinical setting. Given the relative recency of the concept of psychospirituality, and the absence of an extensive literature base, the following clinical examples are offered.

CASE 1

An example is the case of B., a seven-year-old girl who sustained a significant spinal cord injury following a motor vehicle accident, leaving her with quadriplegia. She and her family were quite religious, and her parents were open in sharing their belief that God would help heal their daughter. They went on to share their belief that God works through people on earth and frequently thanked the team members for their help. They carefully explained to the medical team members that it was their practice to pray several times each day and asked that they not be interrupted during these sessions. The team agreed, and the parents became active partners in their child's care, often assisting in her therapies. Her parents were quite religious prior to the accident and were convinced that the Lord would heal their daughter. In keeping with this belief, they asked staff to not say anything in front of B. that could negate this belief, and they went on to pick a date by which the healing would take place and she would again walk. In the meantime, the team spoke with the parents, and they decided that at times, the Lord may work through people on earth and, regarding their daughter, those people might be members of our rehabilitation team.

Also, as was the practice on this rehabilitation unit, shortly after admission, a family-team meeting was scheduled. The parents requested that the team members perform a prayer circle just before the start of the meeting so that "God could bless their work." The day before the meeting was scheduled, a brief discussion was held regarding each team member's opinions and feelings. Following this, the team agreed to the family's request, and a prayer circle was performed. This allowed for some measure of increased comfort on the part of the parents, who were given a rather pessimistic prognosis for recovery. The medical director was able to frame the difficult news within a spiritual paradigm by adding the explanation that it appears that "God has not yet decided it is time to fully heal your daughter." It should be noted here that neither the team nor the physician normally used a spiritual paradigm in explanations to patients or their families. Because the team was able to adapt to the stated spiritual needs of this family, it helped to facilitate the entire family's recovery.

CASE 2

C. was a 19-year-old girl with end-stage renal disease, lupus, and HIV. She had been on hemodialysis since age 10, when complications from lupus almost completely eliminated her renal functioning. C. was well known to our service, having been followed on an as-needed basis since

(Continues)

(Continued)

age 12 due to previous referrals regarding problems with diet adherence. C. was once again referred at age 19 following her diagnosis of HIV due to staff concerns that she was both more anxious and once again non-adherent to her prescribed medical regimen, which now required her to take over 20 different medications per day. Dialysis staff were frustrated, complaining that educational techniques were ineffective, and requested a psychological consult for assistance.

During the interview, C. did express some anxiety and insight into her problem. She understood the importance of taking the medication and understood the negative consequences of taking her medication on an irregular basis. She explained that the problem as she saw it was the size of some of the pills, stating that they were simply too large for her to swallow. She described her experience as her throat "getting tight and small" whenever she attempted to take them. She also shared that this was the first time the staff could provide no other alternative methods of taking the medication (e.g., liquid, smaller pills, etc.). When offered the choice of a relaxation therapy or hypnosis, she surprisingly refused. We had worked well together in the past and successfully utilized other similar behavioral interventions. When asked what the problem was, she explained that she had become more religious since our last meeting and would not do anything that could "invite the devil into me." She had heard that hypnosis and relaxation could "open me up to possession."

After further discussion, it was clear that she would not change her mind. The situation was serious since the staff explained that if her adherence did not improve quickly, she could invite further physical complications. I then asked if she believed the Lord wanted her to stay alive for a while longer. She said she believed he did. Then she was asked if she believed in prayer, which she said she did, and she added that she prayed daily and believed that God answered her prayers. It was then suggested that she use her favorite prayer to ask Jesus to help her body accept the medicine by relaxing and opening her throat, allowing her to swallow her pills and stay healthy. It was explained that in this manner, she might be able to "be well and do God's work." It was hoped that by allowing her to choose her own prayer, it would increase her sense of control and make the intervention more syntonic with her present worldview. Additionally, asking her to directly petition her Lord was a way of respecting her personal view of God. In this example, the fact that C. was already using prayer was utilized for the therapeutic end of increasing her adherence and decreasing her anxiety. By understanding the role of spirituality in her life, it became possible to use her spiritual understanding to help her achieve her therapeutic goals.

After this intervention, with continued follow-up psychotherapy, where she was encouraged to continue to pray, compliance went up dramatically, and she reported being significantly less anxious. She understood the improvement to be the direct result of "Jesus answering [her] prayers." Since this explanation gave her a profound sense of peace and probably would have been resistant to change under any conditions, her attribution was left intact.

CASE 3

T. was a 15-year-old with lupus who had been followed by our service for over three years. Persistent problems existed with compliance, and she was frequently hospitalized. During one of her more painful hospitalizations, we were discussing coping strategies, and she tearfully admitted that she deserved "to be sick and in pain." When questioned further, she stated that she had murdered her sister. Thinking that she was confused by her pain medication, she was reminded that she did not have a sister. She went on to explain that she did when she was younger.

Apparently, at age six, her mother asked her to watch her sister, aged two, while she quickly went to the local market. While alone with her sister, the toddler got hold of some matches, burned herself, and died from her resulting injuries. T. was diagnosed with lupus approximately six months later and always saw her illness as a punishment from God. She tearfully explained that she had no right to stop God's punishment by taking her medications and that she could be well only when God forgave her or was simply done "punishing" her. Unfortunately, shortly after this hospitalization, she and her family were lost to follow-up and never returned to the clinic.

Certainly more research and work needs to be done on incorporating psychospirituality into child and adolescent psychology to better help those children who come into our care. What the above examples have in common is a lack of judgment on the part of the therapist and seeing the patients' religious views as similar to a worldview. It is possible sometimes to use this view to effect psychotherapeutic change.

CONCLUSION

Rehabilitation has a long history of incorporating creative approaches to problems facing individuals with functionally limiting conditions—this is part of its culture and history. This chapter has shown that this trend is continuing. Rehabilitation facilities now have the opportunity to utilize integrative approaches that bring the strengths of separate disciplines together into an individualized treatment for each patient: the incorporation of unique interventions, for example, Tai Chi or pulsed electrical stimulation, and the use of telemedicine and spirituality to improve the relationship between the rehabilitation professionals and the people they serve. Improved communication, trust, and improved outcomes can only facilitate the challenging road to recovery of function.

TOOL KIT FOR CHANGE

Role and Perspective of the Healthcare Professional

1. The rehabilitation professional must stay abreast of new developments in the field and be aware of integrative approaches to assist patients.
2. It is important for rehabilitation practitioners to establish a sense of trust and caring with the patient that goes beyond the application of new areas of knowledge to facilitate a healing relationship and open communication.

Role and Perspective of the Patient/Participant

1. A patient must take an active role in his own health and rehabilitation.
2. A patient must be willing to tell his healthcare workers how an approach is working for him.

Interconnection: The Global Perspective

1. Rehabilitation as a discipline provides a model that can be used to develop a beginning approach to integrate other areas of healthcare.
2. Rehabilitation often provides healthcare for individuals with illness and injury that stretch the limits of traditional health services and technology. Focusing on spirituality and prayer can be an effective way of assisting patients who wish to incorporate it into their own rehabilitation and take a more integrative approach.
3. Telehealth practices can effectively extend the reach of rehabilitation beyond limits imposed by geography and travel time. It can pave the way for delivery of other areas of medicine via telehealth.

REFERENCES

Barlow, A., & Walkup, J. (1998). Developing mental health services for Native American children. *Child and Adolescent Psychiatry Clinics of North America, 7,* 555–577.

Bashshur, R. L. (1997). Critical issues in telemedicine. *Telemedicine Journal, 3,* 113–126.

Bruyere, S., & Peterson, D. (2005). Introduction to the special section on the international classification of functioning, disability and health: Implications for rehabilitation psychology. *Rehabilitation Psychology, 50,* 103–104.

Burke, M., Hackney, H., Hudson, P., Miranti, J., Watts, G., & Epp, L. (1999). Spirituality, religion, and CACREP curriculum standard. *Journal of Counseling and Development, 77,* 251–257.

Casimiro, L., Brosseau, L., Robinson, V., Milne, S., Judd, M., Wells, G., et al. (2002). Therapeutic ultrasound for the treatment of rheumatoid arthritis. *Cochrane Database of Systematic Reviews, 2002*(3), Article CD003787.

DeJong, G., & Sutton, J. P. (1995). Rehab 2000: The evolution of medical rehabilitation in American health care. In P. K. Landrum, N. D. Schmidt, & A. McLean Jr. (Eds.), *Outcome-oriented rehabilitation: Principles, strategies, and tools for effective program management* (pp. 3–42). Gaithersburg, MD: Aspen.

DeLisa, J. A., Currie, D. M., & Martin, G. M. (1998). Rehabilitation medicine: Past, present, and future. In J. A. DeLisa & B. M. Gans (Eds.), *Rehabilitation medicine: Principles and practice* (3rd ed., pp. 3–19). Philadelphia: Lippincott, Williams, and Wilkins.

Friedman, R. H., Kazis, L. E., Jette, A., Smith, M. B., Stollerman, J., Torgerson, J., et al. (1996). A telecommunications system for monitoring and counseling patients with hypertension: Impact on medication adherence and blood pressure control. *American Journal of Hypertension, 9,* 285–292.

Glueckauf, R. L. (2002). Telehealth and chronic disabilities: New frontier for research and development. *Rehabilitation Psychology, 47,* 1–7.

Glueckauf, R. L., Fritz, S., Ecklund-Johnson, E. P., Liss, H. J., Dages, P., & Carney, P. (2002). Home-based videocounseling for rural teenagers with epilepsy: Phase I findings. *Rehabilitation Psychology, 47,* 49–72.

Glueckauf, R. L., Jeffers, S. B., & Sharma, D. (in press). Recruitment and retention of rural and ethnic minority populations in eHealth research: Key issues and emerging developments. *American Journal of Preventive Medicine.*

Glueckauf, R. L., & Ketterson, T. U. (2004). Telehealth for individuals with chronic illness: Research review and implications for clinical practice. *Professional Psychology, 35,* 615–627.

Glueckauf, R. L., Ketterson, T. U., Loomis, J. S., & Dages, P. (2004). Online support and education for dementia caregivers: Overview, utilization, and initial program evaluation. *Telemedicine Journal and e-Health, 10,* 223–232.

Glueckauf, R. L., Pickett, T. C., Ketterson, T. U., Loomis, J. S., & Rozensky, R. H. (2003). Preparation for the delivery of telehealth services: A self-study framework for expansion of practice. *Professional Psychology: Research and Practice, 34,* 159–163.

Glueckauf, R. L., Pickett, T. C., Ketterson, T. U., Nickelson, D. W., & Loomis, J. S. (2006). Telehealth research and practice: Key issues and developments in research. In S. Llewelyn & P. Kennedy (Eds.), *Essentials of clinical health psychology* (pp. 305–331). London: John Wiley.

Glueckauf, R. L., Whitton, J. D., & Nickelson, D. W. (2002). Telehealth: The new frontier in rehabilitation and healthcare. In M. J. Scherer (Ed.), *Assistive technology: Matching device and consumer for successful rehabilitation* (pp. 197–213). Washington, DC: American Psychological Association.

Glueckauf, R. L., Young, M. E., Stine, C., Bourgeois, M., Pomidor, A., & Rom, P. (2005). Alzheimer's Rural Care Healthline: Linking rural dementia caregivers to cognitive-behavioral intervention for depression. *Rehabilitation Psychology, 50,* 346–354.

Goldman, A. (1996). Home care of the dying child. *Journal of Palliative Care, 12,* 16–19.

Gustafson, D. H., Hawkins, R., Boberg, E., Pingree, S., Serlin, R. E., Graziano, F., et al. (1999). Impact of a patient-centered, computer-based health information/support system. *American Journal of Preventive Medicine, 16,* 1–9.

Haas, L. J., Benedict, J. G., & Kobos, J. C. (1996). Psychotherapy by telephone: Risks and benefits for psychologists and consumers. *Professional Psychology: Research and Practice, 27,* 154–160.

Han, A., Judd, M. G., Robinson, V. A., Taixiang, W., Tugwell, P., & Wells, G. (2006). Tai Chi for treating rheumatoid arthritis. *Cochrane Database of Systematic Reviews, 2006*(2), Article 1464-780X.

Henley, L. (1999). A home visit programme to teach medical students about children with special needs. *Medical Education, 33,* 749–752.

Hulme, J., Robinson, V., DeBie, R., Wells, G., Judd, M., & Tugwell, P. (2006). Electromagnetic fields for the treatment of osteoarthritis. *Cochrane Database of Systematic Reviews, 2006*(2), Article 1469-493X

Little, C. V., Parsons, T., & Logan, S. (2000). Herbal therapy for treating osteoarthritis. *Cochrane Database of Systematic Reviews, 2000*(4), Article CD002947.

Mahoney, D. F., Tarlow, B. J., & Jones, R. N. (2003). Effects of an automated telephone support system on caregiver burden and anxiety: Findings from the REACH for TLC Intervention Study. *Gerontologist, 43,* 556–567.

Nicolescu, B. (1996) *The transdisciplinary evolution of learning.* Retrieved June 28, 2006, from http://www.learndev.org/dl/nicolescu_f.pdf

Nierenberg, B., & Sheldon, A. (2001). Psychospirituality and pediatric rehabilitation. *Journal of Rehabilitation, 17,* 87–92.

Peterson, D. (2005). International classification of functioning, disability, and health: An introduction for rehabilitation psychologists. *Rehabilitation Psychology, 50,* 105–112.

Piette, J. D., Weinberger, M., & McPhee, S. J. (2000). The effect of automated calls with telephone nurse follow-up on patient-centered outcomes of diabetes care: A randomized, controlled trial. *Medical Care, 38,* 218–230.

Piette, J. D., Weinberger, M., McPhee, S. J., Mah, C. A., Kraemer, F. B., & Crapo, L. M. (2000). Do automated calls with nurse follow-up improve self-care and glycemic control among vulnerable patients with diabetes? *American Journal of Medicine, 108,* 20–27.

Scherer, M. J. (Ed.). (2002). *Assistive technology: Matching device and consumer for successful rehabilitation.* Washington, DC: American Psychological Association.

Schopp, L., Johnstone, B., & Merrell, D. (2000). Telehealth and neuropsychological assessment: New opportunities for psychologists. *Professional Psychology: Research and Practice, 31,* 179–183.

Telemedicine Information Exchange. (2006). *Telemedicine and telehealth programs.* Retrieved June 12, 2006, from http://tie.telemed.org/programs/browseByLocation.asp

Thorsen, C. (1999). Spirituality and health: Is there a relationship? *Journal of Health Psychology, 4,* 291–300.

Weaver, A., Koenig, H., & Larson, D. (1997). Marriage and family therapists and the clergy: A need for clinical collaboration, training, and research. *Journal of Marital and Family Therapy, 23,* 13–25.

World Health Organization. (1980). *International classification of impairments, disabilities, and handicaps: A manual of classification relating to the consequences of disease.* Geneva, Switzerland: Author.

World Health Organization. (2001). *International classification of functioning, disability, and health (ICF).* Geneva, Switzerland: Author.

Chapter Seven

INTEGRATIVE PROTOCOLS: INTEGRATING PHILOSOPHY AND PRACTICE IN THE REAL WORLD

Marie A. DiCowden, PhD, Frank M. Maye, DOM, ND, Diane Batshaw Eisman, MD, and Eugene Eisman, MD

INTRODUCTION

The current healthcare system in the United States is one of the most technologically advanced in the world. However, barring a crisis that forces an individual to the emergency room, where law mandates that a person be treated, over 45 million people in this country lack access to healthcare on a regular basis (Lambrew, 2004). Moreover, significant health disparities exist among various racial and ethnic groups as well as between genders for a wide variety of health concerns, including cancer, cardiac disease, diabetes, and maternal and infant health (Redmond, Bowman, & Mensah, 2000–2005). While the emphasis in the healthcare delivery system is on acute episodes, it is illness and impairment due to chronic conditions that is the healthcare management and cost challenge of the twenty-first century (Frank, Hagglund, & Farmer, 2004). Statistics about our broken healthcare system abound. Healthcare in the United States is highly sophisticated yet ignores long-term management of health needs; it is extremely costly yet often inhumane to the very people it is designed to serve.

Various studies, over the last five years, on the efficacy and cost-effectiveness of complementary and alternative practices in meeting the chronic health needs of a wider population show promising results that deserve further study (Board on Health Promotion and Disease Prevention, 2005; Herman, Craig, & Caspi, 2005; Pan American Health Organization, 2003). In addition, the role of psychological interventions in efficacious and cost-effective general healthcare interventions has long been well documented (Fiedler & Wright, 1989; Jones, 1979; VandenBos & DeLeon, 1988).

While there has been a great deal written on the need for and prerequisite mechanisms necessary to apply integrative care to heal our own healthcare system in the United States (Faas, 2001; Frank, McDaniel, Bray, & Heldring, 2004), very little has been written about what actually happens when different healthcare providers work together to apply their healing services to a patient and how they solve their differences. In their book *The Primary Care Consultant*, editors James and Folen (2005) have provided a well-documented source of case studies on how to integrate psychological care into issues of pain management, coronary heart disease, HIV/AIDS, diabetes mellitus, insomnia, pediatric disorders, and women's health issues. Numerous journal articles have also documented specific complementary/alternative protocols for a wide variety of health issues from stress and anxiety to cancer and cardiovascular disease (Boon et al., 2000; Wood, Stewart, Merry, Johnstone, & Cox, 2003). This chapter does not attempt to present a wide spectrum of case studies or a definitive empirical approach to integrative protocols for specific diseases or disabilities. This chapter, however, does attempt to present an up close and personal discussion of some of the issues, feelings, and questions present in integrating different philosophies of healthcare professionals and how they affect treatment protocols and outcomes when applied in actual cases in the real world.

In this chapter, three different providers present their perspectives and philosophies of three different types of treatment—allopathic, complementary/alternative (CAM), and behavioral medicine. Their writing styles, like their treating styles, differ. In presenting their approach to integrative care, the reader is given a rare opportunity to sense what real-life discussions among these varied professionals are like. Allopathic physicians refer to large, well-documented, empirical studies—in addition to their own clinical experiences—to move cautiously into the realm of integrative care. CAM providers go to great lengths to explain the long-standing historical and intricate approach to alternative care, especially with traditional Chinese medicine, which is so different in thought process from Western medicine. Behavioral medicine psychologists advocate strongly for the recognition and inclusion of mental and emotional processes in the course of recovery in illness and cite wide-ranging studies that document the need for a more comprehensive approach to healthcare. Each clinician speaks his own language but attempts to translate overlapping concepts and create a new language of integrative medicine.

The first half of the chapter provides that rare glimpse into the intimate processes of such personal expressions as they often present themselves on a team where professionals speak to professionals to state their cases. In real-life discussions the different philosophies, pejorative assumptions, and difficult feelings on all sides must be voiced before any effective coalition of healthcare providers can evolve an effective integrative treatment for a patient seeking help. The second half of the chapter presents three cases, illustrating care that integrates these approaches in different health delivery models.

INTEGRATIVE MEDICINE FROM THE VIEWPOINT OF TWO TRADITIONAL ALLOPATHIC PHYSICIANS

Integrative medicine is a controversial concept to some of us in traditional medicine. We traditionalists have been talked about by those in alternative fields with disdain, as if we lack understanding of our patients and do not look for the real causes of their illnesses and problems. We are lumped into a group often referred to as "allopathic." And we were not given that label in our training. Calling us allopathic may bother some of us who realize that *allo* came from the Greek and means "other." So we are just "other" kinds of physicians...and we always thought we were the real thing! Actually, there have been instances when alternative physicians have proposed things that many of us "other" physicians believe have a tinge of the alchemist about them.

In our particular medical practice, we consider ourselves not just physicians, but holistic physicians, who do not see our patients as a collection of individual body parts, but as people with bodies, minds, and spirits, all of which contribute both to health as well as disease. We recall an episode in medical school when we were making rounds with the surgeons, and one of our young colleagues was asked to present a patient. At one point he alluded to the "gall bladder in room 606" and was thoroughly excoriated by the senior attending physician. Everything stopped while we were all made firmly to understand that we were honored to help in the care of human beings, not organs, and it was not the "gall bladder in room 606," but a person with a name, and that person happened to have a gall bladder that needed attention. And yet we are scientists and require rigorous scientific validation for what we recommend to those under our care. Some treatments and procedures in the history of non-traditional medicine have proven to be harmful. We know that has occurred in traditional medicine, too.

In the past 20 or so years, there has been a move toward so-called evidence-based medicine; that is, no treatment is adopted unless there are double-blind crossover studies to support it. It is recognized that not all areas of medicine have such good documentation, but when such data are available, we are hard-pressed to choose any other form of therapy, and we are certainly put on the defensive if another form of therapy is chosen. This is because we have been badly burned in the past. What we thought was good medicine turned out, after more experience and more testing, to have been harmful to the patient. One example is vitamin E, which has the laudable quality of being an antioxidant. But recent carefully reviewed studies have found that the common high doses of the supplement actually increase mortality (Miller et al., 2005).

Another excellent example of the pitfalls of deviating from the philosophy of evidence-based medicine is our experience with estrogen replacement. There was an observational study (Grodstein et al., 2000; Hulley et al., 1998) involving a large number of nurses. In this Nurses Health Study, half were taking Premarin, and half were not taking any estrogen replacement therapy. It appeared to many physicians that the nurses on the estrogen were getting a tremendous protection from coronary heart disease. Some observers felt that there was up to an 80 percent protection. Premarin was considered a virtual fountain of youth for women. So what if it caused a little bit of breast cancer, some might have thought, look at all the other lives it saved. There were a few who were concerned over the fact that this was an observational study. Were there any other differences between these two groups of women besides their use of Premarin?

As you might guess, women who took estrogen were a bit more likely to visit their physicians on a regular basis, eat a healthier diet, run a few miles each day. In the past couple of years, we finally came around to testing Premarin using time-honored, double-blind crossover studies (Manson et al., 2003). Not only did Premarin *not* offer protection from heart disease, but if the woman had a previous heart attack history, Premarin was seriously detrimental to her health. What we observe is not always what we see when we take a closer look.

When our patients exclaim that their herbal mixtures are natural, and therefore harmless, we tell them about Eugene's experience when he spent a year as a doctor in Vietnam during the war. A woman was having severe spasms of all her muscles and was unable to breathe. A history was finally obtained, and we discovered that she had taken half a cup of a bitter tea prescribed by a Chinese physician. (It was too bitter for her to consume the whole cup.) It turned out to be strychnine—a poison. We treated the patient for strychnine poisoning, and she recovered uneventfully. Even though strychnine is a natural chemical that comes from a plant, it is not harmless. It is poison. While this is an example of how a natural substance can be used inappropriately, there are also other examples of how appropriate natural drugs can actually have toxic effects when combined with other natural medicines and/or with chemical drugs. To believe that every natural chemical is completely safe under all circumstances is as foolish as to believe that every synthetic chemical must be harmful. When we were medical students decades ago, milk and cream were considered excellent treatment for peptic ulcer disease. Now, after careful studies (Johnsen, Forde, Straume, & Burhol, 1994), researchers have learned that the fat and calcium actually increase the amount of acid in the stomach, worsening the ulcer and putting weight on the patient, in addition to clogging up arteries.

Physicians do not have the perfect treatment for many problems and often have to use medicine that is not evidence-based, but we recognize that this is not the ideal situation, even though it may be necessary. On the other hand, we all recognize that many of our viable drugs, such as colchicine, quinine, aspirin, and digitalis, have come from plants. The goal we should strive for, whether we are chiropractic, ancient Chinese, herbal, or allopathic, should be evidence based.

As traditional physicians, we are aware that some of our therapies first appeared in the alternative medicine arena. Once research confirmed their efficacy, they were adopted by allopathic physicians. Undoubtedly, in the future, researchers will continue to test herbal, acupuncture, and chiropractic techniques with the so-called scientific method. Barriers to this type of testing will be the source of money to do all these studies as well as the need to evolve the scientific method itself to address issues that are not easily conceptualized. The pharmaceutical companies spend many millions of dollars studying their drugs to pass Food and Drug Administration muster. While this is not a satisfactory situation, the question remains, Who will supply sufficient funds for such studies?

There are many different types of complementary medicines. The fear has been that these will be used in place of conventional medicine. Integrative healthcare seeks a way to use these modalities along with conventional medicine, to develop a community of healthcare practitioners who work together as a team. The most obvious form of this combined use is in the mind-body area. As an example, one of our patients faced a lengthy surgical procedure. An audio tape was made in conjunction with her psychotherapist. This tape consisted of affirmations, her favorite music, and other supportive readings. The tape looped continuously during the anesthesia induction and through her surgery. The tape was not discontinued until after she awoke in recovery. She needed no pain medicine and was alert and in good spirits. Her procedure ended at 11:30 P.M., and the next morning, she insisted on going home. A few weeks later, she underwent a minor procedure for one hour. No tape was used. She did not have the same postsurgical outcome. Instead, she felt weak, drained, and depressed. Of course, this is only one example; it is observational in nature and hardly does a study make. But it does lead us to want to explore this area in greater depth and indicates the need for greater research in combining mind and body approaches.

As physicians, we must also be open to the religious beliefs of our patients. To reject them outright because of our personal feelings may do the patients great harm. When Eugene was a medical student, one of his patients insisted on stopping his IV antibiotic. We told the patient that his bacterial endocarditis would run out of control and that he would die without his medication. The patient told us that he must stop the IV antibiotic so he could leave the hospital to go and be baptized by total immersion or his soul would be lost. He wanted to go with his minister to the river. How were we to find a compromise and prevent a loss of life? That night, we opened the Hubbard tanks in the physical therapy department, and he was baptized without any interruption of his antibiotic therapy.

In Pleiku, Vietnam, a family insisted on taking their family member home from the hospital. Eugene explained that he was on dialysis for renal failure caused by his malaria. The family insisted that he must be under the care of the village tribal doctor. The solution was simple. I obtained "one case" privileges for their tribal doctor. He came to the hospital, performed his ritual chanting and small burnt offering at the patient's bedside, and the patient did well.

We attended a medical school that stressed treating a patient holistically. Our Saturday mornings were spent in a course the students abbreviated to "Conjoint." Each week, a specific disease entity was studied. The anatomists, physiologists, and biochemists discussed normal functioning. The pathologists took the stage and discussed the abnormal and how disease developed (if they knew). Finally, the patient was interviewed by behavioral scientists and talked about how he felt. Other family members discussed the impact in every way: physical, environmental, financial, spiritual. And finally, a team panel of all of these people reviewed the illness, with questions and suggestions from the students. This was a great start in the education of medical students and long predated the advent of the term *integrative medicine*.

This is the way we need to begin: with cooperation and understanding of our patients' own belief systems. This is the philosophy we were taught as students: to bring the best evidence-based medicine to the care of our patients, while doing our best to understand our patients and consider alternative methods that could benefit their health. Our beloved medical school, the University of Kentucky, is currently involved in an integrative care project. With rigorous scientific thinking, using evidence-based medicine, we can scientifically evaluate complementary medicine modalities, and we can design a module to bring our skills to the true patient-centered practice of medicine.

INTEGRATIVE MEDICINE FROM THE VIEWPOINT OF A COMPLEMENTARY/ALTERNATIVE PRACTITIONER

Integrative medicine is a view of medical intervention from different vantage points on the patient's biologic compass. The center of this circle includes the patient and his symptom presentation. The outer circle, or vantage point, is occupied by a team from different systems of medicine, each contributing his interpretation of the patient's presentation. These views may be quite diverse, with a tendency to be highly opinionated based on the history of excellent education of each practitioner in his own discipline. Integrative teams may consist of allopathic physicians working with psychologists or CAM providers. The quality of integrative medicine is determined by the quality of each member on the team. Naturopaths and Chinese medicine practitioners are primarily representative of CAM practitioners in the United States and are licensed in numerous states. Homeopaths, though not licensed in this country, are also well known for their contributions to CAM literature. Many licensed CAM providers are also trained in homeopathy and incorporate homeopathic treatment into their protocols.

Naturopaths and traditional Chinese medicine physicians are licensed as primary care practitioners in many states. Naturopaths are currently licensed in 14 states plus the District of Columbia (American Association of Naturopathic Physicians, 2006). The American Board of Medical Acupuncture (2006), responsible for licensing traditional Chinese medicine practitioners, reports licensure regulation in 35 states. Rigorous four-year programs, with an extended clinical clerkship, are the promoted standard of care. The National Institute of Health has also funded clinical studies relative to multiple CAM protocols and their efficacy. The general acceptance of these approaches to medicine is being more acknowledged by some traditional physicians. However, the overwhelming skepticism and marginalizing of CAM practitioners, by allopathic medicine in general over the years, often leaves all CAM physicians feeling one down as they begin to work on teams.

Employing a team coordinator provides the best model for integrative teams to pursue excellence. The team coordinator mediates the communication, care planning, and cross training among the disciplines. The coordinator plays an integral role in the team's success. The coordinator can be from any of the disciplines, but the critical characteristic is the coordination, not the discipline (Mingji, 1992). There are well-discussed issues among conventional, psychological, and complementary/alternative practitioner philosophies that need to be resolved. Additionally, CAM practices themselves may diverge and must be mediated. Since CAM practices cover multiple and diverse philosophies, it is important to briefly review some of the major differences of a few select CAM practices found most often in the United States.

Traditional Chinese Medicine

Traditional Chinese medicine contributes a view of human health with physics as its primary science. The electromagnetic function of the patient is evaluated by examining a sophisticated bioenergetic grid called "meridians." Meridians are the electric product of biochemical reactions within the body. Acupuncture and herbal pharmacology are the primary sources of intervention. Balance of all bodily functions is the goal. The basic philosophy is that homeostasis, when achieved, will bring about longevity and good health. Asian-trained physicians are highly skilled in pulse and tongue diagnostics.

Traditional Chinese medicine is commonly referred to as TCM. This philosophy of medicine is 4,000 years old (DeMorrant, 1994), and a rich history of practice has been accepted throughout the Asian Pacific rim for much of this time. During the last 100 years, TCM has been introduced throughout Europe, with possibly the greatest achievements in modernization occurring in Germany and France. Because of the long-standing and intricate theories that undergird TCM, a brief overview is warranted.

TCM internal medical theory is divided into two strategies. The *five element theory* is how the human body and its incorporated emotional body fit into the universal view of life. Based on natural elements found in the world, the five elements are conceptualized as wood, air, fire, water, and metal. The Chinese perceive the universe as an infinite number of microcosms that are all mathematically and conceptually in ratio with a greater macrocosm and each other. Everything in the entire universe can be divided into five categories. This belief system extends to theories of astronomy, agriculture, politics, medicine, and religion. These five element principles are the foundation of all philosophy and are the reason for all TCM physicians to be trained in philosophy before all other subjects.

The five element theory divides the major organ systems of the body into five categories. Each organ is expected to display predictable physical presentations or syndromes. TCM, however, also views psychological presentation and syndromes that are predictable along with the physical presentation. An example would include patients that display anger, which is the corresponding emotion for the liver. Many patients experiencing liver disease will present with anger-related symptoms as well.

The second theory is called the *eight parameter theory*. Once the five element classification is arrived at, the eight parameters can be explored. This theory appears simple, yet it is quite profound and difficult to practice. The following are its subcategories:

1. yin and yang
2. exterior/interior
3. hot/cold
4. excess/deficiency.

Many Western physicians have great difficulty with Chinese medical nomenclature. Chinese medical terminology is organic to the Chinese culture. China has always had a large population. The ability to feed these dependants has demanded a great historical emphasis on agriculture. The Chinese alphabet is pictorial and depicts this agricultural influence. Chinese medical terminology reflects this influence as well. Therefore Chinese medical theory demands an in depth understanding of their philosophy, culture, life, and language.

Yin and yang reflect the concepts of female and male energy that applies to the entire universe. Yin and yang divide all aspects into passive (yin) and active (yang) principles. All organs that move fluids and wastes through the body are considered yang, or active. Subsequently, organs that store fluids or wastes are defined as yin. Each yin and yang organ is coupled with one of another influence, thus forming a circle where five element theory and eight parameter theory are intertwined. Yin organs are found on the left side of the body. Yang organs are found on the right.

Exterior and *interior* refer to acute conditions and chronic conditions, respectively. All bacterial and viral infections are classified as exterior due to their theoretical entrance to the body from outside pathogens. Chronic presentations are due to the disruption of internal body chemistry. Hot and cold represent a TCM focus on organ thermodynamics. Four thousand years of clinical observation have led the Chinese to believe that subtle changes in organ temperature will trigger an organ, or the body as a system, to respond in syndrome presentations that are relatively predictable, although with individual variances. These syndromes, along with their variances, affect a series of 18 radial pulse presentations. The size, shape, and color of the tongue in conjunction with the tongue coating will also reflect these subtle changes. Excess and deficiency concepts represent the electromagnetic influence of the body and all its parts. Electromagnetic energy is a natural aspect of life, and its perpetual series of chemical interactions is always occurring in our environment. The human body is no different. The Chinese refer to this concept as Qi. Although this is oversimplified for purposes of this book, the theory as presented offers a beginning of electromagnetic energy as a subtle interaction of body chemistry and its interaction with universal physics. Once again, pulse and tongue diagnosis will reflect these changes.

The treatment tools the Chinese discovered to be most useful were acupuncture and herbal pharmacology. Each was understood within the philosophy, culture, and language of the Chinese worldview and its corresponding TCM theories. Acupuncture may very well be the first system of microsurgery on the planet. It has evolved over 4,000 years and continues to evolve in current times. Acupuncture may be demystified by the following explanation. The electromagnetic energies throw off a constant biologic interaction that forms a grid in the body. This grid is navigated by means of ley lines or meridians that traverse the body from head to toe and back. Approximately 365 acupuncture points are distributed within this grid. Each point is capable of several functions that affect local and distal points of the body.

Acupuncture points are consistently located by anatomical geometry in all subjects. The 365 points form a keyboard with which a message may be delivered through the body's matrix or connective tissue. From the connective tissue and its fluid matrix the body as a whole is manipulated. This manipulation can be quite profound. In present-day TCM practice, this "acupuncture keyboard" and its connection to the matrix are no longer limited to insertion of gold, silver, or stainless steel needles. Herbal and homeopathic solutions are being injected into acupuncture points with good results. Quite often, less solution is necessary than by intramuscular injection. Allopathic physicians in Germany and China are using Procaine for acupoint injection with positive results in pain management. The discovery of lasers has added another method of stimulating the matrix through the acupuncture keyboard. Low-level lasers, which emit pure light at 800 nanometers or 670 nanometers, also show good results in reducing inflammation and pain (De Morrant, 1994). Subsystems of acupuncture are located on the hand, scalp, and ear. These subsystems have been used for both pain management and some neurological conditions associated with pain or impaired motor function.

Herbal pharmacology has evolved alongside acupuncture. Several thousand formulas exist, with approximately 1,000 being in popular use by herbalists trained in TCM. TCM pharmacology uses the tincture principle. This allows for a relatively direct, quick, and safe delivery for the patient. The tincture can be further diluted into a tea or granules. Plants, minerals, and animal parts are all used to formulate some of the most complex herbal pharmacologic decoctions on the planet. A formula comprises anywhere from 3 to 20 herbs in various gram amounts. One to two herbs usually are the basis of syndrome rectification. The remaining herbs support the overall function of the body or provide relief of side effects.

All herbs, minerals, and animal products are evaluated and prescribed by their individual functions within the five element and eight parameter diagnostic system. This allows formulas to be modified either to support the overall diagnosis or correct a side effect, for example, loose stool. TCM herbal pharmacology does have effects on body chemistry, and therefore serious consideration of allopathic drug and herbal interactions must be considered when prescribing herbs.

An interesting example that quite often presents itself is the depression frequently presented by postoperative cardiac patients taking Plavix and Coumidin. Cardiologists are rightfully concerned with secondary events that could complicate treatment or end in fatal consequences. Should a cardiologist and TCM pharmacologist integrate their protocol, consideration could be given to the addition of a formula, that is, Si Wu Tang or Bu Zhong Yi Qi Tang. The dosage of either formula is begun with an 80 percent reduction in dosage. More frequent visits to both practitioners, along with more frequent pro thrombin tests, may be successful in safeguarding the patient and also relieving his depression.

The integrative usage of traditional Chinese medicine in China along with allopathic medicine is called *Fu Zheng therapy*. This term may prove interesting to those interested in key-wording the internet to explore the success with which it has been implemented in Asia. The Society of Integrative Oncology utilizes this approach. Here in North America, many prestigious U.S. medical schools are members of this society (Harvard, the Mayo Clinic, Johns Hopkins, etc.).

Naturopathy

Naturopaths study all the natural systems of medicine. They believe in the cause and effect relationship of disease. Their mission is one of investigating and teaching. Naturopathic medicine includes the study of allopathic pharmacology, Western laboratory testing, western pathology, and biochemistry. Many naturopathic physicians employ sophisticated electrically amplified voltage (EAV) and bioresonance equipment to aid them in discovering the cause of conditions. Naturopaths are trained in pharmacologic considerations. A primary emphasis in pharmacologic considerations is based on natural elements and differs in that respect from allopathic or TCM pharmacology.

Because of this emphasis on natural chemistry, naturopaths also place a great deal of emphasis on detoxification of the body systems and on decreasing general inflammation.

Detoxifying the body, the mind, and the environment are all considered important. Overall systemic health of the person is supported while reducing the cause of specific presenting symptoms. Naturopaths are trained to refer specific, acute, and highly toxic illnesses to specialists in the primarily allopathic healthcare system and to work in conjunction with the allopathic system.

The relationship of a person to his environment is also considered crucial to healing. The naturopathic philosophy also focuses on the spiritual, emotional, and physical experiences important to the patient. All the experiences intertwine and are best viewed, the naturopath believes, in totality. The mind-body-spirit connection may be most accurately reflected in the delicate neural chemistry of the brain. Future breakthroughs in healthcare may be best accomplished by integrative practitioners, trained to witness and document these neurochemical changes in disease and treat them as naturally as possible.

Homeopathy

Homeopaths view disease as a condition caused by many different environmental and genetic factors. Extensive history taking is necessary to determine the correct course of treatment. Homeopathy is based on the principle that like cures like. Diluted medicines can therefore alleviate conditions that tincture levels of the same medicine can cause. Homeopathy is quite common in India, Germany, and Great Britain. The royal family has maintained a homeopath as their primary physician.

Homotoxicology is a hybrid of allopathic medicine and homeopathy. It is a widely accepted method of integrative medical delivery found more in Europe than in the United States at this time. The system was developed in 1952 by Hans Heinrich-Reckeweg, MD. Dr. Heinrich-Reckeweg was allopathically trained in Germany with a strong family background in classical homeopathy and a deep understanding of TCM. Different from classical homeopathy, homotoxicity requires that its medications be categorized by indications similar to allopathic treatment. Similar to classical homeopathy as well as TCM theory, potency by tincture and or dilution of pharmacology is the delivery system. Homeopathic medicines are combined in various potencies and used to treat allopathic indications and modulate body chemistry. Germany has taken the lead in the greatest advances in this field (Society of Homotoxicology, 2006). Recently, also, Drs. Bianchi, Perra, and Malzac of Guna Pharmaceuticals in Italy have successfully isolated and diluted intracellular components and developed homeopathic medicines at various potencies. The following have been isolated: 15 interleukins, 6 cell growth factors, 3 inteferons, hypophysis, hypothalamus, thalamus, Dehydroepiandrosterone (DHEA), cortisol, progesterone, DNA, RNA, melatonin, various amino acids, and vitamins. Use of lower dilutions of certain intracellular components open cell receptor responses to a smoother transition for other chemical interventions (Bianchi, Perra, & Malzac, 2005). Such discoveries have the potential to impact all inflammatory diseases as well as autoimmune ailments.

INTEGRATIVE MEDICINE FROM THE VIEWPOINT OF A BEHAVIORAL MEDICINE PERSPECTIVE

Behavioral medicine has developed as a specialty area over the last 20 years (McKegney & Schwartz, 1986). Behavioral factors play a pivotal role in acute care adherence, management of chronic illness, and lifestyle changes. Statistics cite that up to 70 percent of illnesses seen in primary care practitioners' offices have a psychological component (Gatchel & Oordt, 2003), and 85 percent of all health issues have a significant psychological component (American Psychological Association, 1995). In addition, the 10 leading causes of death in the United States are attributable to behavioral factors (Frank, Hagglund & Farmer, 2004).

In addition to behavioral medicine, psychological adjustment in relationships and the more traditional concept of mental health are also important. Dean Ornish, in his breakthrough program in treating patients with cardiac disease, required group therapy with his patients and their spouses as part of their rehabilitation protocol. This therapy was in addition to exercise and physical, medical, and nutritional interventions. When results were in and the elements in recovery analyzed, group therapy with the patients and their spouses was one of the most important factors that predicted prognosis and long-term health outcomes (Ornish et al., 1998). Mounting research reveals that the practice of mind-body interventions and attention to relationships are an important part of treating the whole person through behavioral medicine.

Traditional allopathic practitioners lament that the requirements of present-day healthcare delivery allow only about 15 minutes per visit. While research shows us that female physicians tend to spend slightly more time with patients (two minutes more per visit) and engage in more positive support and psychosocial counseling with patients (Roter, Hall, & Aoki, 2002), this still leaves little time to address the emotional and behavioral issues that are so important to a patient's health. More and more internal medicine practitioners, pediatricians, and family medicine caregivers are turning to behavioral medicine specialists to provide this care, both within their office and through referral. However, while the need for such assistance is acknowledged, providing such care is still not the norm.

Complementary/alternative practitioners address emotional and behavioral issues through most CAM philosophies. However, there is a notable lack of collaboration between both CAM providers and psychologists on a systematic basis within the context of their professional organizations. It is left primarily to individual practitioners on both sides of the fence to establish personal relationships, which often evolve into more formalized professional referrals and support.

There is a vast array of literature that documents the benefits of mind-body practice in well-accepted, peer-reviewed scientific journals. However, similar to the lack of coordination of allopathic, CAM, and behavioral medicine interventions in practice, there is also a dearth of knowledge of this literature among allopathic and CAM providers in general. Many psychologists publish within their own sphere and in so doing fall prey to the fallacy of preaching to the choir. Over the last several decades, however, one particular mind-body intervention that has crossed discipline boundaries regarding its effectiveness is progressive relaxation therapy and the relaxation response (Benson, 1975; Benson & Proctor, 1985). Numerous journal articles and books have been published regarding the effects of progressive relaxation in managing stress-related diseases (Benson & Stark, 1997; Benson & Stuart, 1993; Lutgendorf et al., 2000). Research has more recently expanded to attempt to reveal and understand the different processes underlying relaxation and meditation (Walsh & Shapiro, 2006). There is evidence that as little as 20 minutes of meditation daily can decrease blood pressure and decrease the level of blood sugar (Casey & Benson, 2005). Decrease of blood flow in dental surgery has also been documented through the use of deep relaxation and holds potential for other types of surgery as well (Ayer, 2005).

Employing guided imagery along with relaxation and meditative interventions has also proven highly successful. Research in this field has developed over the last 30 years. There is strong documentation and double-blind studies that indicate the efficacy of employing imagery in treatment with cancer patients undergoing chemotherapy (Collins & Dunn, 2005; Sheikh, 2003). Data also reveal that patient images and beliefs about the expectations of efficacy regarding a drug or particular medical procedure holds high predictive value to the actual benefits of the drug or procedure in some cases (DePascalis, Chiaradia, & Carotenuto, 2002; Galli, Riccio, & Guidetti, 2004; Vase, Robinson, Verne, & Price, 2005). In practice, focusing on patient expectations goes further than the physician simply reassuring the patient. While such reassurance is important, the course of recovery from a disease or disability often challenges the coping skills of patients and can play on their anxieties and fears. This is where the services of a behavioral medicine specialist are best employed. Working on issues to maintain adherence to prescribed treatment regimens over time, and developing positive imagery and coping skills, the patient can learn to develop and enhance the therapeutic effects of both allopathic and CAM interventions.

Pain management is another area where behavioral medicine can make a significant difference in treatment. Studies have shown that mental imagery and repetition of behaviors and various scenarios can have the same effect as actual en vivo interventions in some cases. Furthermore, through altering neural chemistry via visualization, potency of medications can be mobilized. In some cases the need for medications can even be reduced or eliminated (Holroyd et al., 2001). Learning such techniques, however, takes knowledge of psychological interventions as well as time for patient learning and rehearsal. The behavioral medicine specialist can assist the patient in developing these skills through individual and group therapy. The new health and behavior codes accepted by Medicare over the last 10 years to document and bill for such interventions are an acknowledgment of the importance of such types of interventions (American Psychological Association, 2005).

In patients with chronic diseases (e.g., HIV/AIDS and cancer) and long-term disabilities (e.g., spinal cord injury and brain trauma), psychologists have been providing integrative care with allopathic physicians for many years (Rusk Institute, 2006; Wolsko, Eisenberg, Davis, & Phillips, 2004). Now there is a growing use of mind-body interventions by behavioral medicine specialists in primary care. This is particularly prevalent in working with elderly patients, pediatric patients, and patients with cardiac problems or diabetes (James & Folen, 2005).

Because of their specific training in cognitive and emotional health and neuropsychology, behavioral medicine specialists have much in-depth knowledge to bring to the care of the patient and to other members on the treatment team. In addition to patient interventions per se, the behavioral medicine specialist can play a unique role in moving the patient forward in the course of recovery. Helping the patient cognitively understand and process multiple treatment options—and make decisions about his own healthcare in the midst of often emotional circumstances—is a particular skill that a psychologist brings to bear in behavioral medicine treatment. Additionally, because of the knowledge of group dynamics, the behavioral medicine specialist is often the glue that holds the treating team together and facilitates communication among team members, and with the patient and family, while integrative medical treatment plans are being developed and implemented. Treating the whole person means more than treating mental health and physical health needs. It means recognizing that an individual's mind and body are not separate—and that health providers have an obligation to treat the whole person as more than the sum of the parts. To do this most effectively, integrative medicine providers must incorporate not only what they know in their particular disciplines, but they must be willing to discover what they do not know and, when new knowledge is credibly presented, to revise their treatments and intervention strategies accordingly for the good of the patient.

INTEGRATIVE TREATMENT AND OUTCOMES: CASE STUDIES

Combining the multiple philosophies of various healthcare practitioners is a challenge. Translating these philosophies into practical interventions to create a synergy that promotes the patient's health and achieves efficacious outcomes is an even greater challenge. The current healthcare system does not have a definitive method for delivering coordinated and integrated healthcare to the whole person in the mainstream allopathic tradition. It is even harder to find ways to coordinate treatment provided by holistic practitioners in concert with allopathic medical care.

This section presents three case studies as examples of how integrative medicine can be delivered. The first case study involves delivery of both allopathic and CAM services by different practitioners who worked independently and coordinated minimally. The second case study presents a treatment and its outcomes when services from the allopathic system, CAM, and behavioral medicine were provided individually but coordinated in an interdisciplinary setting by an integrative team. The third case discusses the delivery of allopathic care, CAM, and behavioral medicine services provided by an integrative team in an interdisciplinary setting but where services were provided, at various points, in a transdisciplinary model.

CASE STUDY 1

Social History

Mr. L. is an 80-year-old man. He is an accountant and attorney who continued to practice until two years ago. He survived political exile

(Continues)

(Continued)

from two countries. The patient was successful in his home country as a young man. Each time he has had to reestablish himself in a new country, he has managed to use his abilities to do quite well. His history, including his residency in the United States, reveals him to be financially successful, with an intact family. He is also a contributor to his local community of residence.

Medical History

Mr. L. first sought medical care in the United States approximately 20 years ago due to cardiac problems. He has had angioplasty, cardiac bypass surgery, an aortic resection, and an intestinal resection. The patient returned to his normal family, community, and work life after each medical treatment. The patient is currently taking Plavix, Toprol, and Nexium to manage health issues related to these procedures. Approximately 12 years ago, Mr. L. was diagnosed with metastatic prostate cancer. He sought allopathic care and received chemotherapy. He was treated by his oncologist with Taxotere.

Presenting Problem

Two years ago, Mr. L. began a severe struggle with fecal incontinence approximately nine times per day. This interfered significantly with his daily life. Despite continuing to be somewhat active while undergoing treatment for his cancer, Mr. L. now no longer worked, abandoned his community involvement completely, and limited extended family interactions. He also became very depressed. Mr. L. was homebound and dependent on sanitary assistance.

Integrative Treatment

Mr. L. sought assistance from a series of gastroenterologists with impressive credentials. They exhausted all testing and various allopathic protocols to resolve his incontinence. However, his fecal incontinence continued, and Mr. L.'s depression deepened.

It was at this point that the patient sought treatment from a traditional Chinese medicine practitioner who was also trained in homeopathy. Mr. L. chose to pay for this treatment out of pocket. The TCM practitioner—a believer in integrative medicine—spoke, with the patient's permission, to the treating gastroenterologist and oncologist to coordinate past history and ongoing treatment. All physicians were pleasant yet guarded given the current climate of medical healthcare delivery when dealing with the alternative medical practitioner. All physicians, however, shared a genuine appreciation of the elderly patient—a resourceful, successful gentleman—who had, until the onset of severe incontinence, continued to live a productive and quality life.

The goals of TCM were to (1) return normal bowel control to the patient and (2) relieve his depression. Coordinating herbals with the patient's treating allopathic physicians, Mr. L. was given 1 cubic centimeter of tonico compositim sublingually every day to assist in relieving his depression. The patient received no other antidepressant medication. Additionally, the patient was given a combined protocol of scalp and body acupuncture and moxibustion every other day for four months. Moxibustion (a slow burning of medicinal herbs held over acupuncture points) was applied to three of a total of seven acupuncture points. The moxibustion was applied for five minutes over each acupuncture point. Moxibustion was also applied bilaterally for five minutes over each kidney, where no acupuncture needles were used. The goal of this treatment was to increase the patient's abdominal muscle control and restore the necessary vital energy to maintain peristaltic movement for digestion and elimination.

The homeopathic remedy Ubichinon was prescribed at 1 cubic centimeter three times per week. It included podophyllum peltatum 4X, which is helpful in correcting fecal incontinence. It also helps to buttress cellular respiration in the Krebs cycle to aid the patient's internal functioning. All other allopathic treatments remained the same.

Clinical Outcome

Within two weeks of beginning the tonico compositim and the other combined protocols, Mr. L.'s depression began to lift. At approximately two months, Mr. L.'s fecal incontinence began to subside. At four months, the patient's bowel movements returned to normal. Mr. L. continued the homeopathic remedy for one year. At that time he continued to report normal bowel movements and stated that he was not depressed. The patient's cancer was in remission, and while he did not return to work, Mr. L.'s quality of life had significantly improved. He no longer was homebound and did not need sanitary assistance. He also returned to some activities with his extended family and in the community.

CASE STUDY 2

Social History

Ms. H. is a 58-year-old female. She has been married twice and has one daughter and a four-year-old granddaughter. She is the primary social contact for her 92-year-old mother, who is diagnosed with Alzheimer's and lives in a nursing home. Her relationship with her family, both her mother and her daughter, is antagonistic. From time to time, there are periods where she and her daughter are not in contact. Regardless of the emotional climate with her mother, however, Ms. H. goes to the nursing home every weekend to have breakfast with her.

Ms. H. lives alone. She was adopted as a young child and had a brother, who was also adopted from another family. Her brother, who became a physician, died approximately 20 years ago. Mrs. H. became an artist and attended a special high school and college art program for her training. She was also active in playing sports throughout her life.

Medical History

Ms. H. had a previously unremarkable medical history. However, she was diagnosed with Arnold Chiari syndrome, which only became apparent as an older adult. Arnold Chiari is a rare malformation of the brain that is characterized by abnormalities where the brain meets the spinal cord. Part of the brain protrudes into the spinal canal and interferes with the flow of cerebrospinal fluid to and from the brain. At age 51, Ms. H. had surgery to relieve pressure from the buildup of cerebrospinal fluid that was not circulating properly. Postoperatively, she was referred by her neurosurgeon to an interdisciplinary rehabilitation setting with an integrative medicine program. The patient was taking morphine, Neurotin, and clonipine.

Presenting Problem

At initial referral, the patient was barely ambulatory, walking only a few steps with maximum assistance. She was in a great deal of pain, very anxious, depressed, and needed home assistance. Ms. H. was fortunate, however, to have a private health insurance plan that covered her for the prescribed treatments to reestablish her physical and emotional functioning and quality of life. The treatments covered by her plan included traditional rehabilitation physical services, behavioral medicine. and acupuncture.

Integrative Treatment

The patient was seen three times a week for physical therapy and occupational therapy. Working toward goals to reestablish strength, endurance, coordination, and balance, Ms. H. was able eventually to walk with Lofstrand crutches and regain her independence at home. Pain management, however, was much harder.

Pain was addressed through the use of scalp and auricular acupuncture treatments given on a weekly basis. Stimulation of body acupuncture points was contraindicated due to periodic bouts of edema in the extremities. Physical goals for the patient were to (1) reduce inflammation, (2) decrease neuropathic pain, and (3) restore organ balance and vital energy. Overall goals of acupuncture were to augment physical therapy and assist in restoring the patient to more independence in her daily life.

The patient was also seen for individual psychotherapy to address her depression, anxiety, and isolation. Cognitive behavioral interventions and supportive therapy were utilized to assist the patient in mediating fears and anger that interfered with her adherence to medical treatment and medication regimens and that also kept her from transferring skills learned in rehabilitation into the outside world. Behavioral medicine interventions of visual imagery and progressive relaxation were also employed in pain management.

Each discipline provided treatments individually and in concert with the patient's prescribing physician. However, in addition, the team met on a weekly basis to discuss the patient's progress physically and emotionally. The team, along with the patient, also coordinated a treatment care plan that prioritized which goals would be addressed and in what order. In this manner, each clinician was able to emphasize working on the patient's particular problem simultaneously but from a multimodal intervention plan. Coordinated treatment, through an integrative care plan and weekly rounds, allowed all disciplines to focus simultaneously on such diverse goals as improving Ms. H.'s walking, eliminating her fears of falling, increasing her ability to dress and undress, increasing her independence at home and in the community, and decreasing her isolation and depression. The patient was treated with this coordinated integrative approach intensively for one year. Thereafter, ongoing care

(Continues)

(Continued)

has been provided on a regular basis to maintain gains and prevent deterioration.

Clinical Outcome

Ms. H. continues to live independently in the community five years after her surgery. She uses crutches at home and a motorized scooter in the outside world. She has an adaptive, wheelchair-accessible van that she drives to and from her daily activities. She has gained a level of self-assertiveness that has allowed her to have more productive relationships with her family. She is also more involved in the community, making new friends at the pool and at the Starbucks that she frequents. While pain management continues to be an issue, ongoing acupuncture and behavioral medicine interventions have allowed her to decrease significantly her dependence on narcotic medication. She reports that her pain has been reduced by 60 percent. The team continues to assess her follow-up on a monthly basis to address any changes in her needs and prevent deterioration. While Arnold Chiari syndrome has left this patient with a serious disability and a prognosis of prolonged deterioration as she ages, integrative treatment in an interdisciplinary setting may well add to her longevity as well as to the quality of her life.

CASE STUDY 3

Social History

Mr. C. is a 27-year-old man, married, with a two-year-old child. His wife is expecting their second child in three months. The patient's wife is on maternity leave from her job, and Mr. C. is currently the sole support of his family. He completed his master's degree but has been working as a waiter in a restaurant to supplement income while looking for a job in his chosen field. Extended family live in another state approximately 3,000 miles across the country.

Medical History

The patient's past medical history is unremarkable, with the exception of an emergency appendectomy when he was a child.

Presenting Problem

At work, Mr. C. slipped on liquid in the kitchen of the restaurant where he was employed while carrying a full tray of dishes. Both feet went out from under him, and he fell flat on his back. He was diagnosed with herniated discs at L5–S1. He had debilitating sciatica and has not been able to return to work. He could not sit, stand, or lie down for any length of time greater than 45 minutes. His gait was stiff and altered. He could not pick up his child. He rated his pain as 8 out of 10 for 80 percent of the time. Two neurosurgeons recommended surgery, and one predicted an onset of paralysis and possible loss of bowel and bladder functions if surgery was not performed soon.

Integrative Treatment

For the first two weeks, the patient was initially treated for his symptoms with conservative physical therapy. Hot packs and functional electrical stimulation were applied. He also received passive range of motion. During this time he underwent a thorough medical workup, and a care plan, which included surgery, was developed by his neurosurgeon. He was prescribed Vicodan and Flexaril to manage pain and for muscle relaxation. Despite the second opinion recommending surgery, the patient decided against the operation and continued conservative treatment of physical therapy as prescribed by his doctor. Five months later, after the birth of their second child, the patient, his wife, and two children decided to move across country to be closer to their families.

The patient elected to begin an integrative treatment protocol for his condition. His workers' compensation benefits, which followed him from the other state, paid for this treatment. A care plan was developed, and the treatment was provided in an interdisciplinary setting that included CAM and behavioral medicine. As the care plan developed over time, it eventually provided that some services be combined in a transdisciplinary protocol. Team members included a neurosurgeon, a TCM practitioner, and a behavioral medicine psychologist. The patient was prescribed traditional physical therapy three times a week to provide core trunk strengthening as well as massage and manual manipulation. He was also given a home exercise program to supplement his clinic visits.

Individual therapy was provided to address the emotional sequelae of the numerous changes in the patient's life, including his physical changes

(Continues)

(Continued)

in activity, pain, relocation across country, reinvolvement with extended family, work, and birth of his second child. The patient also was provided with a protocol for visual imagery and relaxation for pain management in addition to maintaining his regimen of Vicodan and Flexaril. Additionally, the patient began a course of acupuncture for pain management. Shortly after beginning both behavioral medicine and acupuncture, the protocol for these treatments was combined. Acupuncture needles were inserted at the appropriate acupuncture points for the patient's condition. During the 30 minutes in which the patient lay on the table with the needles inserted, he received a relaxation and visual imagery protocol to address the pain and physical responses of his body. At the end of the behavioral medicine intervention, the acupuncture needles were removed.

Within several months of transdisciplinary treatment, the patient was able to begin to eliminate narcotics for pain management. At that time, an herbal blend for reduction of inflammation and for analgesic effects was provided in coordination with the patient's physician. Additionally, the patient began an active intestinal detoxification program. This program combined use of herbals and nutritional changes to eliminate toxins and promote overall vitality. One year after his injury, and seven months after the initiation of integrative treatments, a program of kundalini yoga was also added. Team rounds on a weekly basis, with all disciplines participating, continuously adjusted Mr. C.'s program. He was discharged from care one year after beginning integrative treatments.

Clinical Outcome

The patient reported "major pain relief" within five months of beginning integrative treatments. From an initial intense pain rating of 8 out of 10, the patient now rated his pain as 3 out of 10 for 90 percent of the time, although on "bad" days it would escalate again to 8 out of 10. As a result of herbal and nutritional interventions, the patient also lost 10 pounds, which further improved his overall health status. By the completion of treatments, Mr. C. was completely off all medications and reporting his pain as 0 out of 10. He was working full-time, enjoying an active family life with his wife and two small children, and engaged in community events.

Throughout the course of treatment, the patient reported relief with the addition of each new modality in the treatment protocol. Mr. C. would then attain a greater level of functionality before ultimately plateauing.

A coordinated change in the treatment plan among all disciplines was essential to continue to fine-tune his program and continue enhancing the patient's course of recovery. For example, combining acupuncture and behavioral medicine interventions as a transdisciplinary intervention in the same session was reported as providing quicker and more complete relief of pain than the two treatments provided separately.

During a follow-up study, the patient was interviewed approximately 10 years postinjury. He reported that in the ensuing 10 years, he had continued in good health and had also taken up jogging. His only medical status change was a recent notification by his primary care physician that his cholesterol was mildly elevated. Mr. C. had still managed to avoid surgery. He stated that he had only two "flare-ups" with back problems since completing his integrative treatments. The first incident occurred eight years postinjury. He rated the pain as 5 out of 10 and did not seek treatment, but reinstituted his home program of stretching and exercises. The pain subsided after 8–10 weeks. The most recent pain incident occurred in the last year prior to the follow-up. Pain had recurred at an 8 out of 10 rating. The patient took only ibuprofen and sought medical treatment. He was given a prescription for six weeks of physical therapy. Presently, the patient is working at a highly demanding job in his chosen profession. He is now the father of three children and works extensively in the community as well.

CONCLUSION

Shifting of Primary Roles

The integrative team has the ability to shift primary roles. Each member's contribution can change based on the patient's presentation (Ken, 1995). The acute condition, for example, bacterial infection, demands the most sophisticated and technologically efficient intervention to prevent the rapid onset to critical status. Full-spectrum or highly targeted antibiotics will be best delivered and monitored by allopathically trained physicians. Some patients may demand the close monitoring of hospitals equipped to provide the best testing and verification.

Once the infection has been controlled and the patient's symptoms alleviated, and diagnostic tests indicate that basic health has been restored, primary roles may shift. Approximately two to six weeks after the initial infection, thought should be given to the homeopathic detoxification of the antibiotics so as to prevent toxic overload and or suppression of symptoms deeper within the body. This may also be a good time to introduce preventative medicine through the practice of naturopathy or TCM. These disciplines have a rich history in maintaining homeostasis.

Critical care is the exclusive world of allopathic primary care. Life-threatening or life-changing illnesses call for highly advanced testing and evaluation. Aftercare is also important, and it is here where alternative opportunities are valuable. Chronic conditions, including many autoimmune diseases, have a psychosomatic component. For some time the literature has indicated an emotional presentation in as many as 70 percent of chronic disease sufferers (Mingji, 1992). It is this array of ailments that provides the most fertile ground for all the disciplines to learn and share their healing arts and science.

Working Together

Integrative medicine applied in the real world of today's healthcare system has a long road to travel before it is the accepted norm. There are many issues to be addressed among the various philosophies of practitioners, in addition to determining appropriate clinical interventions and appropriate delivery systems. Financial hurdles for obtaining such treatment must also be overcome. However, given the results of studies appearing in respected peer-reviewed journals that evaluate protocols ranging from herbals and acupuncture to visual imagery and brain chemistry, integrative medicine warrants a closer examination of how such an approach may enhance our current healthcare delivery. The philosophies are diverse, as noted by the differing perspectives of the clinicians at the beginning of this chapter. The manner in which various services are coordinated and offered to the patient can also serve to enhance the efficacy of treatments or create situations where some treatments are actually contraindicated. Integrative medicine protocols need to be carefully evaluated and even more carefully implemented.

The three case studies presented here provide a view, albeit limited, of how thoughtful integrative care can be used to benefit the whole person. These studies show the application of integrative care with a young adult, a middle-aged person, and an elderly individual. They also indicate how systematically applied integrative interventions can benefit treatments in diverse clinical scenarios, for example, chronic disease, congenital deficits, and acute orthopedic/neurological injury. It is well worth noting that funding in each of these cases was also diverse. Traditionally, integrative care from complementary/alternative practitioners is reported as being paid for by the patient out of pocket. While that was the situation in one case reported, the other two were funded by a major health insurance company and by a major insurance carrier of workers' compensation. While the last two sources of funding are relatively rare, it is an indication of how the larger viewpoint of treating the whole person is beginning to be acknowledged by the insurance industry, at least in some cases.

As in all three cases cited, a major caveat for providing integrative medicine is that the integrative services need to be coordinated among all healthcare providers. Whether the coordination is minimal, for example, a phone call placed to the various practitioners at their respective offices, or more involved, with coordination systematized under one roof at regularly held team meetings, and even within treatment sessions, the interweaving of goals, medicines, and psychological approaches is essential.

Treatment of the whole person through effective, integrative protocols requires the same things that any good relationship requires in everyday living. First, all parties must be willing to take responsibility—this means the patient as well as all healthcare providers; second, there must be a respect for differing viewpoints and a willingness to learn from one another; third, active communication about these differences must occur in the context of respect; fourth, trust among the treating colleagues providing integrative medicine, as well as with the patient, must be established; fifth, there must be a commitment by the team of professionals to work through differences in service of a higher goal—that goal being an enhanced level of human caring for the person they are entrusted to heal.

TOOL KIT FOR CHANGE

Role and Perspective of the Healthcare Professional

1. Healthcare professionals must be open to working with, and learning from, caregivers in other disciplines that can provide good evidence-based and clinical practice procedures beyond their own.
2. Active communication about the patient and differing treatments must occur among the team professionals.
3. Health practitioners need to be flexible and show respect for the patient and for modes of healing beyond their own.

Role and Perspective of the Patient/Participant

1. The patient must be an active team member in the management of his own healthcare.
2. While the patient is encouraged to bring up all issues and modes of treatment that he has considered, once the patient has chosen an integrative team with which to work, the patient must have patience in following integrative team recommendations rather than mixing and matching other approaches not yet incorporated into the integrative treatment protocol.

Interconnection: The Global Perspective

1. Integrative medicine services need to be coordinated among all healthcare providers.
2. Working on a team extends the knowledge base available to help the patient and, in some cases, can enhance efficacy of treatments when they are delivered together rather than in isolation.
3. The integrative team has the ability to shift primary roles as needed to best assist the patient in healing. Acute care may require the preeminence of the allopathic physician. Chronic, or long-term, follow-up may require that other integrative practitioners take a primary role.

REFERENCES

American Association of Naturopathic Physicians. (2006). Licensed states and licensing authorities. Retrieved November 12, 2006 from http://www.naturopathic.org/viewbulletin.php?id=118.

American Board of Medical Acupuncture. (2006). Purposes of the american board of medical acupuncture. Retrieved November 12, 2007 http://www.dabma.org.

American Psychological Association. (1995). *Public perceptions of the value of psychological services.* Washington, DC: Author.

American Psychological Association. (2005). Medicare milestone: All carriers now cover health and behavior services. Retrieved November 12, 2006, from http://www.apapractice.org/apo/health_and_behavior.html#.

Ayer, W. (2005). *Psychology and dentistry.* New York: Haworth Press.

Benson, H. (1975). *The relaxation response.* New York: William Morrow.

Benson, H., & Proctor, W. (1985). *Beyond the relaxation response.* Berkeley: University of California Press.

Benson, H., & Stark, M. (1997). *Timeless healing.* New York: Scribner.

Benson, H., & Stuart, E. (1993). *Wellness book: The comprehensive guide to maintaining health and treating stress-related illness.* New York: Scribner.

Bianchi, I., Perra, A., & Malzac, J. L. R. (2005, January). Use of cytokines in homeopathy. *La Biologica Medica,* 43–50.

Board on Health Promotion and Disease Prevention, Institute of Medicine. (2005). *Complementary and alternative medicine in the United States.* Washington, DC: National Academies Press.

Boon, H., Stewart, M., Kennard, M. A., Gray, R., Sawka, C., Brown, J. B., et al. (2000). Use of complementary/alternative medicine by breast cancer survivors in Ontario: Prevalence and perceptions. *Journal of Clinical Oncology, 18,* 2515–2521.

Casey, A., & Benson, H. (2005). *Harvard Medical School guide to lowering your blood pressure.* New York: McGraw-Hill.

Collins, M., & Dunn, L. (2005). The effects of meditation and visual imagery on an immune system disorder: Dermatomyositis. *Journal of Alternative and Complementary Medicine, De Morant, G.S.(1994) Chinese Acupuncture, trans. Lawrence Grinnel. 11,* 275–284.

De Morant, G. S. (1994) *Chinese Acupuncture,* trans. Lawrence Grinnel.

DePascalis, V., Chiaradia, C., & Carotenuto, E. (2002). The contribution of suggestibility and expectation to placebo analgesia phenomenon in an experimental setting. *Pain, 96,* 393–402.

Faas, N. (2001). *Integrating complementary medicine into health systems.* Gaithersburg, MD: Aspen.

Fiedler, J. L., & Wright, J. B. (1989). *The medical offset effect and public health policy: Mental health industry in transition.* New York: Praeger.

Frank, R., Hagglund, C., & Farmer, J. (2004). Chronic illness management in primary care: The cardinal symptoms model. In R. G. Frank, S. H. McDaniel, J. H. Bray, & M. Heldring (Eds.), *Primary care psychology* (pp. 259–275). Washington, DC: American Psychological Association.

Frank, R., McDaniel, S., Bray, J., & Heldring, M. (Eds.). (2004). *Primary care psychology.* Washington, DC: American Psychological Association.

Galli, F., Riccio, B., & Guidetti, V. (2004). The effect of placebo and neurophysiological involvements. *Journal of Headache and Pain, 5,* 374–377.

Gatchel, R., & Oordt, M. (2003). *Clinical health psychology and primary care: Practical advice and clinical guidance for successful collaboration.* Washington, DC: American Psychological Association.

Grodstein, F., Manson, J. D., Colditz, G. A., Willett, W. C., Speizer, F. E., & Stampfer, M. J. (2000). A prospective, observational study of postmenopausal hormone therapy and primary prevention of cardiovascular disease. *Annals of Internal Medicine, 133,* 933–941.

Herman, P. M., Craig, B. M., & Caspi, O. (2005). Is complementary and alternative medicine (CAM) cost effective? A systematic review. *BioMed Central Complementary and Alternative Medicine, 5,* 11. Retrieved August 26, 2006, from http://www.pubmedcentral.nih.gov/articlerender.fcgi?tool=pubmed&pubmedid=15932647

Holroyd, K., O'Donnell, F., Stensland, M., Lipchik, G., Cordingley, G., & Carlson, B. (2001). Management of chronic tension-type headache with tricyclic antidepressant medication, stress management therapy, and their combination: A randomized controlled trial. *Journal of the American Medical Association, 285,* 2208–2215.

Hulley, S., Grady, D., Bush, T., Furgerg, C., Herrington, D., Riggs, B., et al. (1998). Randomized trial of estrogen plus progestin for secondary prevention of coronary heart disease in postmenopausal women: Heart and estrogen/progestin replacement study (HERS) research group. *Journal of the American Medical Association, 280,* 605–613.

James, L. C., & Folen, R. A. (Eds.). (2005). *The primary care consultant.* Washington, DC: American Psychological Association.

Johnsen, R., Forde, O. H., Straume, B., & Burhol, P. G. (1994). Aetiology of peptic ulcer: A prospective population study in Norway. *Journal of Epidemiology and Community Health, 48,* 156–160.

Jones, K. (Ed.). (1979). Report of a conference on the impact of alcohol, drug abuse, and mental health treatment on medical care utilization. *Medical Care, 17*(Suppl), 1–82.

Ken, C. (1995). Traditional Health Systems and Public Policy. Protocols of Botanical Medicine. *Journal of Alternative and Complimentary Medicine (Vol. 2 No. 3),* 405–409.

Lambrew, J. (2004). *Uninsured America.* Retrieved August 26, 2006, from http://www.americanprogress.org/issues/2004/08/b173900.html

Lutgendorf, S., Logan, H., Kirchner, H., Rothrock, N., Svengalis, S., Iverson, K., et al. (2000). Effects of relaxation and stress on the capsaicin-induced local inflammatory response. *Psychosomatic Medicine, 62,* 524–534.

Manson, J. D., Hsia, J., Johnson, K. C., Rossouw, J. E., Assaf, A. R., Lasser, N. L., et al. (2003). Estrogen plus progestin and the risk of coronary heart disease. *New England Journal of Medicine, 349,* 523–534.

McKegney, F. P., & Schwartz, C. E. (1986). Behavioral Medicine: Treatment and Organizational Issues. *General Hospital Psychiatry. 8 (5)*:330-39.

Miller, E. R., Pastor-Barriuso, R., Dalal, D., Riemersma, R. A., Appel, L. J., & Guallar, E. (2005). Meta-analysis: High-dosage vitamin E supplementation may increase all-cause mortality. *Annals of Internal Medicine, 142,* 37–46.

Mingji, P. (1992). Cancer treatment with Fu Zheng Pei Ben principle: Cancer using an integrative approach. *BiotherapeuticIndex,* Winter 2006, 1–74.

Mokdad, A., Marks, J., Stroup, D, & Gerberding, J. (2004). Actual causes of death in the United States, 2000. *Journal of the American Medical Association, 291,*1238–1245.

Ornish, D., Scherwitz, L., Billings, J., Gould, K., Merritt, T., Sparler, S., et al. (1998). Intensive lifestyle changes for reversal of coronary heart disease. *Journal of the American Medical Association, 280,* 2001–2007.

Pan American Health Organization. (2003). *Traditional, complementary, and alternative medicines and therapies: Evaluation Plan of Work 2000–2001 and Plan of Work 2002–2003.* Washington, DC: Author.

Redmond, L. J., Bowman, B. A., & Mensah, G. A. (Comp.). (2000–2005). *Health disparities: A selected bibliography from the National Center for Chronic Disease Prevention and Health Promotion.* Atlanta, GA: Centers for Disease Control.

Roter, D., Hall, J., & Aoki, Y. (2002). Physician gender effects in medical communication: A meta-analytic review. *Journal of the American Medical Association, 288,* 756–764.

Rusk Institute. (2006). *About us.* Retrieved November 12, 2006, from http://www.med.nyu.edu/about/overview/nyuhc/rusk.html

Sheikh, A. A. (2003). *Healing images.* Amityville, NY: Baywood.

Society of Homotoxicology. (2006). Retrieved from http://www.biopathica.co.uk/Society.htm

VandenBos, G., & DeLeon, P. H. (1988). The use of psychotherapy to improve physical health. *Psychotherapy, 25,* 335–343.

Vase, L., Robinson, M., Verne, G., & Price, D. (2005). Increased placebo analgesia over time in irritable bowel syndrome (IBS) patients is associated with desire and expectation but not endogenous opioid mechanisms. *Pain, 115,* 338–347.

Walsh, R., & Shapiro, S. (2006). The meeting of meditative disciplines and Western psychology. *American Psychologist, 61,* 227–239.

Wolsko, P., Eisenberg, D., Davis, R., & Phillips, R. (2004). Use of mind–body medical therapies: Results of a national survey. *Journal of General Internal Medicine, 19,* 1497–1525.

Wood, M. J., Stewart, R. L., Merry, H., Johnstone, D., & Cox, J. (2003). Use of complementary and alternative medicine in patients with cardiovascular disease. *American Heart Journal, 145,* 806–812.

Chapter Eight

INTEGRATIVE HEALTHCARE AND MARGINALIZED POPULATIONS

Martha E. Banks, PhD, Lydia P. Buki, PhD, Miguel E. Gallardo, PsyD, and Barbara W. K. Yee, PhD

> Everyone has the right to a standard of living adequate for the health and well-being of himself and of his family, including food, clothing, housing and medical care and necessary social services, and the right to security in the event of unemployment, sickness, disability, widowhood, old age or other lack of livelihood in circumstances beyond his control (United Nations, 1948, Article 25[1]).

INTRODUCTION

Good health is not only beneficial for individuals and their families, but is also an important contributor to sound economic policy (National Academy on an Aging Society, 1999; Rowe & Kahn, 1998). Although health improvements have been made in segments of American society, significant health disparities remain. Ethnicity-specific data have indicated that mortality is significantly higher among Native Hawaiians, Samoans, African Americans, American Indians, and Alaska Natives than among non-Latino whites (Leigh & Huff, 2006). Many site-specific cancers are considerably higher among ethnic minorities, including (1) higher cervical cancer incidence rates among Vietnamese and Hispanic women, (2) higher lung cancer deaths among black, American Indian and Native Alaskan, Hispanic, and Asian males, and (3) the highest stomach cancer incidence rates among Vietnamese, Korean, Japanese, and Hawaiian people (Miller et al., 1996). And while many immigrant populations are healthier than those who are native-born, with behavioral and lifestyle changes that take place during the acculturation process, health advantages of immigrants may disappear after a lifetime of living in the United States (Hernandez & Charney, 1998).

The health and healing process is affected by institutional, social, community, cultural, and individual variables. In this chapter we explore these variables as they relate to marginalized populations and integrative healthcare service delivery. In the first part of the chapter, we present an overview of the health status of various marginalized populations: African Americans, American Indians and Alaska Natives, Asian Americans, Native Hawaiians and other Pacific Islanders, and Latinos. In addition, we examine the issues surrounding marginalization as a function of gender, ability status, and immigration status. Finally, we examine the influence of individuals' cultural contexts and cultural explanatory models on healthcare utilization.

The second half of the chapter attends to the promise of integrative healthcare in the effort to eliminate health disparities. In this section we present two contrasting models of integrative healthcare delivery: nontargeted and targeted models of care. We also explore issues related to the use of complementary and alternative medicine and discuss the status of cultural competence in healthcare. The chapter closes with recommendations for enhancing integrative healthcare service provisions to marginalized populations.

HEALTH STATUS OF MARGINALIZED POPULATIONS

Nearly 60 years after the United Nations declared adequate medical care as a human right, there are still such wide disparities within the United States that the Agency for Healthcare Research and Quality has been mandated to provide an annual report evaluating progress made in closing these gaps (Smedley, Stith, & Nelson, 2003; U.S. Department of Health and Human Services, 2002, 2005). While at one time, socioeconomic status was presumed to account for all healthcare disparities, it is now clear that ethnicity, gender, and ability status are also critical variables (Lillie-Blanton & Lewis, 2005; Smedley et al., 2003).

Byrd and Clayton (2003) documented the U.S. history that has included separate and unequal healthcare based on ethnicity; the result is continued disparity in healthcare delivery, with members of marginalized populations receiving minimal care. In addition, members of nondominant populations who have the means to afford quality healthcare do not receive the same treatment as their dominant peers. Bierman, Lurie, Collins, and Eisenberg (2002) noted that "racial and ethnic disparities in health outcomes have been observed among persons with similar health insurance, within the same system of care, and within the same managed care plan" (p. 92). In contrast with the everyday experience of many ethnic minorities, healthcare should be available, accessible, acceptable, and of good quality and must meet ethical standards and be culturally appropriate (Carmalt & Zaidi, 2004).

ETHNICITY

Members of marginalized ethnic groups in the United States are at high risk for inadequate or inappropriate healthcare. Factors contributing to this high risk pattern are multiple and interrelated in complex ways. According to Shavers and Shavers (2006), some of these factors include "provider bias against racial/ethnic minorities, uncertainty in their interactions with minority patients, beliefs or stereotypes regarding the health behavior of minority patients and patient response to perceived provider mistreatment or other negative racial experiences" (pp. 391–392). Next, we will provide contextual information about health disparities for the four major ethnic/racial minority groups in the United States: (1) African Americans, (2) American Indians and Alaska Natives, (3) Asian Americans, and (4) Latinos.

African Americans

Historically, people of African descent in the United States had been kidnapped by people of European descent and treated as inhuman property from the 1600s until the mid-1800s. Laws were introduced that relegated people of African descent to subhuman status, including Constitutional designation as "three fifths of all other Persons" (U.S. Constitution, Article I, Section 2, as cited in Rothenberg, 1992, p. 264). With the abolition of slavery, new laws were enacted continuing abridgment of the rights of people of African descent, mostly through codified segregation such as the Black Codes (DuBois, 1935). This oppressive environment was also evident in the medical arena; during this time, African Americans were treated separately or not allowed access to healthcare. By 1910, renowned biostatisticians had predicted that the observed health disparities would lead to the extinction of African Americans by the end of the twentieth century (Byrd & Clayton, 2003). Whereas segregated education was publicly acknowledged as unequal and ultimately outlawed in the 1950s, disparities in healthcare were not considered a national priority until the 1990s. Moreover, serious health abuses were perpetrated against African Americans prior to this recognition. Specifically, between 1932 and 1972, the U.S. Public Health Service conducted an investigation later known as the Tuskegee Study, in which 399 African American men who had syphilis were left untreated and were simply observed until their deaths (Freimuth et al., 2001). This study, which is the longest nontherapeutic study in medical history, reflects the societal context of the time, and its legacy is still with us today (Freimuth et al., 2001).

Among the many barriers to adequate healthcare services are institutional and provider biases. In the healthcare setting, there is a tendency to group together all people of African descent, regardless of immigration status, education, and other social demographics. This tendency, based on unfounded assumptions, results in the provision of inferior healthcare services by virtue of ignoring individual variables that affect the healing process. Another bias includes a stereotype that African Americans do not expect to receive good healthcare and will not cooperate with treatment (Good, DelVecchio, Good, & Becker, 2003). The cost of healthcare is another barrier to receipt of adequate healthcare services. Chumney, Mauldin, and Simpson (2006) found that African American health costs were significantly higher than those of European Americans in South Carolina due to lack of ambulatory and preventive healthcare. Despite the knowledge that access to healthcare is critical, hospitals that traditionally have served African Americans are being closed: "The closing of hospitals serving predominantly black communities is controversial and often found to be driven more by the racial composition of the hospitals' neighborhoods than by economic conditions" (Leigh & Jimenez, 2002, p. 133).

American Indians and Alaska Natives

Health of Native Americans and Alaska Natives was negatively impacted as Europeans in the seventeenth, eighteenth, and nineteenth centuries introduced new illnesses (e.g., measles, smallpox) while displacing people. Some tribes, such as the Patuxet people, were exterminated by these diseases; other tribes were more fortunate and experienced death rates between 50 percent and 60 percent (Stannard, 1992). In the twentieth century, through treaty agreements, legislation was passed to provide health services to Native Americans and Alaska Natives. One system of healthcare is the Indian Health Service (IHS), which is funded annually *at the discretion of Congress* (Joe, 2003). In recent years, the IHS has been allowed to accept Medicaid funding. However, the funding of IHS has been seriously inadequate, resulting in rationing and lack of healthcare for many Native Americans and Alaska Natives (Schneider, 2005). This has been particularly problematic as specific facilities have limited services available only to members of certain tribes, precluding people from other tribes who have married into those tribes from receiving care (Joe, 2003).

Joe (2003) described some of the challenges faced by Native Americans and Alaska Natives seeking health treatment. For people with traditional values, healthcare and implementation of treatment recommendations are not based on individual decisions, but involve consultation with family and tribal healers. Clients are perceived as "difficult" by culturally insensitive healthcare providers who do not appreciate the importance of taking the time to include significant others in the determination of the appropriateness of treatments. Because clients are often seen alone, additional appointments are needed to carry out an effective treatment plan in consultation with others in the patient's life. Other barriers to healthcare include language, lack of choice of quality healthcare providers, and stereotyping by providers (e.g., assumptions that all health concerns are related to substance abuse). Moreover, institutional issues, such as problems with recruitment and retention of physicians, result in ongoing understaffing of IHS facilities. According to Kim (2000), a 50 percent vacancy rate for physicians existed at one Navajo facility for five months in 1998. During these times of vacancy, pressure is placed on hired physicians to work longer hours, further compromising their willingness to work in the facility and critically affecting quality of care (Kim, 2000). These and other issues related to institutionally mandated and staffed care, and to the provision of care in rural areas, combine to create a critical need for improvement of healthcare services available to American Indians and Alaska Natives.

Asian Americans

Asian American populations are diverse, encompassing individuals with origins in 20 countries with different languages and geopolitical histories (Ong, 2000). Within this diverse group, a large majority of Asian Americans are foreign born (63%) and have limited English proficiency (41%; Asian and Pacific Islander Health Forum, 2000). Consequently, limited English proficiency, culture, immigration with lack of citizenship (25.7% for Asian and Pacific Islanders vs. 2.9% for the U.S. population), and insurance coverage are significant barriers to healthcare access for many, but particularly for older Asian populations. Underutilization of health services is exacerbated by lack of a regular physician and a complex healthcare system with significant access barriers.

Despite these barriers, Asian Americans have high life expectancy rates; in California the rate of life expectancy from birth was highest among all racial groups at 86.5 years for Asian females and 80.9 for Asian males in 1990 (Leigh & Huff, 2006). The leading causes of mortality are heart disease, malignant neoplasms, cerebrovascular diseases, diabetes, and unintentional injuries. Although heart disease is the leading cause of death for males and females across ethnicities, it is not the leading cause of death for Asian American women. Malignant neoplasms are the leading cause of mortality for Asian American women. The lower incidence of heart disease among Asian Americans, especially women, contributes to better health outcomes. There are high rates of certain cancers in Asian populations (i.e., lung cancers in Vietnamese, Cambodian, and Hmong males; colorectal, liver, and cervical cancers among Vietnamese women; see Miller et al., 1996) as well as an alarming growth in the rates of breast cancer among Japanese and Chinese American women who were born in the United States or are long-term U.S. residents. Among documented health disparities, the rate of dementia among Asian American elders appears to be comparable to non-Latino whites; however, older Asian Americans have a higher rate of vascular dementia and a lower rate of Alzheimer's dementia, although this ratio may be changing (see Manly & Mayeux, 2004). Other health disparities include lower rates of health insurance, health access, and health screening and disease prevention among Asian American populations (Leigh & Huff, 2006). For instance, immigrant Vietnamese, Cambodian, and Hmong women have low breast and cervical cancer screening rates as compared to non-Latino whites or African American women (Kagawa-Singer & Pourat, 2000; National Asian Women's Health Organization, 2000).

In the National Latino and Asian American Study, Alegria et al. (2006) found that Chinese, Filipino, and Vietnamese plus other smaller groups of Asian Americans have lower rates of mental illnesses, but they also reported that they were less likely to seek treatment for mental illness (Meyers, 2006). These individuals felt that they would experience unfair treatment, and 63 percent of participants attributed this anticipatory treatment discrimination to racial and linguistic bias factors. In addition, cultural factors appear to hide true prevalence rates for stigmatizing mental health conditions or problems that are considered private family matters such as domestic abuse. Culture also influences the efficacy of standardized mental health therapeutic approaches. For instance, Chen and Davenport (2005) found that cognitive behavioral therapy works better with Chinese American clients when adapted to conform to Chinese values, beliefs, and cultural characteristics. Cognitive behavioral therapy appears useful when cultural and other modifications are made, such as educating clients about the therapeutic process to decrease anxiety, lessening the use of personal questions in the initial session, teaching about assertiveness in certain situations, and making therapeutic adaptations to handle a tendency to control strong emotions and possible somatization.

Native Hawaiians and Other Pacific Islanders

Similar to Asian Americans, this group is diverse and encompasses individuals of diverse origins, such as Native Hawaiian, Samoan, Tongan, Guamanian or Chamorro, Fijian, and other Pacific Islanders (Braun, Yee, Browne, & Mokuau, 2004). Unfortunately, data for this group are sparse and are typically combined with those of Asian Americans. In turn, the health of some immigrant Asian Americans has obscured the relatively poorer health outcomes for Pacific Islanders.

Data from California obtained in 1990 shows that the life expectancy from birth for Native Hawaiian and Pacific Islanders (70.5 for males and 77.8 for females) is significantly shorter than that of their non-Latino white counterparts (males at 75.4 and females at 80.5; Leigh & Huff, 2006). Consistent with this trend, data from Hawaii suggest that Native Hawaiians have significantly higher mortality rates for most causes of death when compared to other ethnic groups (Braun et al., 2004). Leading causes of mortality in this population are heart disease, malignant neoplasms, cerebrovascular diseases, and diabetes.

Investigators have attributed this health disparity to (1) advanced disease at diagnosis, (2) higher rates of underlying contributing factors such as hypertension and obesity, (3) cultural and socioeconomic barriers, such as poverty, that result in lower health care access, and (4) health behaviors such as higher smoking rates and inferior nutrition. For example, Native Hawaiian women have the second highest incidence rate of breast cancer and the highest cancer death rate in comparison to other ethnic groups in Hawaii. Cultural values influence their health perceptions, health practices, health remedies, and health utilization. A Native Hawaiian belief is that illness is related to the loss of mana (spiritual or divine power). This loss of mana comes from a disruption in the harmonious relationships between people, ancestor spirits, the environment, or the land (Pukui, Haertig, & Lee, 1972). For Native Hawaiians, illness is overcome and a state of wellness reestablished by improving harmony between themselves and other people, among themselves and the spirit realm, or any other disharmonious relationships. Therefore, to treat illness and achieve wellness, the disharmonious relationships between people, spirits, environment, and land must be addressed. Other Pacific Islander cultures, such as Samoan and Chamorro, also believe in the integration of the individual, family, community, and spiritual realms. These holistic worldviews frame health beliefs and perceptions that influence health and service utilization.

Although there is a scarcity of mental health research with Native Hawaiian and other Pacific Islanders, it appears that stigma, discrimination, and social stereotyping (with negative consequences such as low self-esteem, demoralization, and depression) are associated with lower educational attainment, poverty, poorer health behaviors, such as smoking, and mental health disparities as compared to other ethnic groups in Hawaii. In addition, adolescents and older Native Hawaiians have the highest rates of suicide in Hawaii. Discrimination, negative stereotyping, breakdown of traditional support systems, and poorer educational outcomes contribute to a higher level of depression and produce negative health and mental health outcomes (see the review in Braun et al., 2004).

Latinos

Latinos are a heterogeneous group with different immigration and migration patterns, with roots in at least 21 countries (Centers for Disease Control and Prevention, 1994). The main groups have origins in Mexico (64%), Puerto Rico (10%), Cuba (3%), Dominican Republic (3%), and El Salvador (3%), although immigrants have also come from other Central American and South American countries (U.S. Census Bureau, 2005a). Latinos of various ancestries bring with them possible differences in cultural norms, language, beliefs, expectations, quality of formal education experiences, and reasons for immigrating to the United States. All these factors contribute to differences in lifestyle, socioeconomic status, and incidence of chronic illness across groups.

It is critical to examine the social and environmental contexts of the Latino community to understand the medical and mental health needs of this population. On examination, it becomes clear that institutional, social, cultural, and individual variables combine to place the community at risk for disease and unhealthy behaviors. For example, in 2004, the uninsured rate for Latinos was approximately three times as high (32.7%) as the rate for non-Latino whites (11.3%; U.S. Census Bureau, 2005a). Moreover, of approximately 43 million Latinos living in the United States, 31 million speak Spanish (U.S. Census Bureau, 2005a); among adult Latinos, almost half (47%) are primarily Spanish speaking (Pew Hispanic Center, 2004), making language an additional barrier to adequate healthcare for millions of individuals. The pressure to acculturate and assimilate also influences the physical and psychological well-being of Latinos as well as social stereotyping, given that Latinos live in a culture based on Eurocentric values and norms.

Additional barriers to health promotion include insufficient access to quality medical services, lack of transportation, insufficient insurance coverage, lack of access to providers with the language skills necessary to treat the community, culturally insensitive care on the part of the provider, cultural health beliefs that negatively influence uptake of health promotion behaviors, and low levels of health literacy (Buki, 1999; Buki, Borrayo, Feigal, & Carrillo, 2004; National Council of La Raza, 2004; North Carolina Institute of Medicine, 2003). Consequently, disease prevention and health promotion are important public health measures that must be implemented to remedy the increasing healthcare deficits that large segments of the community face (Gonzalez Castro & Hernandez, 2004).

The top five leading causes of death among Latinos in the United States are heart disease, cancer, unintentional injuries, stroke, and diabetes (National Center for Health Statistics, 2004). Overall, Latinos have higher prevalence rates of the following conditions and risk factors: chronic obstructive pulmonary disease, HIV/AIDS, obesity, suicide, teenage pregnancy, and tuberculosis. Many of these conditions are associated with lifestyle factors (e.g., diet, exercise) that are amenable to intervention. In the delivery of interventions, it is important to acknowledge the worldviews held by the various subgroups within the population. For example, in Mexican culture, there is no clear separation between physical and mental illnesses; therefore a balance must be achieved between an individual and the environment, or the chances of acquiring a disease will increase (Santana-Martin & Santana, 2005). Factors that contribute to the manifestation of illness include emotional, social, physical, and spiritual elements: "The causes of illness are God's will or unacceptable behavior" (Santana-Martin & Santana, p. 168). In addition, physical disabilities may be seen as more acceptable than mental disabilities. For example, in some Mexican cultures, there is no word for *disability;* individuals who have disabilities are seen as fully functioning members of Mexican society. In comparison with a Western, patriarchal society, where independence is highly valued, a Mexican matriarchal value system provides a cultural context and environment that fosters a sense of care, dependence, preservation, and the creation of life (Santana-Martin & Santana, 2005). Consequently, in Mexican culture, when a health professional diagnoses one member of the family, an entire community and family are diagnosed. In turn, family members with disabilities are unlikely to be placed in institutional healthcare agencies, but rather, they will live at home until their deaths.

It is not uncommon for Latinos to employ holistic home and folk remedies to treat certain illnesses in the family before attempting to use forms of healing defined and constructed by Western culture and society. For this reason it is imperative that healthcare providers address the needs of the Latino community in a culturally sensitive manner by implementing a collaborative healing approach between providers and patients.

GENDER

Women experience more barriers to healthcare than men do; this has resulted in significant health disparities along gender lines (Brett & Hayes, 2004; Leigh & Huff, 2006; Salganicoff, Ranji, & Wyn, 2005). The barriers involve not only the individual woman's health, but also that of people for whom she has a caregiving responsibility (Ackerman & Banks, 2007; Nabors & Pettee, 2003): "The health care system is falling short for many groups of women, particularly those who are already sick. For many of these women, obtaining the full range of services they need to improve or maintain their health is a formidable challenge at best and for many simply not achievable" (Salganicoff et al., 2005, p. 48). This is particularly a problem for women who are members of nondominant ethnic groups (Leigh & Huff, 2006).

Salganicoff et al. (2005) highlighted a number of concerns about healthcare delivery to women in the United States.

- In evaluating women's health needs, it is critical to consider age and heath status. Many disorders previously associated with older women (e.g., arthritis, hypertension, and diabetes) are now prevalent in younger women.
- Although on the surface it appears that women with insurance have greater access to healthcare, there are serious high costs that serve as barriers to many women. This is particularly noticeable in the costs of prescription medication.

Many women do not fill costly prescriptions, or split doses, to keep the treatment as affordable as possible.

• Prevention counseling is minimal for women, despite evidence that counseling about smoking or alcohol use, calcium and bone health, sexual health, and intimate partner violence help to promote good health. In addition, there has been a decline in the use of traditional early detection measures such as mammography, pap tests, and blood pressure tests.

• Women are at higher risk of having fragmented care because many women have multiple providers and have short relationships with these doctors. These doctors typically do not share information about the patient, which further compromises care.

ABILITY STATUS

People with disabilities struggle with many difficulties in the healthcare arena. Many have chronic illnesses, which can be a barrier to quality healthcare (Salganicoff et al., 2005). Attitudes of healthcare professionals also impair the process of assessment, treatment, and referral (Corbett, 2003; Dotson, Stinson, & Christian, 2003; Mukherjee, Reis, & Heller, 2003; Poulin & Gouliquer, 2003; Williams & Upadhyay, 2003). Banks and Ackerman (2006) described the severe economic limitations faced by people with disabilities that add another barrier to access to quality healthcare. Moreover, although many people are concerned with hospitalization as a consequence of diagnosis of serious illness, people with disabilities are at risk for involuntary hospitalization due to inaccurate assessment or discrimination based on misperception of ability (Banks, 2007). Inpatient settings can pose particular safety risks to people with disabilities due to so-called excused violence perpetrated by staff or other patients (McCarthy, 1998).

IMMIGRANT POPULATIONS

Foreign-born individuals (i.e., immigrants) are a diverse group that constitute 12 percent of the total U.S. population, with people from Latin America comprising 53 percent of all immigrants in the United States (U.S. Census Bureau, 2005b). Not only are their nationalities varied, but so are their reasons for immigrating to this country, educational backgrounds, income levels, extent of professional training, ability to speak the English language, and levels of acculturation. For example, some immigrants may be political refugees who fled civil war in their countries of origin; these individuals may be reluctant to seek and accept healthcare from a government-run facility. Others may have immigrated due to economic circumstances and, not speaking the language and with limited skill sets, work in the agricultural fields or in low-skill labor, occupations that typically do not offer any type of health insurance or time off for preventive healthcare yet expose workers to various chemicals and unsafe working conditions. On the other hand, highly trained professionals may come to the United States to work in international banks, the healthcare industry, and other high-profile organizations. In working with the immigrant population, it is important to keep in mind the diversity inherent in the group as well as the possibility that individuals may have different levels of acculturation.

Acculturation refers to the process of psychological and behavioral change that results from long-term contact with another culture (Berry, 1980; Berry & Sam, 1997; Stonequist, 1935, 1937). Recent conceptualizations of acculturation suggest that acculturation is bilinear; that is, people may exhibit various degrees of acculturation not only related to their host culture (e.g., the United States), but also to their native culture (e.g., Mexico, China). In addition, the concept of acculturation is multidimensional. According to Zea, Asner-Self, Birman, and Buki (2003), acculturation encompasses three distinct subscales: (1) cultural identity (people's sense of belonging to a culture, (2) cultural competence (people's knowledge about a culture), and (3) language competence (people's knowledge of their country of origin language and/or the host country's official language).

Research suggests that health outcomes in immigrant populations may differ as a function of acculturation levels and gender. For example, López-Gonzalez, Aravena, and Hummer (2005) found that health behaviors (i.e., alcohol consumption and smoking) of less acculturated immigrant women are more positive than those of immigrant women with higher levels of acculturation. On the other hand, acculturation did not discriminate between these health behaviors in men. Similarly, researchers have examined the Latino mortality paradox, given that Latinos in the United States have a lower socioeconomic status profile than non-Latino whites, but a lower all-cause mortality rate. Findings suggest that that this paradox may be explained, in part, by level of acculturation and gender (Abraído-Lanza, Chao, & Flórez, 2005). In some cases, however, conclusions about the relationship between acculturation and health behaviors have been difficult to make due to the use of flawed assessment measures (Abraído-Lanza, Armbrister, Flórez, & Aguirre, 2006). Nonetheless, taken together, this research points to a need for healthcare providers to consider not only the influence of acculturation on health outcomes, but also how acculturation may differ across population subgroups (López-Gonzalez et al., 2005). In turn, different levels of acculturation may be associated with different health practices and different levels of adherence to traditional health beliefs, requiring different interventions for health promotion at various levels.

Adding to the complexity of work with immigrant populations is the need to have an interpreter when patients are limited English speakers. Interpreters are often nurses, physicians, family members or friends, or other hospital employees, the majority of whom have received no formal training for this task (Baker, Hayes, & Fortier, 1998; Echemendia & Julian, 2002). It is clear that any distortion of information during the medical interview may have serious negative consequences (e.g., misdiagnosis, obtaining unnecessary tests, having difficulty comprehending instructions for treatment, receiving overall poor quality of care, having a higher cost of care, and fostering poor patient-provider relationships; Dower, 2003).

To address the need for accurate and ethical interpretation services, several standards have been developed specifically for medical interpretation. According to Baker et al. (1998), a particularly useful set of standards is that developed by the Massachusetts Medical Interpreters Association (MMIA). The MMIA states the following:

> These standards of practice...recognize the importance of the medical encounter in establishing a therapeutic connection between provider and patient. The formulation of a therapeutic relationship is especially difficult when parties cannot communicate directly, and it becomes even more complex when different culturally based belief systems are involved. A competent interpreter can mediate these barriers by attending not only to the linguistic but also to the extra-linguistic aspects of communication. (Massachusetts Medical Interpreters Association, 1995)

The standards include guidance for (1) setting up and explaining the role of the interpreter at the outset of a medical encounter, (2) transmitting information accurately and completely, (3) managing the flow of communication among all participants in the encounter, (4) encouraging doctor and patient to address each other directly, and (5) assisting with closure activities (e.g., patient follow-up and referral instructions). By attending to issues related to culture, such as language barriers and cultural beliefs, the promise of integrated healthcare will have a greater chance of being realized.

CULTURAL EXPLANATORY MODELS

Cultural explanatory models (CEM), a term used by medical anthropologist Arthur Kleinman (Kleinman, Eisenberg, & Good, 1978), refers to socioculturally based belief systems that individuals hold. Beliefs held by health professionals who follow a biomedical model are based on empirical, observable, measurable, objective, individualistic, absolute, and rational tenets. On the other hand, lay individuals' CEMs are vague, dynamic, have emotional meaning, and are embedded in a person's sociocultural context (i.e., cultural beliefs, socioeconomic factors, and community social networks; Rajaram & Rashidi, 1998). CEMs relate to the way individuals conceptualize an illness, its causes, signs and symptoms, modes of prevention and diagnosis, treatment, prognosis, and roles and expectations of the patient. Therefore the goal of healthcare encounters, disease detection, or health promotion may vary across cultures and individuals. For example, assumptions may differ about roles and expectations of the patient and the healer across cultures. In traditional Chinese medicine, healers did not get paid if the patient became sick.

In contrast with traditional Western conceptualizations of health promotion that focus on rational-cognitive considerations, the growing health behavioral literature (Snider & Satcher, 1997) suggests that emotional-affective considerations (Millar & Millar, 1995) may be equally important in promoting health. In fact, traditional theoretical models of health behavior have been criticized on the grounds that they emphasize the role of rationality in health promotion behaviors. In a review of the literature, Rajaram and Rashidi (1998) discussed shortcomings of the health belief model (Rosenstock, 1974), theory of reasoned action (Fishbein & Ajzen, 1975), protection motivation theory (Rogers, 1983), and subjective expected utility theory (Edwards, 1954). Common themes among these models are perception of risks and benefits, perceived severity of illness, and perceived efficacy of personal action. Viewed from a cultural perspective, shortcomings include the following: (1) models are primarily based on cognition and do not include emotional aspects of help seeking and affect; (2) risk perceptions are viewed as separate from an individual's sociocultural context; (3) risk perceptions are based on a Western medical model such that a patient's knowledge about a condition is compared with established biomedical and epidemiological norms, resulting in a deficit approach; and (4) the influence of gender, race, and social class has not been integrated sufficiently into the models.

An integrated, universal health promotion healthcare strategy would be more consistent with worldviews of health held by many, would improve behavioral motivation to pursue health, would lead to closing the gap in life-threatening health disparities, and would foster improvement in individuals' health across this nation. Specifically, a culturally relevant collaborative or integrative approach to healthcare delivery addresses two major deficits in the current system: (1) the challenges in physicians' sensitivity to cultural issues in the presentation of medical concerns and (2) the challenges that physicians have in identifying underlying psychological manifestations in the presentation of physical ailments. In addition, an integrative model of care leads to a more efficient system of care, with fewer stigmas attached to receiving mental health services, while fostering the development of closer relationships between primary care providers and patients.

INTEGRATIVE HEALTHCARE

Integrative healthcare reflects a combination of traditional European-influenced allopathic treatment, complementary and alternative medicine

(CAM), and behavioral health treatment (see Jones, 2005, for a classification of health treatments). The European-influenced allopathic treatment primarily involves a medical model where the illness resides in the patient, with a specific healthcare expert working toward curing/removing the disease using drugs or surgery that are incompatible with the diagnosed disease. Modern healthcare portrays this as a partnership in which the client takes responsibility for prevention and cooperation with the prescribed treatment, which often involves self-administration of medication. Under this model, the mind (mental health) is considered separate from the body (physical health). However, the social context of the doctor-patient relationship has changed with the implementation of managed care, increased public access to health information, and awareness of malpractice (Fredericks, Odiet, Miller, & Fredericks, 2006). With the advent of behavioral medicine, mental health approaches have been integrated into traditional European-influenced treatment protocols. Three examples of integrative healthcare will be discussed, and ways in which these systems can provide culturally responsive care will be presented.

Integrative healthcare includes a combination of both medical and behavioral health services (Kenkel, DeLeon, Mantell, & Steep, 2005). As many patients in primary care settings continue to deal with underlying psychological concerns, such as stress, anxiety, depression, and other health-related issues, the importance of incorporating psychological healthcare providers as part of primary medical settings is essential.

Overall, initial reports indicate that integrated models of healthcare delivery address the most salient issues facing the current healthcare delivery model today (Kenkel et al., 2005). To duplicate these services, it is important to understand the infrastructure of already existing collaborative models of care to further expand this growing area for primary care physicians and psychological service providers.

The most effective models of integrative healthcare are provided when mental health providers share the same space as primary care physicians. This allows for all providers in charge of healthcare services to patients to collaborate more efficiently, see clients conjointly, and determine treatment plans in a more timely manner than when access to providers involves separation in time and space (Aitken & Curtis, 2004). Blount (2003) reviewed 60 integrated healthcare studies and found that integrated care improved clinical outcomes, increased client and provider satisfaction, and improved cost-effectiveness. Integrated care is a fast-growing area that is currently being implemented in family practice, internal medicine, obstetrics, and pediatrics (Aitken & Curtis, 2004). Integrated models of delivery are identified as either nontargeted or targeted. Nontargeted practices include more general services to a broader array of clients, whereas targeted practices provide services to those who are experiencing a specific concern (e.g., cancer; Aitken & Curtis, 2004).

Nontargeted Model of Care

In this model, mental health providers assume a case management approach to mental health concerns, and physicians are the primary care providers for patients. Mental health providers assess for mental illness, connect clients to appropriate services, and provide time-limited treatment (Aitken & Curtis, 2004). Additionally, to establish a more egalitarian power structure, most models create a paradigm shift for both physicians and mental health providers by equalizing the terminology used. For example, in one setting, all professional staff are called "clinicians": physicians are called "primary care clinicians," and mental health providers are called "behavioral health clinicians" (Aitken & Curtis, 2004). In another model, mental health providers are called "healthcare providers" or "consultants" (Kenkel et al., 2005).

Lesser (2000) described a nontargeted model of care in which comprehensive family medical care and mental health services are provided to a diverse community. The practice consists of a physician, two social workers, a psychologist, a consulting psychiatrist, and a nurse practitioner. The mental health services provided include individual, group, and family counseling; support groups; psychoeducational groups; and case management. As a result of this collaborative service delivery, clients have fully utilized the mental health service component.

Another model of nontargeted healthcare delivery was presented by Munsey (2006). The author described the workings of an ongoing collaboration between a psychology doctoral training program and a local community center predominantly serving the poor and uninsured or underinsured. In the model used in this setting, psychologists treat the mental health needs of the patients, allowing physicians to spend more time and energy with the patients' medical issues; approximately 80 percent of the patients seen in this setting have behavioral health needs (Munsey, 2006). The model represents ongoing efforts by the American Psychological Association's Education Directorate and local communities and provides graduate training for students in psychology to learn how primary care settings function and to better prepare them for the changing healthcare delivery system. This model operates like most other integrated healthcare models: instead of providing the traditional 50-minute sessions off-site, psychologists occupy the same physical space as other healthcare providers and coordinate in 15-minute blocks with the time physicians see patients to ensure prompt consultation whenever needed. Physicians and psychologists also schedule several time blocks throughout the day when they can see patients jointly. In addition, psychologists work together with physicians on psychotropic medication management. Overall, the model appears to be filling a great need for services among poor, underinsured individuals who may not otherwise receive the mental health treatment necessary to lead medically and psychologically healthy lives.

Targeted Model of Care

An example of a targeted model of care can also include a combination of nurses, social workers, counselors, and psychologists who provide counseling, education, and case management. Most mental health providers are located in-house or on contract to provide frequent on-site treatment. Much like in the nontargeted models, there is ongoing collaboration among professionals. McQuellon, Hurt, and DeChatelet (1996) provided an example of a targeted cancer patient program comprising a psychologist, a director, two master's-level counselors, and 25 volunteers. The program also has 75 community volunteers who provide fundraising support for the program. The overall goal of the program is to provide psychological services to cancer patients and their families through an orientation program and individual, group, and family counseling. In addition, case management services are provided, along with psychoeducational programs and child care. The psychologists' primary responsibilities include, but are not limited to, consultation, research, individual and group counseling, program coordination, psychological evaluation, and supervision of practicum and internship students.

Nontargeted and targeted models are a start to remedying the challenges in providing comprehensive, destigmatized services to ethnic and racial populations, but simply integrating services is not enough. To be culturally responsive, collaborative models must ensure that their service delivery model represents the populations they serve and that providers are culturally trained.

Complementary and Alternative Medicine

CAM is identified by Keith, Kronenfeld, Rivers, and Liang (2005) as including acupuncture, nutritional advice, massage therapy, herbal remedies, biofeedback, meditation training, homeopathic therapy, spiritual healing, hypnosis, and/or traditional cultural medicine. While these treatment approaches are considered nontraditional by people of European descent, many are integral to treatment that is culturally relevant to members of marginalized populations in the United States (e.g., acupuncture is a traditional Chinese medical technique). These CAM approaches do not include, however, religious healing traditions (such as prayer, shamanism, or distance healing) that are very likely to be used by large numbers of people, but are not documented as healthcare (Jones, 2005; Yoon, 2006). Although these treatments have roots in several cultures, Keith et al. (2005) found that "whites were most likely to use CAM therapies, followed by Asians, Hispanics, and African Americans, in that order" (p. 27); however, they were unable to discern patterns that might indicate why there were such ethnic differences.

It is important to understand that for many people, traditional healing is the only sensible approach to treatment. Joe (2003) noted that while this is critical, there is a negative history based on European-imposed values:

> The role of traditional tribal healing is especially important in health promotion because the concept of health for most tribes is wellness centered, enforced by social rules of behavior and taboos intended to help prevent illness or misfortune. Use of traditional tribal healing and its practitioners, however, was not always accepted by non-Indian healthcare providers. In fact, some healing practices were outlawed by the federal government in the late-nineteenth century at the urging of missionaries who deemed such practices as barbaric and un-Christian. (pp. 538–539)

To continue some traditional healing practices, it is critical that attention be paid to the environment to ensure the survival of plants and herbs used for treatment:

> The loss of access to traditional environments or ecosystems and the historical suppression of religious and medical practices also threaten the body of knowledge developed from plants and herbs. The fact that the IHS endorses the use of traditional healing practices in combination with Western medicine to treat patients in its facilities—for example, most Indian hospitals allow smoke detectors to be disconnected so that the practice of smudging can occur—is a cooperative activity that may help mitigate this. Sharing facilities in this manner not only may help foster and preserve American Indian/Alaska Native heritage, but also may expose IHS health professionals to non-Western healing practices from which they may be able to learn. (Leigh & Huff, 2006, p. 7)

In sum, a holistic health worldview appears across many ethnic communities in this country and around the world (Pachuta, 1993; Ramaswami & Sheikh, 1993), yet a disease- and specialty-oriented healthcare system in Western countries may account for some of the health disparities in the United States. A holistic or more integrated delivery of healthcare may improve healthcare overall and, in particular, the health of those who disproportionately suffer from poorer outcomes.

CULTURAL COMPETENCE IN HEALTHCARE

There is documented evidence that healthcare providers receive inadequate training with respect to cultural issues (Weissman et al., 2005). With only brief introductions to "cultural competence," practitioners are at risk for making impersonal misdiagnoses based on inaccurate application of learned stereotypes (Good et al., 2003). In fact, research suggests that the lack of culturally sensitive care provided to ethnic and racial individuals negatively impacts quality of care, leads to misunderstandings in the medical encounter, and further extends health disparities (Nápoles-Springer, Santoyo, Houston, Pérez-Stable, & Stewart, 2005).

Cross, Bazron, Dennis, and Isaacs (1989) described a culturally competent system of care in which a healthcare system incorporates, at all levels, the inclusion of cultural factors. The model includes six stages or levels: (1) cultural destructiveness, (2) cultural incapacity, (3) cultural blindness, (4) cultural precompetence, (5) cultural competence, and (6) cultural proficiency. A culturally destructive system of care adheres to attitudes, policies, and procedures that actively deny the cultural realities of individuals and groups, in other words, one that purports that one ethnicity/race is superior to another. An example of this system includes denying people access to their natural helpers or healers (Cross et al., 1989). A culturally incapacitated system, on the other hand, includes a system that does not actively engage in cultural destructiveness, but simply does not have the capacity or resources to help ethnic and racial communities. These agencies are biased in that they believe in the superiority of dominant culture helping practices. Incapacitated systems remain insensitive to multicultural individuals and may enforce racist policies, discriminate in their hiring policies, and lower expectations of their ethnic and racial clients (Cross et al., 1989).

Culturally blind systems function under the universality worldview, or the belief that we are all the same and that culture makes no difference. The practices in the system reflect the belief that all dominant practices can be applied to everyone in an equally effective way. The challenge in this system is that services are seldom effective for unacculturated or unassimilated individuals. These systems encourage assimilation, blame the victims for their problems, and ignore cultural strengths (Cross et al., 1989). Ethnic and racial individual problems are viewed from a culturally deprived model, in which providers believe that these individuals lack cultural resources, and institutional racism interferes with the proper training of staff and culturally relevant delivery of services. These systems tend to view themselves as culturally liberal and responsive, but their narrow ethnocentric perspective is reflected in their attitudes, policies, and practices.

In contrast, culturally precompetent models have taken the initial steps toward cultural responsiveness. These systems recognize their weaknesses, make attempts to improve them, hire minority staff, initiate training for staff in the area of cultural sensitivity, and recruit ethnic/racial individuals at all levels of the organizational structure. The accomplishment of one goal in this system may provide a sense that the system has prematurely reached its goal, and therefore efforts toward further growth may stop. Additionally, these systems may give up after an unsuccessful attempt at accomplishing one goal.

A culturally competent model of care accepts and respects difference, continuously expands on its cultural knowledge and resources, and adapts its services to reflect the needs of the communities it serves. The system views cultural groups as distinctly different, with specific subgroup characteristics. In addition, mechanisms are in place for providers to continuously seek consultation from the ethnic and racial communities they serve and to provide support to staff who work in cross-cultural environments. Finally, a culturally proficient model of care holds culture in high regard. These systems provide leadership in the areas of research and in the development of new culturally responsive intervention strategies and therapeutic approaches. Staff in this system are hired because of their expertise in the area of culturally sensitive and responsive practices. Culturally proficient systems advocate for improved relations among cultures throughout society and between society and the systems of care.

As the previous sections show, for the healthcare delivery system to adequately meet the needs of the growing culturally diverse populations, it must (1) redesign its current practices and (2) encourage the development of integrated healthcare delivery systems that are culturally sensitive and responsive. To encourage the development of one without the other will continue to leave underrepresented groups feeling misunderstood, misdiagnosed, untreated, and in poor health.

ENHANCING INTEGRATED HEALTHCARE FOR MARGINALIZED POPULATIONS

Clearly there is a great need to enhance the healthcare services provided to marginalized populations. Below, we discuss three important facets of such an endeavor: the promotion of integrated healthcare, enhanced training, and research.

Promoting Integrated Healthcare

A 2005 report from the Institute of Medicine indicated that integrative approaches to healthcare are being used by hospitals with a specific emphasis on cancer treatment (Committee on the Use of Complementary and Alternative Medicine, 2005). In that report, however, it was noted that there was a lack of information about how such programs were reaching members of marginalized populations. To gauge the effectiveness of programs such as these in reaching underserved populations, it is critical that information on race/ethnicity, gender, and ability status be obtained and used in the preparation of statistical reports.

Another area that must be addressed is the implementation of health policy that supports the notion that integrated healthcare delivery systems and subsystems may be essential to closing gaps in health outcomes. Moreover, attention must be directed to the issue of inequity between reimbursement for physical health conditions as compared with expenditures for treatment of mental health conditions. Parity in reimbursement for physical health and mental health conditions must be addressed at the policy level. Ultimately, although cost is always of concern, costs could be capped, no matter whether physical or mental health services are used. Those who suffer from mental health conditions should not be treated as "less than." In fact, a significant health disparity is the lack of equity in funds used for research and treatment of mental illnesses.

Training

The diversity of healthcare professionals, including the previously European American–dominated medical field, has increased dramatically in some areas of the United States since the early 1990s. Although this is encouraging, there is an ongoing need to increase the number of people from marginalized populations in the healthcare professions (Noonan & Evans, 2003; Smedley, Stith, & Bristow, 2004). Moreover, the training received by healthcare providers has been inadequate and slow to change: "Failure to attend to social context may not only have adverse consequences in case formulation and treatment decision-making, but may also contribute to the disenfranchisement of ethnic minority populations relative to their healthcare" (Good et al., 2003, p. 608).

Good et al. (2003) noted that as of late, medical training programs include information on cultural competence but neglect to examine the interaction of healthcare with institutional and aversive racism (Dovidio, Gaertner, Kawakami, & Hodson, 2002). Healthcare professionals have complained that they were trained to focus only on specific presenting medical problems to *quickly* diagnose and treat; they found the real-world problems faced by members of marginalized populations to be distracting and disruptive to the "simple" diagnostic process. As a result, they failed to refer such "difficult" clients for the newest treatments (Good et al., 2003). An integrated healthcare model is likely to ameliorate some of these documented problems.

Research

Importantly, research must examine the health outcomes for minority populations under integrated healthcare systems. There must be more evidence-based research on integrated healthcare, and a special effort is needed to provide data on the promise of integrated healthcare to close the gap in disparities in mental health services.

CONCLUSION

As the number of ethnically and racially distinct individuals continues to grow throughout the United States, it has become increasingly important that we address the lack of appropriate healthcare, the role of culture in healthcare practices and attitudes (Betancourt & Ananeh-Firempong, 2004; Penn, Kar, Kramer, Skinner, & Zambrana, 1995; Shi & Stevens, 2005), the role of CAM (Keith et al., 2005; Silenzio, 2002), and affordable access to healthcare for all. Additionally, as the population has diversified, the literature has addressed the need to examine providers' biased and racist attitudes toward certain ethnic and racial groups *and their cultural health practices,* as this impacts diagnoses, treatment methodologies employed, and the development of culturally responsive, inclusive, and sensitive approaches to healthcare (Johnson, Saha, Arbelaez, Beach, & Cooper, 2004; Nápoles-Springer et al., 2005; Ridley, Chih, & Olivera, 2000). Without this framework and understanding, health disparities in the United States will continue to flourish, and the economically challenged and culturally diverse will continue to suffer (Betancourt & Ananeh-Firempong, 2004).

TOOL KIT FOR CHANGE

Role and Perspective of the Healthcare Professional

1. Training in cultural sensitivity for the healthcare provider must go beyond an introduction to stereotypes and include education about the historical precedents for inequitable treatment of individuals from different cultures.
2. Healthcare providers must be given the opportunity to examine and understand the biases they bring to the healthcare setting.
3. Healthcare providers must be willing to challenge their own understanding and training in addressing the healthcare of individuals from cultures different from the provider's own.

Role and Perspective of the Patient/Participant

1. Patients must attempt to communicate about their own individual needs and issues with their healthcare provider.
2. If healthcare providers are not responsive, patients should seek an alliance with friends, family, or community advocates whenever possible to address the communication of healthcare needs and issues.
3. Patients need to be willing to participate in research that is culturally relevant to both healthcare recipients and providers.

Interconnection: The Global Perspective

1. Cultural sensitivity needs to be built into all aspects of healthcare.
2. Research on health and healthcare must be continued and expanded. Research on traditional European-influenced allopathic treatment, psychological care, and CAM, both separately and in combination, is needed.
3. Research must go beyond client satisfaction and examine actual health outcomes to address health disparities.

REFERENCES

Abraído-Lanza, A. F., Armbrister, A. N., Flórez, K. R., & Aguirre, A. N. (2006). Toward a theory-driven model of acculturation in public health research. *American Journal of Public Health, 96,* 1342–1346.

Abraído-Lanza, A. F., Chao, M. T., & Flórez, K. (2005). Do healthy behaviors decline with greater acculturation?: Implications for the Latino mortality paradox. *Social Science and Medicine, 61,* 1243–1255.

Ackerman, R. J., & Banks, M. E. (2007). Caregiving. In V. Muhlbauer & J. C. Chrisler (Eds.), *Women over 50: Psychological perspectives.* New York: Springer.

Aitken, J. B., & Curtis, R. (2004). Integrated health care: Improving client care while providing opportunities for mental health counselors. *Journal of Mental Health Counseling, 26,* 321–331.

Alegria, M., Takeuchi, D. T., Canino, G., Duan, N., Shrout, P., Meng, X-L., et al. (2006). Considering context, place and culture. The National Latino and Asian American Study. *International Journal of Methods in Psychiatric Research, 13,* 208–220.

Asian and Pacific Islander Health Forum. (2000). *Asian and Pacific Islander socioeconomic status: U.S. immigration and citizenship data.* Retrieved October 1, 2006, from http://www.apiahf.com/cic/state_ins.asp?stateID=00

Baker, D. W., Hayes, R., & Fortier, J. P. (1998). Interpreter use and satisfaction with interpersonal aspects of care for Spanish-speaking patients. *Medical Care, 36,* 1461–1470.

Banks, M. E. (2007). Women with disabilities, domestic violence against. In N. A. Jackson (Ed.), *Encyclopedia of Domestic Violence.* New York: Taylor and Francis.

Banks, M. E., & Ackerman, R. J. (2006). Health disparities: Focus on disability. In K. J. Hagglund & A. W. Heinemann (Eds.), *Advances in disability and rehabilitation research* (pp. 45–70). New York: Springer.

Berry, J. W. (1980). Acculturation as varieties of adaptation. In A. Padilla (Ed.), *Acculturation: Theory, models, and some new findings.* Boulder, CO: Westview.

Berry, J. W., & Sam, D. (1997). Acculturation and adaptation. In J. W. Berry, M. H. Segall, & C. Kagitcibasi (Eds.), *Handbook of cross-cultural psychology: Social behavior and applications* (2nd ed., pp. 291–326). Boston: Allyn and Bacon.

Betancourt, J. R., & Ananeh-Firempong, O. (2004). Not me! Doctors, decisions, and disparities in health care. *Cardiovascular Review, 25,* 105–109.

Bierman, A. S., Lurie, N., Collins, K. S., & Eisenberg, J. M. (2002). Addressing racial and ethnic barriers to effective health care: The need for better data. *Health Affairs, 21,* 91–102.

Blount, A. (2003). Integrated primary care: Organizing the evidence. *Families, Systems, and Health, 21,* 121–133.

Braun, K., Yee, B. W. K., Browne, C. V., & Mokuau, N. (2004). Native Hawaiian and Pacific Islander elders. In K. E. Whitfield (Ed.), *Closing the gap: Improving the health of minority elders in the new millennium* (pp. 9–34). Washington, DC: Gerontological Society of America.

Brett, K. M., & Hayes, S. G. (2004). *Women's health and mortality chartbook.* Washington, DC: DHHS Office on Women's Health. Retrieved October 9, 2006, from http://www.cdc.gov/nchs/data/healthywomen/coverplus.pdf

Buki, L. P. (1999). Early detection of breast and cervical cancer among medically underserved Latinas. In M. Sotomayor & A. García (Eds.), *La familia: Traditions and realities* (pp. 67–85). Washington, DC: National Hispanic Council on Aging.

Buki, L. P., Borrayo, A. E., Feigal, B., & Carrillo, I. Y. (2004). Are all Latinas the same? Perceived breast screening barriers and facilitative conditions. *Psychology of Women Quarterly, 28,* 400–411.

Byrd, W. M., & Clayton, L. A. (2003). Racial and ethnic disparities in healthcare: A background and history. In B. D. Smedley, A. Y. Stith, & A. R. Nelson (Eds.), *Unequal treatment: Confronting racial and ethnic disparities in health care* (pp. 455–527). Washington, DC: National Academies Press.

Carmalt, J., & Zaidi, S. (2004). *The right to health in the United States of America: What does it mean?* Brooklyn, NY: Center for Economic and Social Rights. Retrieved October 9, 2006, from http://cesr.org/ushealthright

Centers for Disease Control and Prevention. (1994). *Chronic disease in minority populations.* Atlanta: Author.

Chen, S. W. H., & Davenport, D. S. (2005). Cognitive-behavioral therapy with Chinese American clients: Cautions and modifications. *Psychotherapy: Theory, Research, Practice, Training, 42,* 101–110.

Chumney, E. C. G., Mauldin, P. D., & Simpson, K. N. (2006). Charges for hospital admissions attributable to health disparities for African-American patients: 1998–2002. *Journal of the National Medical Association, 98,* 690–694.

Committee on the Use of Complementary and Alternative Medicine, American Public Board on Health Promotion and Disease Prevention. (2005). *Complementary and alternative medicine in the United States.* Washington, DC: National Academies Press.

Corbett, C. A. (2003). Special issues in psychotherapy for minority deaf women. In M. E. Banks & E. Kaschak (Eds.), *Women with visible and invisible disabilities: Multiple intersections, multiple issues, multiple therapies* (pp. 311–329). New York: Haworth Press.

Cross, T. L., Bazron, B. J., Dennis, K. W., & Isaacs, M. R. (1989). *Towards a culturally competent system of care* (Vol. 1). Washington, DC: Georgetown University Child Development Center / CASSP Technical Assistance Center.

Dotson, L. A., Stinson, J., & Christian, L. (2003). "People tell me I can't have sex": Women with disabilities share their personal perspectives on health care, sexuality, and reproductive rights. In M. E. Banks & E. Kaschak (Eds.), *Women with visible and invisible disabilities: Multiple intersections, multiple issues, multiple therapies* (pp. 195–209). New York: Haworth Press.

Dovidio, J. F., Gaertner, S. E., Kawakami, K., & Hodson, G. (2002). Why can't we just get along?: Interpersonal biases and interracial distrust. *Cultural Diversity and Ethnic Minority Psychology, 8,* 88–102.

Dower, C. (2003). *Health care interpreters in California.* San Francisco: UCSF Center for the Health Professions.

DuBois, W. E. B. (1935). *Black reconstruction.* New York: Harcourt Brace Jovanovich.

Echemendia, R. J., & Julian, L. (2002). Neuropsychological assessment of Latino children. In F. R. Ferraro (Ed.), *Minority and cross-cultural aspects of neuropsychological assessment* (pp. 181–203). Heereweg, Netherlands: Swets and Zeitlinger.

Edwards, W. (1954). The theory of decision making. *Psychological Bulletin, 51,* 380–417.

Fishbein, M., & Ajzen, I. (1975). *Belief, attitude, intention, and behavior: An introduction to theory and research.* Reading, MA: Addison-Wesley.

Fredericks, M., Odiet, J. A., Miller, S. I., & Fredericks, J. (2006). Toward a conceptual reexamination of the patient-physician relationship in the new millennium. *Journal of the National Medical Association, 98,* 378–385.

Freimuth, V. S., Quinn, S. C., Thomas, S. B., Cole, G. E., Zook, E., & Duncan, T. (2001). African Americans' views on research and the Tuskegee syphilis study. *Social Science and Medicine, 54,* 797–808.

Gonzalez Castro, F., & Hernandez, N. T. (2004). A cultural perspective on prevention interventions. In R. J. Velasquez, L. M. Arellano, & B. W. McNeill (Eds.), *The handbook of Chicana/o psychology and mental health* (pp. 371–397). Mahwah, NJ: Lawrence Erlbaum.

Good, M.-J., DelVecchio, J. C., Good, B. J., & Becker, A. E. (2003). The culture of medicine and racial, ethnic, and class disparities in healthcare. In B. D. Smedley, A. Y. Stith, & A. R. Nelson (Eds.), *Unequal treatment: Confronting racial and ethnic disparities in health care* (pp. 594–625). Washington, DC: National Academies Press.

Hernandez, D. J., & Charney, E. (Eds.). (1998). *From generation to generation: The health and well-being of children in immigrant families.* Washington, DC: National Academies Press.

Joe, J. R. (2003). The rationing of healthcare and health disparity for the American Indians/Alaska Natives. In B. D. Smedley, A. Y. Stith, & A. R. Nelson (Eds.), *Unequal treatment: Confronting racial and ethnic disparities in health care* (pp. 528–551). Washington, DC: National Academies Press.

Johnson, R. L., Saha, S., Arbelaez, J. J., Beach, M. C., & Cooper, L. A. (2004). Racial and ethnic differences in patient perceptions of bias and cultural competence in health care. *Journal of General Internal Medicine, 19,* 101–110.

Jones, C. H. (2005). The spectrum of therapeutic influences and integrative health care: Classifying health care practices by mode of therapeutic action. *Journal of Alternative and Complementary Medicine, 11,* 937–944.

Kagawa-Singer, M., & Pourat, N. (2000). Asian American and Pacific Islander breast and cervical carcinoma screening rates and Healthy People 2000 objectives. *Cancer, 89,* 696–705.

Keith, V. M., Kronenfeld, J. J., Rivers, P. A., & Liang, S. Y. (2005). Assessing the effects of race and ethnicity on use of complementary and alternative therapies in the USA. *Ethnicity and Health, 10,* 19–32.

Kenkel, M. B., DeLeon, P. H., Mantell, E. O., & Steep, A. E. (2005). Divided no more: Psychology's role in integrated health care. *Canadian Psychology, 46,* 189–202.

Kim, C. (2000). Recruitment and retention in the Navajo area Indian Health Service. *Western Journal of Medicine, 173,* 240–243.

Kleinman, A., Eisenberg, L., & Good, B. (1978). Culture, illness, and care: Clinical lessons from anthropologic and cross-cultural research. *Annals of Internal Medicine, 88,* 251–258.

Leigh, W. A., & Huff, D. (2006). *Women of color health data book: Adolescents to seniors* (3rd ed., NIH Publication No. 06-4247). Bethesda, MD: Office of Research on Women's Health, National Institutes of Health.

Leigh, W. A., & Jimenez, M. A. (2002). *Women of color health data book* (2nd ed., NIH Publication No. 02-4247). Bethesda, MD: Office of Research on Women's Health, National Institutes of Health.

Lesser, J. F. (2000). Clinical social work and family medicine: A partnership in community service. *Health and Social Work, 25,* 119–126.

Lillie-Blanton, M., & Lewis, C. B. (2005, March). *Policy challenges and opportunities in closing the racial/ethnic divide in health care.* Washington, DC: Kaiser Family Foundation.

López-Gonzalez, L., Aravena, V. C., & Hummer, R. A. (2005). Immigrant acculturation, gender, and health behavior: A research note. *Social Forces, 84,* 581–593.

Manly, J. J., & Mayeux, R. (2004). Racial and ethnic disparities in health and mortality among the U.S. elderly population. In N. B. Anderson, R. A. Bulatao, & B. Cohen (Eds.), *Critical perspectives on racial and ethnic differences in health in late life* (pp. 95–141). Washington, DC: National Academies Press.

Massachusetts Medical Interpreters Association. (1995). *MMIA standards of practice.* Retrieved May 20, 2006, from http://www.mmia.org/standards/standards.asp

McCarthy, M. (1998). Sexual violence against women with learning disabilities. *Feminism and Psychology, 8,* 544–551.

McQuellon, R. P., Hurt, G. J., & DeChatelet, P. (1996). Psychosocial care of the patient with cancer: A model for organizing services. *Cancer Practice, 4,* 304–311.

Meyers, L. (2006). Asian-American mental health. *Monitor on Psychology, 37,* 44–46.

Millar, J. G., & Millar, K. (1995). Negative affective consequences of thinking about disease detection behaviors. *Health Psychology, 14,* 141–146.

Miller, B. A., Kolonel, L. N., Bernstein, L., Young, J. L., Jr., Swanson, G. M., West, D., et al. (1996). *Racial/ethnic patterns of cancer in the United States 1988–1992.* Bethesda, MD: National Cancer Institute.

Mukherjee, D., Reis, J. P., & Heller, W. (2003). Women living with traumatic brain injury: Social isolation, emotional functioning, and implications for psychotherapy. In M. E. Banks & E. Kaschak (Eds.), *Women with visible and invisible disabilities: Multiple intersections, multiple issues, multiple therapies* (pp. 1–26). New York: Haworth Press.

Munsey, C. (2006). Making integrated health care a reality. *Monitor on Psychology, 37,* 24–26.

Nabors, N. A., & Pettee, M. F. (2003). Womanist therapy with African American women with disabilities. In M. E. Banks & E. Kaschak (Eds.), *Women with visible and invisible disabilities: Multiple intersections, multiple issues, multiple therapies* (pp. 331–341). New York: Haworth Press.

Nápoles-Springer, A. M., Santoyo, J., Houston, K., Pérez-Stable, E. J., & Stewart, A. L. (2005). Patients' perceptions of cultural factors affecting the quality of their medical encounter. *Health Expectations, 8,* 4–17.

National Academy on an Aging Society. (1999). Is demography destiny? *Public Policy and Aging Report, 9,* 1–14.

National Asian Women's Health Organization. (2000). *A profile: Cervical cancer and Asian American women.* Retrieved October 3, 2006, from http://www.nawho.org/pubs/NAWHOCC.pdf

National Center for Health Statistics. (2004). *Health, United States, 2004 with chartbook on trends in the health of Americans.* Washington, DC: U.S. Government Printing Office.

National Council of La Raza. (2004, February). *State of Hispanic America 2004: Latino perspectives on the American agenda.* Washington, DC: Author.

Noonan, A. S., & Evans, C. A. (2003). The need for diversity in the health professions. *Journal of Dental Education, 67,* 1030–1033.

North Carolina Institute of Medicine. (2003). The challenge of health promotion and health literacy in North Carolina's Latino population. In *NC Latino health 2003* (pp. 117–124). Durham: Author. Retrieved October 9, 2006, from http://www.nciom.org/projects/latino/latinopub/C8.pdf

Ong, P. M. (Ed.). (2000). *The state of Asian Pacific America—Transforming race relations: A public policy report* (Vol. 4). Los Angeles: LEAP Asian Pacific American Public Policy / UCLA Asian American Studies Center.

Pachuta, D. M. (1993). Chinese medicine: The law of five elements. In A. A. Sheikh & K. S. Sheikh (Eds.), *Eastern and Western approaches to healing: Ancient wisdom and modern knowledge* (pp. 64–90). New York: John Wiley.

Penn, N. E., Kar, S., Kramer, J., Skinner, J., & Zambrana, R. E. (1995). Panel VI: Ethnic minorities, health care systems, and behavior. *Health Psychology, 14,* 641–646.

Pew Hispanic Center. (2004). *Survey briefs: Assimilation and language.* Retrieved March 20, 2006, from http://pewhispanic.org/files/factsheets/11.pdf

Poulin, C., & Gouliquer, L. (2003). Part-time disabled lesbian passing on roller blades or PMS, Prozac, and essentializing women's ailments. In M. E. Banks & E. Kaschak (Eds.), *Women with visible and invisible disabilities: Multiple intersections, multiple issues, multiple therapies* (pp. 95–108). New York: Haworth Press.

Pukui, M. K., Haertig, E. W., & Lee, C. A. (1972). *Nana I Ke Kumu* (Vol. 1). Honolulu, HI: Hui Hanai.

Rajaram, S. S., & Rashidi, A. (1998). Minority women and breast cancer screening: The role of cultural explanatory models. *Preventive Medicine, 27,* 757–764.

Ramaswami, S., & Sheikh, A. A. (1993). Buddhist psychology: Implications for healing. In A. A. Sheikh & K. S. Sheikh (Eds.), *Eastern and Western approaches to healing: Ancient wisdom and modern knowledge* (pp. 91–123). New York: John Wiley.

Ridley, C. R., Chih, D. W., & Olivera, R. J. (2000). Training in cultural schemas: An antidote to unintentional racism in clinical practice. *American Journal of Orthopsychiatry, 70,* 65–72.

Rogers, R. W. (1983). Cognitive and physiological processes in fear appeals and attitude change: A revised theory of protection motivation. In J. Cacioppo & R. Petty (Eds.), *Social psychophysiology* (pp. 153–176). New York: Guilford Press.

Rosenstock, I. M. (1974). Historical origins of the health belief model. *Health Education Monographs, 4,* 328–335.

Rothenberg, P. S. (1992). *Race, class, and gender in the United States: An integrated study* (2nd ed.). New York: St. Martin's Press.

Rowe, J. W., & Kahn, R. L. (1998). *Successful aging.* New York: Pantheon Books.

Salganicoff, A., Ranji, U. R., & Wyn, R. (2005). *Women and health care: A national profile—Key findings from the Kaiser Women's Health Survey.* Washington, DC: Kaiser Family Foundation.

Santana-Martin, S., & Santana, F. O. (2005). An introduction to Mexican culture for service providers. In J. H. Stone (Ed.), *Culture and disability: Providing culturally competent services* (pp. 161–186). Thousand Oaks, CA: Sage.

Schneider, A. (2005). Reforming American Indian/Alaska Native health care financing: The role of Medicaid. *American Journal of Public Health, 95,* 766–768.

Shavers, V. L., & Shavers, B. S. (2006). Racism and health inequity among Americans. *Journal of the National Medical Association, 98,* 386–396.

Shi, L., & Stevens, G. D. (2005). Vulnerability and unmet health care needs. *Journal of General Internal Medicine, 20,* 148–154.

Silenzio, V. M. B. (2002). What is the role of complementary and alternative medicine in public health? *American Journal of Public Health, 92,* 1562–1564.

Smedley, B. D., Stith, A. Y., & Bristow, L. R. (2004). *In the nation's compelling interest: Ensuring diversity in the health care workforce.* Washington, DC: National Academies Press.

Smedley, B. D., Stith, A. Y., & Nelson, A. R. (Eds.). (2003). *Unequal treatment: Confronting racial and ethnic disparities in health care.* Washington, DC: National Academies Press.

Snider, D. E., & Satcher, D. (1997). Behavioral and social sciences at the Centers for Disease Control and Prevention. *American Psychologist, 52,* 140–142.

Stannard, D. E. (1992). *American holocaust: The conquest of the New World.* New York: Oxford University Press.

Stonequist, E. V. (1935). The problem of the marginal man. *American Journal of Sociology, 41,* 1–12.

Stonequist, E. V. (1937). *The marginal man: A study in personality and culture conflict.* New York: Russell and Russell.

United Nations. (1948, December 10). *Universal declaration of human rights.* Retrieved October 9, 2006, from http://www.unhchr.ch/udhr/lang/eng.pdf

U.S. Census Bureau. (2005a). *Facts for features and special editions: Hispanic heritage month: September 15–October 15.* Retrieved September 22, 2005, from http://www.census.gov/Press-Release/www/releases/archives/facts_for_features_special_editions/005338.html.

U.S. Census Bureau. (2005b). *Foreign-born population tops 34 million, U.S. Census Bureau estimates.* Retrieved March 28, 2007, from http://www.census.gov/Press-Release/www/releases/archives/foreignborn_population/003969.html

U.S. Department of Health and Human Services, Agency for Healthcare Research and Quality. (2002, March). *AHRQ focus on research: Disparities in health care* (AHRQ Publication No. 02-M027). Retrieved June 15, 2005, from http://www.ahrq.gov/news/focus/disparhc.htm.

U.S. Department of Health and Human Services, Agency for Healthcare Research and Quality. (2005, December). *2005 national healthcare disparities report.* Rockville, MD: Author.

Weissman, J. S., Betancourt, J., Campbell, E. G., Park, E. R., Kim, M., Clarridge, B., et al. (2005). Resident physicians' preparedness to provide cross-cultural care. *Journal of the American Medical Association, 294,* 1058–1067.

Williams, M., & Upadhyay, W. S. (2003). To be or not be disabled. In M. E. Banks & E. Kaschak (Eds.), *Women with visible and invisible disabilities: Multiple intersections, multiple issues, multiple therapies* (pp. 145–154). New York: Haworth Press.

Yoon, S. L. (2006). Racial/ethnic differences in self-reported health problems and herbal use among older women. *Journal of the National Medical Association, 98,* 918–925.

Zea, M. C., Asner-Self, K. K., Birman, D., & Buki, L. P. (2003). The Abbreviated Multidimensional Acculturation Scale: Empirical validation with two Latino/a samples. *Cultural Diversity and Ethnic Minority Psychology, 9,* 107–126.

Chapter Nine

INTEGRATIVE HEALTHCARE AND EDUCATION FOR CHILDREN: A HEALTHCARE COMMUNITY PERSPECTIVE

Marie A. DiCowden, PhD, Mark L. De Santis, PsyD, and Tristan Haddad DiCowden, MS

CHANGING ISSUES AND NEEDS IN CHILDREN'S HEALTH AND EDUCATION

Over the next 20 years, the numerical majority of the population of the United States will consist of an aggregate mix of various racial and ethnic groups that are today considered minorities (Hernandez, 2004). South Florida presents a microcosm of the changing demographics of the United States. The Miami community, in particular, presents a unique challenge in addressing the needs of children and families that are foreign-born. In the last 10 years, the population of Miami-Dade County grew by 16 percent to 2,250,000. The Hispanic population increased by 36 percent. Currently, immigrants and people of color make up over 60 percent of the Miami-Dade population ("Market Research," 2006), reflecting the overall growing trend in the remainder of the United States.

This growth has put tremendous pressure on the health and educational infrastructure of the south Florida area. In May 2002 the Miami-Dade Immigrant Health Task Force reported that 25 percent of the population in the county did not have health insurance. A disproportionate share of the uninsured were people of color and immigrants (Doonan, 2002). And just two years earlier, the U.S. Department of Education (2000) cited Miami as "one of the busiest 'gateway' points for new immigrants as well as a center of southern migration." This source also reported that Miami-Dade education officials stated that 41 percent of their schools were at least 150 percent over capacity. Eighty-four thousand students had to attend school in portable classrooms, and it was estimated that it was necessary to build one elementary school a month just to keep up with the influx of new immigrants (U.S. Department of Education, 2000).

Miami-Dade is the fourth largest school district in the United States. As of November 2005, it had a student enrollment of 421,467. It is also the largest district in the country with a minority population in school. Sixty percent of students are of Hispanic origin, 28 percent are African American, and 3 percent listed as nonwhite of other minorities (U.S. Census Bureau, 2005–2006). Add to this the fact that Florida has 375,000 students with special education needs. Eleven percent of the students with special needs reside in Miami-Dade County, and most come from immigrant families. The combined educational and healthcare needs are staggering. In addition to the sheer need for services, cultural competence as to how such services are delivered becomes increasingly important. The manner in which people from different cultures perceive and address the meaning of special education needs, illness, and rehabilitation varies (U.S. Public Health Service, 2006).

Miami-Dade also covers one of the largest geographical areas of any school district in the country. This creates problems educationally: "Recent studies strongly suggest that size does matter and that students, teachers, parents and taxpayers are all better off where school districts are smaller in size. . . . Negative impacts of large school districts outweigh the positive" (Schmidt & Schlottman, 2006, p. 7). Size also creates problems in healthcare. Jackson Memorial Hospital, a teaching hospital for the University of Miami School of Medicine, is located in the center of Miami. It is the primary receiving hospital for the uninsured, regardless of in what section of Miami-Dade County they reside—assuming they can arrive at the emergency room. The sheer size of land as well as the population of the district create serious problems for quality delivery of educational and healthcare services (Nieves, 2003).

Children with special needs suffer the greatest losses from declining quality in education and healthcare. Overcrowded classrooms, improper diagnoses, lag in assessments, poorly trained teachers, and fragmented rehabilitation services all militate against a child's increase in functioning cognitively, physically, and emotionally. To help address the needs of this population, Florida established the John McKay Scholarship program in 1999. The McKay Scholarship is a state- and federally funded voucher program. It allows students with special education needs with an individualized education plan (IEP) to attend a school that may best meet their needs. This can be a different public school from their assigned home school or a state-approved private school.

Over the last six years, the movement to institute vouchers for education has created a vociferous debate. Proponents of the voucher system have cited the increased personal attention and enhanced quality of education that students can receive in private schools through voucher-funded programs (Howell & Greene, 2005; Greene, 2001a, 2001b, 2003; Greene & Forster, 2003; Greene,

Peterson & Du, 1998; Rouse, 1998). Opponents claim that vouchers take much-needed funds out of public schools and that this decreases the quality of overall public education. Additionally, they say that there is no proof that voucher-funded programs actually provide a better education for the children who make use of the system.

These laws have also created serious concern about the private religious schools that receive public funding for education. Opponents see such funding as a violation of the separation of church and state. In some cases, for example, the Florida Constitution, public funding to religious institutions is directly or indirectly prohibited to maintain separation of religious and state matters. Consequently, in Florida, where the statewide voucher program was instituted, court battles on this issue have ensued. In January 2006, the Florida Supreme Court held that vouchers to enable parents to remove their children from so-called failing schools were unconstitutional. However, legal opponents of vouchers for failing schools did not challenge the right of parents to use vouchers for special needs students. In fact, no case has challenged the McKay Scholarship legislation. The leaders of opponents to vouchers have indicated, in public press statements, that they have no intention of challenging vouchers for special needs children (Klas, 2006). Apparently, there is a general acknowledgment that children with special needs require more than traditional schooling can provide.

At the same time, however, the concepts of mainstreaming and inclusion are important in education. There has been as much controversy about full inclusion over the last 20 years as there has been about vouchers for education. The Information Center on Disabilities and Gifted Education of the Council for Exceptional Children Web site (http://www.ideapractices. org) lists an extensive bibliography and a number of links to other Web sites discussing the pros and cons of inclusive school programs. They introduce the Web site by citing from the *Handbook for Successful Inclusion* (Kochbar, West, & Taymans, 1999):

> Age- and grade-appropriate placement is the most controversial component of inclusion because it is based on ideals, values, and goals that are not congruent with the realities of today's classrooms. Proponents of full inclusion assume that the general education classroom can and will be able to accommodate all students with disabilities, even those with severe and multiple disabilities. They assume that such students can obtain educational and social benefits from that placement. Those who oppose full inclusion argue that, although methods of collaborative learning and group instruction are the preferred methods, the traditional classroom size and resources are often inadequate for the management and accommodation of many students with disabilities without producing adverse effects on the classroom as a whole. Some special education experts, however, believe that some students are unlikely to receive appropriate education without placement into alternative instructional groups or alternative learning environments, such as part-time or full-time special classes or alternative day schools.

Discussion of inclusion on the Wisconsin Education Association Council Web site (Stout, 2001) indicates a prime concern that inclusive settings "ensure that sufficient licensed practitioners are employed to address the social, emotional, and cognitive needs of all students. In inclusive settings, reduced class sizes and/or increased numbers of teachers in the classroom are necessary." They go on to state that "real inclusion involves restructuring of a school's entire program." The John McKay Scholarship program provides the mechanism for just such a restructuring to occur in Florida schools.

The Manhattan Institute Study's *Vouchers for Special Education Students: An Evaluation of Florida's McKay Scholarship Program* (Greene & Forster, 2003) is one study that has attempted to examine the impact of vouchers on the structure of education for children with special needs. This is a significant study since the Florida Special Education Program is the second largest in the country, with 375,000 eligible students. The Manhattan Institute report found that behavior problems and victimization of special education students dropped when students were placed in private, voucher-funded programs. It also indicated that delivery of services identified on IEPs increased significantly. Satisfaction of parents with special needs children and satisfaction of the students themselves also increased when the children attended voucher-funded schools. Satisfaction for children with special needs was 32.7 percent for those who attended public schools and 92.7 percent for McKay participants.

Literature from the fields of both psychology and education indicates that children with special needs require a broad-based approach to address behavioral management, emotional issues, and specific learning styles. The principles and organization of services such as behavior modification, individual and group psychotherapy, and other needed services coordinated within the school setting contribute significantly to the child's successful learning and adaptation (Roberts, Jacobs, Puddy, Nye, & Vernberg, 2003). Cognitive behavior modification, group therapy, and social skills training within the school setting have long been documented as effective and essential to decrease aggression, hyperactivity, and impulsivity and to increase academic progress, prosocial behavior, and the emotional well-being of students with special needs (Kulic, Horne, & Dagley, 2004; Lovaas, 1987; Mize & Ladd, 1990; Robinson, Smith, Miller, & Brownell, 1999; Schectman, Gilat, Fos, & Flasher, 1996). Low student-teacher ratios and integrated individualized curricula for special needs children also contribute to students' increased academic performance. Smaller classes allow teachers to focus more on the individual child's strengths and weaknesses. An integrated curriculum enhances learning by breaking down barriers and helping children think in a broader context. Three to four years of such treatment shows pervasive and enduring changes, particularly with minority, poor, male students. But with all students, such a teaching approach helps children gain knowledge and skills to better solve the problems that occur in life and to achieve academically (Achilles, Egelson, & Finn, 1998; Barnes, Brinster, & Fahey, 2005; Hatch & Smith, 2004; Salyer, Curran, & Thyfault, 2002; Stull, 2004).

ONE MODEL PROGRAM: THE HEALTHCARE COMMUNITY ACADEMY PROGRAM

Bearing in mind the changing issues in healthcare and education that children with special needs face, this chapter presents one model, funded by combining education and health dollars, that successfully meets those needs. The Biscayne Academy operates as part of the Biscayne Institutes of Health and Living, Inc. The Biscayne Institutes is a private agency based on the model of a HealthCare Community. This model provides a fully accredited rehabilitation and healthcare program for adults and children under one roof. The Biscayne Academy is a full-service school operating within that model.

The special education services are embedded in the larger HealthCare Community model. Because the Biscayne Institutes must meet national ac0creditation standards for rehabilitation, the Biscayne Academy is also held to these standards. Biscayne Academy is part of the integral fabric of this larger community-based health program. As a result, it provides certain advantages to children with special needs who are enrolled. Physical, occupational, and speech therapists as well as psychologists, neuropsychologists, and social workers are employed full-time, as are the teachers of Biscayne Academy. All personnel are available on an ongoing basis and are actively integrated into the daily school life of the students.

Occupational and physical therapists provide one-on-one treatment for children who need such services. Additionally, they take part on a weekly basis in the physical education of the students as a group and are available to assist on field trips. Because the Biscayne Institutes is a healthcare facility, they are able to work on goals that transfer beyond the classroom into the community and the world at large. Speech therapy is available individually as well as in the classroom, when appropriate. Psychologists and social workers run weekly groups as part of the standard curriculum to address social skills and emotional problems that may interfere with a child's ability to cope and learn. Testing of special education students provides not only cognitive and emotional testing as required, but also extensive neuropsychological testing when indicated. Individual therapy and behavior modification under the auspices of a licensed psychologist are also provided as part of the curriculum for students who need such help and in consultation and cooperation with their parents.

Education is provided cost-effectively with the backup of a full team of healthcare professionals, as is so often required by children with special needs. Additionally, team members are available for ongoing consultation with one another and with teachers and parents. The IEP becomes an individualized whole person care plan. Interdisciplinary team meetings at Biscayne Academy are held on a weekly basis to adjust the program for the needs of each student. Consequently, children go home at the end of their school day with all educational and rehabilitation services provided. They do not have to go to other healthcare providers who may not know the entire history and treatment needs of a child. Children and parents are relieved from spending extended hours, after school, attending additional health appointments that tax the child's and parents' resources of time and energy.

A restructured, integrative learning system, such as the HealthCare Community model provides, integrates education and healthcare. It emphasizes the development of the child as a whole person, intellectually, emotionally, behaviorally, and physically. It also allows for a placement that is the best fit for the child's learning style, as agreed on both by parents and professionals. Additionally, the model is community based. This leads to a wider variety in curriculum as well as experiences in the community at large that are geared for successful outcomes. Field trips as well as community events that bring in families and the public allow students to learn coping skills that transfer outside the classroom. Because these experiences are geared for success, they provide for positive inclusion experiences in the real world. The HealthCare Community model embraces the philosophy so often embraced by advocates of inclusion, that "education is part of, not separate from, the rest of children's lives" (Stout, 2001).

The built environment also emphasizes a real-life approach. The school and the HealthCare Community model for rehabilitation do not look like traditional schools or healthcare facilities. The building is embedded in the heart of a mixed residential and commercial area. It is surrounded by lush foliage and is approached by an avenue lined with overarching foliage that has been described as a "tunnel of trees." There is a fountain in the garden courtyard that leads to the academy entrance. Internally, classrooms are lighted and designed to provide a sense of comfort as well as learning. While the gym has adaptive equipment, for example, parallel bars, there is also traditional wellness equipment, as found in neighborhood gyms. The HealthCare Community also has a sauna and steam room behind the gyms. Individual offices of clinicians who work with the students in speech or individual therapy are decorated with couches, artwork, and rugs that simulate a home environment. The "auditorium" is actually a large, carpeted, round room that overlooks the garden and the fountain through glass walls. When empty, this room is used for dances and physical activities, including yoga. When there is a formal program or graduation, the room is set up with chairs and appropriate equipment. It is within this community-based setting that the particulars of the Biscayne Academy program unfold.

The Integrative Program

Demographics

Fifty children attend the Biscayne Academy Monday through Friday for the school year. The academic program begins the end of August and extends through early June. The diagnoses of the children that attend range from traumatic brain injury, spinal cord injury, cerebral palsy, Asperger's syndrome, and pervasive developmental disorders and learning disabilities to rare cases, for example, congenital acorpus callosum. The children's ages range from 6 to 21 years. Classes are provided from the first grade through high school. The school is able to award a regular diploma to graduating seniors. Fifty percent of the children are African and Haitian American. Twenty-five percent are Hispanic, and the remaining twenty-five percent are white. These children also come from a combination of intact families, step-parent families, and single-parent families. Seventy-five percent of all children are from immigrant families and are from families whose earnings put them in lower socioeconomic brackets. IQs range from the category of moderate mental retardation through high average. Neuropsychological functioning ranges from severely impaired in a minimum number of cases, to diffuse, moderately impaired functioning, and through normal functioning with a pattern of discrete deficits.

Assessment and Placement

All children applying for entrance to Biscayne Academy are considered for admission on a case-by-case basis. Children and adolescents who are floridly psychotic, ventilat or-dependent, or have documented violence and/or gang-related association are not considered appropriate for this outpatient, integrative model.

Diagnostic information is obtained by clinical interview, review of past academic/medical records, and formal assessment involving various test protocols. All children are administered an achievement test, the Wide Range Achievement Test 3 (WRAT-3; Wilkinson, 1993), on admission as well as at the beginning and end of each academic year. Teachers provide this testing under the direction and training of a psychologist. The WRAT-3 assesses phonetic decoding skills in oral reading and basic math skills. This particular test is chosen as it is most suitable to the population where English is often a second language in the home. Intelligence tests, for example, the Wechsler Intelligence Scale for Children III and the Test of Non-verbal Intelligence 3, may be administered if current test results are not already available in educational or medical records. Additionally, various personality tests may also be administered to the children. On the basis of age and potential diagnosis, tests administered include the House, Tree, Person Drawing Test; the Incomplete Sentence Blank; the Minnesota Multiphasic Personality Inventory for

Adolescents; Children's Depression Inventory; Beck Depression Inventory 2; Beck Anxiety Inventory; and the Thematic Apperception Test. In certain cases, full neuropsychological test batteries are also administered, inclusive of the personality measures. Neuropsychological testing may include the full Halsted-Reitan battery, the Wide Range Assessment of Memory and Learning, and the Bender Motor Visual Gestalt test.

After initial assessment, children are placed in ungraded classrooms. Placement criteria are based on age, cognitive ability, physical developmental size, and social maturation. All factors are considered by the education and rehabilitation team. No more than 10 children are assigned to each classroom. Children with more intense needs, but who qualify for one-to-one aides, are placed according to the above criteria, taking into account the increase in function that an aide can provide environmentally.

Curriculum

The Biscayne Academy uses an integrative approach to meet the varied needs of its students. The curriculum for learning is based on multisensory stimulation. All attendees of the school receive an individualized version of the Florida Sunshine Curriculum, a prescribed curriculum traditionally taught in Florida public schools. An integrated care plan is completed for each student, where individualized curriculum goals are recorded. The goals recorded include academic, behavioral, emotional, social, medical, and rehabilitative goals. This care plan is similar to what is known in public schools as an IEP. However, the goals are more wide ranging and integrate education, physical and emotional learning, and development.

The first part of the school day exists to meet the academic curriculum goals of each student. An individualized language arts program begins the day. Depending on the need, some students are exposed to the Reading Mastery Program, focused on increasing letter and sound recognition, while others work on decoding skills, reading comprehension, and reading fluency. Others are part of a literature program focused on reading and reviewing classic literature. Sandpaper letter feeling, handwriting, transferring from board to paper, creative writing, and journaling are also part of the language arts program. Students participate in the writing process on a daily basis. After the language arts block is complete, each child works on an individualized math program. The students explore math using a variety of media. Students are challenged through educational software, manipulatives, and hands-on activities to reinforce mathematical concepts. The science process skills (observing, classifying, measuring, inferring, predicting, and communicating) are used daily in science class, and each child is given the opportunity to use these skills as he explores each new assignment, again with an emphasis on hands-on and in vivo activities. In social studies, assignments are given to each student based on his highest level of functioning. Social science projects focus not only on facts, but on relationships and cultural issues. Historical and current events are emphasized. Students are encouraged and supported to become active in the community. Life-based assignments are given in good citizenship activities, including working with the homeless, sponsoring Earth Day events, education about the voting process, and other community-based programs. The local Kiwanis Club is also highly involved in supporting the students at Biscayne through initiating student-run Kiwanis Clubs to assist in community service.

The second part of the day focuses on alternative programs as part of the curriculum. Adaptive yoga is one facet of the innovative curriculum. Students participate in breathing techniques and poses (asanas) to increase endurance and flexibility. Accompanying yoga, mind awakening is used to teach focus and concentration. Students are challenged to meditate and learn visualization techniques for healing and goal setting. Computer-based programs are used on a daily basis to stimulate learning in all subjects and increase fine motor control and coordination. Afternoon time in the computer lab is scheduled in addition to any morning in-class computer assignments. The year-round art program includes Opera Day, with a performance by the Florida Grand Opera, theater workshops by Gold Coast Theater, artist workshops run by artists in the community, and weekly art and music classes. Social activities are equally included in the alternative programming of the school. Students receive group therapy and club time and participate in all-school events, social and community based, to help foster positive interpersonal relationships.

An integral part of the curriculum is the learning environment. Classrooms are arranged so that the environment makes the maximum use of sensory stimulation. Natural lighting and color are used to appeal to the senses and increase learning. All the classrooms at the Biscayne Academy have either windows, glass doors, and/or skylights to allow natural light to filter into the room. Incandescent lamps are also used for soft lighting. All-spectrum light filters are encouraged if it is necessary to use supplemental fluorescent lights. The color of paint in the classrooms is a soft, neutral color. The color is intended to have a soothing effect, as this conscious use of color can help create an environment for healing. Seating arrangements of each classroom are intended to maximize both individual time for student studies as well as group work time. The classrooms have traditional desks; however, they also are furnished with beanbag chairs, carpet squares, and sectioned areas of the room outfitted for individual freedom in the learning process.

Integrative Treatments

In addition to the cognitive learning programs, the children are provided various forms of treatment based on their specific problems. The determination of specified treatment is based on the child's intellectual, cognitive, physical, and emotional functioning. The range of treatments available includes both individual and group psychotherapy provided by psychologists and social workers as a regular part of the curriculum. Social work also supplies additional assistance inclusive of family services, home visits, support with obtaining concrete services, and consultation with teachers regarding age-appropriate activities. In addition, the children are provided with physical therapy, occupational therapy, and speech therapy on an individualized basis. The physical and occupational therapists also provide the regular physical education program to the students as a group and assist on field trips. All personnel are dynamically integrated into the daily life of the student.

Specific individual psychotherapy and group therapies are provided to the students based on age and cognitive and emotional functional levels. Individual psychotherapy focuses on many different issues. These include specific behavioral problems, stress reactions, posttraumatic stress disorder, phobias, anosonosgia, bereavement, depression, and issues specific to each child's disabilities. The individual treatments that are utilized include behavioral, cognitive behavioral, insight-oriented, biblio-, play, and/or supportive therapy. Selection of the treatments for each child is based on several factors inclusive of cognitive functioning, age, level of comprehension, and diagnosis.

Group therapy typically involves increasing social skills, group cohesiveness, and self-advocacy. The group therapy is an integral part of the learning curriculum. All groups are held simultaneously at a specified day and time of the week. The group demographics are controlled by the size of the group and the age of the child combined with his cognitive and emotional functioning. Information from individual and group psychotherapy treatments are reviewed within specific ethical parameters with the team during integrative rounds. This allows for titration and modification of the treatments based on feedback from the various disciplines.

For certain individuals, cognitive retraining is utilized to address right and left brain dysfunction. Left hemisphere cognitive retraining typically involves verbal skills, for example, journaling, procedural memory exercises, academic skills, attention/concentration, planning, abstract reasoning, goals, and self-identification of barriers and strengths. Right hemisphere cognitive retraining involves tasks that focus on visual scanning, visual discrimination, visual organization, attention/concentration, and spatial orientation.

Behavior Modification

In addition to all the aforementioned treatments and treatment modalities, all children are placed on an encompassing behavior modification program from the moment they enter the academy until they leave at the end of the day. This is inclusive of break times, treatment times, lunch, and field trips. The objectives of the behavior modification program are to develop positive interpersonal skills, provide a sense of accomplishment, and improve self-esteem.

To provide a sense of consistency for the behavior modification program, there is an interdisciplinary staff training that takes place prior to the start of the academic year. It is reviewed several times throughout the year. The training is given to schoolteachers, physical therapists, physical therapy assistants, occupational therapists, speech therapists, social workers, psychologists, neuropsychologists, certified nursing assistants, volunteers, and any professional students that may be on internship or rotation in various disciplines.

A baseline measurement of each student's behavior is obtained during the first week of school. The baseline establishes the number of positive behaviors that the student exhibits throughout the day. Once this has been established, the student body is informed of the rules and regulations regarding the behavior modification program. The behavior modification program is then implemented the second week.

The behavior modification program can be viewed as a modified token economy. There is a point system where the child can earn up to three points per session. There are seven sessions per day during the school week. Therefore the maximum number of points that can be earned per day is 21. This results in a maximum number of 105 points per week that can be earned. The beginning minimum number of daily points that are required to qualify for a reinforcer is determined and increases exponentially throughout the school year. This is communicated to the children verbally and in writing. It is also posted in the classrooms. A minimum of 10 points per day are required for the two weeks following the baseline period. It increases to 11 points for weeks four through six, to 12 points per day for weeks six to nine. Then it converts to a one-point increase per day for each successive month. During the last two months of school, May and June, students are required to earn a minimum of 19 points per day to qualify for a reward.

Students can earn three points per session based on the following conditions: (1) good talking (respect for others' feelings); (2) getting along (respect for others' bodies and their belongings); and (3) good cooperation (respect for authority complying with tasks required). One point is earned by the student for each of these behaviors during each of the sessions each day. It is emphasized to the children and staff that the children *earn* these points, rather than that the points are taken away by the teachers or therapists for infractions. If the child is uncooperative, he will receive two warnings prior to a "time away." The time away is simply a two-minute period where the child is separated from the individual or group activity. He may be placed in a separate section in the room or made to sit just outside of the classroom or therapist's office door. The child may also receive a "time-out" if he continues to be uncooperative. Immediate time-outs are given for use of swear words or for physical aggression. The time-out procedure consists of placing the child in a designated time-out room, which reduces extraneous stimulation, for 10 minutes. The 10-minute time period initiates once the child is quiet. The person that places the child in the time-out room monitors and removes the child at the end of the time-out period.

If the student is successful at obtaining the minimum number of required points for the week and has not earned a time-out, then the child will be able to obtain what is referred to as Fun Friday. Fun Friday occurs on Friday afternoon from 1:00 to 3:00 P.M. The child may elect to participate in certain fun activities, for example, viewing a film or playing with various games, including child-appropriate video games, and engaging in the pet therapy program. Additionally, throughout the week, there are several earned incentives and privileges that the child may obtain from the teacher based on the number of points earned in a particular day. These privileges may include being line leader, choosing the music the class will listen to at lunch, designation as "teacher's helper," and so on. However, if the child does not earn the minimum number of points or receives a time-out during the week, then the child spends Friday afternoon in a structured academic activity instead of being rewarded by engaging in a fun activity.

Throughout the day, children who also require physical, occupational, or speech therapy are scheduled for appointments with these disciplines. The staff member treating the child also follows the behavior modification program. This allows for a more cohesive behavioral and learning experience. By the time the child has completed the school day, all academic, physical, and psychological therapies have been completed with a coordinated approach. This allows the child more time in the home environment and decreases the need for parents to travel to multiple sites to obtain needed services for the child. Stress is lessened for the child and the whole family. In addition, parents are instructed in the use of behavior modification at home, and performance at school and home is communicated to increase consistency.

How the Team Works

The various disciplines integrate their independent information into a team approach that views the individual as a whole entity. At the outset of each academic year, an integrative care plan is developed for each child by the team in conjunction with the parents. The team meets weekly to review the progress of the students. The integrated care plan is fine-tuned as to how each of the diverse disciplines is approaching the educational and rehabilitation goals for the child. Goals are set for one-, two-, or three-month time periods in which they are to be completed. If a goal is not met, an explanation of why the goal is not achieved must be documented. The goal is then revised, if feasible, to allow the child to attempt again to successfully implement the objectives.

Monthly summaries are provided to parents, physicians, and other appropriate parties with permission of the parents. In addition, report cards are also sent home every nine weeks. Functional data for cognitive, emotional, behavioral, and physical skills are collected for each child by the appropriate discipline. Measures using the Combi are taken at the beginning and end of each academic year. A transition to the International Classification of Functioning–Children and Youth form is currently being implemented.

OUTCOMES

Data Collection

Several measures are used to track the efficacy of this model. Outcome measurements in academic skills, emotional and physical functioning, activities of daily living, and behavioral adjustment are tracked as part of the normal implementation of the program. Changes in scores on the WRAT-3 in the fall and spring of each academic year, administered by trained teachers and psychologists, are tracked and indicate changes in students' abilities for phonemic decoding and basic math skills. Alternate versions are utilized so that a test/retest method for outcome measurement can be used. This allows for the collection of the data in the fall to serve as a baseline and provides a control for the data that is collected in the spring. All students who have measurable verbal ability participate in the WRAT-3 assessment.

All the children, regardless of functional level, are also assessed using the Combi, a standardized combination of the Functional Independence Measures (FIM) and Functional Assessment Measures (FAM) appropriate for this population.

The COMBI rating scales have scores that range from one to seven. A functional measure rating of one means that the individual needs total assistance, while a rating of seven means that the person has complete independence. Scores in between are based on percent of assistance that is required by the child to complete a task. Interrater reliability of the COMBI demonstrated good to excellent intraclass correlation coefficients, which supports the use of the measurement device in rehabilitation facilities (Donaghy & Wass, 1998). Another study conducted by Hawley, Taylor, Hellawell, and Pentland (1999) showed that the COMBI and two derived subscales maintain a high internal reliability when using untransformed ratings in a clinical and research population of patients with brain injuries.

The Combi scales are the currently accepted standard for rehabilitation assessment in rehabilitation healthcare. Standardized scoring methods and training are normed nationally to address issues of consistency and reliability (Hawley et al., 1999; COMBI, 2007, The Center for Outcome Measurement in

Brain Injury, para.1).These scales are used to assess students at the beginning and the end of the academic year by trained occupational therapists, physical therapists, social workers, teachers, psychologists, and neuropsychologists. Standardized training on these measures occurs yearly for staff. Interrater reliability training, conducted at the facility, is in accordance with the standards provided by the Center for Outcome Measurement in Brain Injury.

Additionally, specific individual goals are set for each child by the whole team in various areas, inclusive of physical rehabilitation, emotional functioning, behavioral compliance, and academic achievement. Goals range from such items as "Patient will make needs known appropriately in program at least once a session" to "Patient will walk without cane with standby guard for 30 feet" and "Patient will increase independent reading comprehension by 10 percent over baseline as measured by improved in-class test scores." Goals are assessed, as to whether or not they have been achieved, at a predesignated time of one, two, or three months from the date the goals are set.

Results for the Wide Range Achievement Test 3

The information obtained from the WRAT-3 reading and arithmetic sections together with the FIM/FAM ratings and individual goals attained are used to analyze the functioning of the children throughout the academic year. Along with individual tracking of each child's performance compared to his own baseline, group scores are also analyzed for changes.

The WRAT-3 analyses include all children in one group. Separate analyses are run for standard scores and grade level scores in reading and arithmetic scores derived from the WRAT-3. Results indicate consistent improvement over time. Data analyzed (2003–2004) revealed highly significant results. An analysis of variance (ANOVA) performed on WRAT-3 scores indicated an increase in grade level scores for both reading and math that are significant at $p \leq 0.001$ (Figure 1), while standard scores indicated significance at the $p \leq 0.01$ level (Figure 2).

According to their prior school records and test data, the majority of these children made little or no progress in basic academic skills while attending public school. However, in a program that integrated physical, emotional, and academic care, these children made highly significant progress in both reading and arithmetic, regardless of age or disability. Overall, as a group, Figure 1 indicates that the children's grade level scores advanced almost one full grade level while attending the nine-month Biscayne Academy program. The children's standard reading scores improved by more than three and one-half points, while their arithmetic standard scores improved by almost five points.

Specifically, 19 percent of the children increased from two to four grade levels in reading during the academic year. Two students increased by two grade

Figure 1
Reading and arithmetic grade level scores, Biscayne Academy,
September 2003–June 2004

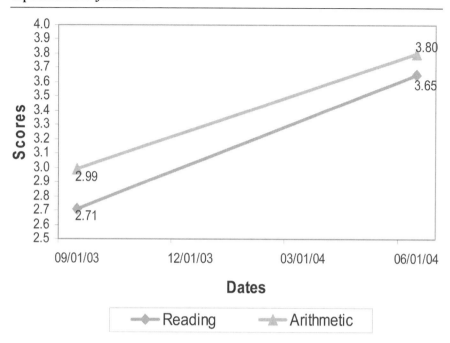

Figure 2
Reading and arithmetic standard scores, Biscayne Academy,
September 2003–June 2004

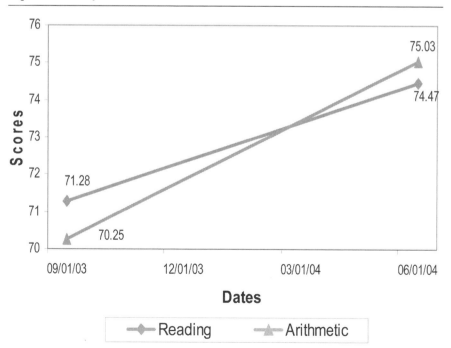

levels; two students by three grade levels; and two students by four grade levels in reading. As for arithmetic, 34 percent of all students made gains of two to three grade levels. Specifically, eight students increased arithmetic scores by two grade levels, while three students increased by three grade levels during the course of nine months. Only four students that showed multiple grade level increases in arithmetic were the same as those students showing multiple grade level increases in reading. This finding reveals that while the overall group made significant increases in reading and arithmetic, 53 percent of all students tested made multiple grade level advances in reading and/or arithmetic.

Results for the Combi

Because of the variability in physical functioning of children and the broad range of diagnoses, the data for the Combi are divided into either a low-functioning group or a high-functioning group. Low-functioning groups are children whose highest level of independence in any area at baseline is scored at three or below. The high-functioning group comprises children with scores over three in every area. Scores on the Combi-assessment demonstrate

Figure 3
Biscayne Academy low-functioning students

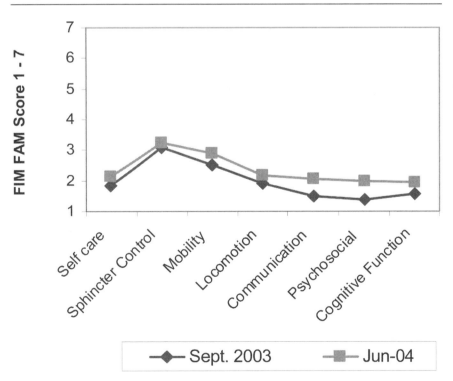

Figure 4
Biscayne Academy high-functioning students

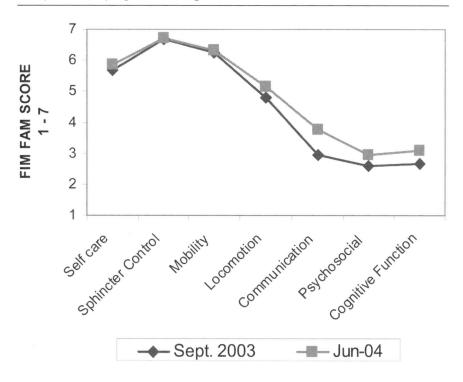

increases in all areas for both low-functioning (Figure 3) and high-functioning groups (Figure 4).

Results were analyzed into the two groups to better replicate the physical and cognitive disparity of the functional levels of the students. There were 33 children in the high-functioning group and 16 in the low-functioning group. High-functioning students were those with mild mental retardation, learning disabilities, Asperger's syndrome, attention deficit disorders, mild traumatic brain injury, or psychosis. Low-functioning students were those diagnosed with autism, cerebral palsy, Rett's syndrome, anoxia, and acorpus callosum.

Results for Individual Goals

The results of the children's successful completion of individual goals for this same sample year (2003–2004) are as follows: 75 percent of the goals were achieved in the physical ability domain; 94 percent in the cognitive domain; 91 percent in the emotional domain; and 95 percent in behavioral improvement. All the domains exceeded the 75 percent achievement objective utilized as determining a successful outcome in accreditation standards.

When a child's individual function in all areas is measured at the beginning of the academic year and is used as a baseline measure of self-efficacy, comparing his individual performance in all areas at the end of the year, significant results are noted. Findings for children enrolled in the Biscayne Academy indicate that an integrated health and education program can provide the basis for an efficacious comprehensive program that treats the child as a whole person. When functional, emotional, and behavioral needs are appropriately addressed and coupled with an individualized curriculum, gains in basic academic skills, such as reading and arithmetic, can show dramatic improvement. Self-efficacy measures do not provide matched group samples against which to compare the child's changes, nor do they provide specific causal explanations to specific determining factors responsible for that change. However, when the performance gains of these same children are compared to their prior static performance over time in the public schools, as reported in school records, it is evident that marked changes occurred when the child participated in the HealthCare Community integrative model. These changes were not previously effected in prior fragmented systems.

Children and parents also report high satisfaction with the results at Biscayne. This is indicated not only by parent and student feedback, but by the number of students who continue their enrollment at Biscayne Academy from year to year. Biscayne Academy's results are a direct outgrowth of the HealthCare Community model. This model combines the best of education with the best of healthcare. Access to full-service, community-integrated care that treats the child as a whole person should be the gold standard, especially for children with special needs.

Case Studies

Given that the study separates low-functioning and high-functioning children, case examples of children with low functioning and high functioning are presented to emphasize their success in this type of model.

CASE 1

S., the first child presented, was determined to be low functioning. He came to the institute with a diagnosis of developmental delay at the age of seven. The child was nonverbal, except for high-pitched, loud vocal screams. When given structure, he would urinate and defecate. He had a very difficult time initially with the behavior modification program and, while in the time-out room, would urinate and defecate and attempt to play with his excrement. The teachers and therapists also observed unusually hostile behavior toward his caregivers when they brought him to the program or came to pick him up at the end of the day.

This information was reviewed with his parents and grandparents in the course of parent conferences. Rather than being a "slow learner" or "rebellious" and in need of physical punishment, as his caregivers had believed, it was explained that S. had a severe problem that was most likely neurologically based. In addition to the behavior modification program at the institute, a home-based behavior modification program consistent with the school-based program was developed, taught to the caregivers, and implemented. Referrals were also made to psychiatry and neurology for medication evaluation and imaging studies.

Results of testing indicated a diagnosis of acorpus callosum based on the imaging studies. A titration to his treatment was made both psychologically and academically while initiating pharmaceuticals. After several months of treatment, the child was beginning to speak and read. He also was able to participate in standardized academic achievement testing (WRAT-3), which he was originally incapable of taking. His behaviors became significantly more manageable at the school and at home to the point that he was able to accept structure, no longer urinated or defecated inappropriately, and became successful in the behavior modification program, earning points and rarely needing a time-out. S.'s conceptual formation and learning will always be low; however, his socialization and ability to learn rudimentary reading and communication skills are essential to more independent functioning and improved quality of life for both himself and his family.

CASE 2

T. is deemed to be currently high functioning. He is a 20-year-old student who has been attending Biscayne's program for five years. His initial traumatic brain injury occurred at age 14. T. was involved in a go-cart accident in his neighborhood. Medical records indicated hematomas in the right frontal and right parietal areas with subfalcine herniation; a Glasgow Coma Scale of 7; diffuse cerebral edema; pneumocephalus; and a right frontal temporal skull fracture.

(Continues)

(Continued)

Prior to the accident, T. had no significant developmental problems or medical history. School records and test data suggest premorbid functioning in the low average range. Following the accident, he exhibited difficulty with selective attention, working memory, impulsiveness, socialization, and maladaptive behaviors, including aggressiveness. His intelligence assessment postinjury fell into the borderline range of functioning.

T. came to Biscayne Academy at age 15 after inpatient rehabilitation, which included speech and occupational therapy. Initial intake also revealed that he had blurred vision, impaired judgment, poor insight, and nightmares. Over the course of attending Biscayne, T.'s functional levels increased dramatically. Reading comprehension is now at high school level. WRAT-3 testing scores went from initial testing at the sixth-grade level to high school in reading; from initial fourth-grade levels in spelling to fifth-grade levels; and from initial fifth-grade arithmetic to sixth-grade level. He continues to receive a specialized and individualized program specific to his diagnosis and symptomatology. Today, he is currently the treasurer of an adolescent chapter of a local Kiwanis Club, providing services in the community to those less fortunate than himself. He serves a strong leadership role in his class. T. also currently owns and runs a part-time landscaping business while continuing to attend school on a full-time basis. He is working on preparation for classes at the local community college in business through the combined effort of Biscayne and the college program for students with special needs.

Data, Dollars, and Diversity

Cost-Effectiveness

The global, integrated approach to combining education and healthcare in the community is made possible because the Biscayne Academy is integrated into the larger Biscayne HealthCare Community model. Monies provided for education through the McKay voucher program are not restricted as to how the institution spends them in educating the child. However, because the amount allotted for each child varies on a matrix, depending on a preassigned list of diagnosed needs set by the local public school authority, voucher dollars cover only a fraction of the cost of such individualized, integrated care. But when these dollars are combined with healthcare dollars from all programs within the Biscayne HealthCare Community, the impact of the education vouchers is highly leveraged.

Over time, the programs build synergistically and become integral to the success of one another as efficiency increases. This results in generally decreasing costs. A financial analysis of the academy program over the last four years indicates that, implemented as a part of the Biscayne HealthCare Community, services for 50 students daily were sustained in the academy program at the following levels of hourly cost/reimbursement efficiency:

$16.30 per hour of treatment 2004
$14.82 per hour of treatment 2003
$16.23 per hour of treatment 2002
$29.33 per hour of treatment 2001.

The Biscayne HealthCare Community academy program integrates education and healthcare. It provides one model for meeting the needs of children who face special challenges. The model treats the child as a whole person and is both efficacious and cost-effective. It combines overhead for both educational and rehabilitation programs from an administrative perspective, while also providing a highly effective clinical program. Funding streams are combined from the Department of Education, Medicaid, the Florida State Brain and Spinal Cord Injury Program, private insurance, and self-pay. This makes for a more coordinated use of dollars. The professional education and health providers, the assessment of needs and the individualized care plan, and communication between the parents and the treating team are more coordinated. The resulting outcome data reveal that the dollars spent achieve a bigger bang for the buck and translate into real life gains for the child. Monies spent are more effective for behavioral changes, cognitive changes, physical changes, emotional changes, and academic changes. Carryover into the real world and from year to year also improves.

Challenges and Limitations

There are practical challenges to implementing such a model. The model cannot meet the needs of all children with special needs, as indicated in the admissions criteria. Additionally, educational and healthcare vocabularies are different among the different disciplines. Professionals must spend time learning to communicate and translate communications into each others' languages. Diagnostic and intervention terminology varies. Conceptual approaches in the classroom may differ in some respects from individual treatment approaches. Underlying philosophies and strategies must be shared and honed. Timing of different intervention programs and therapies need to be continually reviewed and discussed. And most importantly, team relationships need to be built on trust and mutual respect for the child and each other.

Because each child differs in respect to strengths and weaknesses, each child must be individually supported within the community as a whole. The community approach is one of inclusion. And as discussions of inclusion elucidate, to have a truly inclusive program, a classroom needs to emphasize (Stout, 2001)

- higher-order thinking skills
- integrated curricula
- interdisciplinary teaching
- multicultural curricula
- life-centered curricula.

Next Steps

However, an integrated curriculum, interdisciplinary teaching, multicultural life approaches, and an emphasis on higher-order thinking skills are the concepts that the HealthCare Community as a whole is based on. This philosophy clearly makes a difference in the lives of the children with special needs that it serves. It sets a model for meeting the challenges of some of the most complex challenges a child has to face developmentally. And because it works with the most vulnerable in our society, it leads to a logical conclusion that if these same concepts are applied to the integrated education and healthcare of children without special challenges, how much more could they achieve?

The next stage of development for the HealthCare Community is to develop the curriculum to meet the individual needs of students who do not have special needs but who want to achieve a more global education. Ironically, as children without special needs are incorporated into the Biscayne Academy and helped to achieve their highest level of functioning, it provides an opportunity for a dynamic reverse inclusion model. This reverse inclusion model, based on the current Biscayne Academy model, can continue to provide guided opportunities for children, with and without special needs, to learn to swim upstream together, to enhance individual and group functioning, and to cope with challenges at all levels. Children of all ages and abilities can be taught in a more community-based environment, learning tolerance and acceptance and still achieving individual goals. Like salmon, who are stronger for swimming upstream to spawn, the HealthCare Community concept of "upstreaming" allows each child to draw on the strengths he possesses and learn to cope to the best of his ability.

TOOL KIT FOR CHANGE

Role and Perspective of the Healthcare Professional

1. Treating children's health means treating children in the context of their community and school network. Active, regular communication among healthcare professionals, the school, and the family is required.

2. Within 20 years the numerical majority of the population in the United States will be an aggregate of various minorities. This includes an expanding population of children who are themselves from other cultures or are children of immigrants from other cultures. The healthcare provider must be sensitive to cultural issues and to a larger definition of health for children that includes the community and school networks.

3. Depending on the individual child, the best teaching style for information about health, academic learning, and life functioning may vary. Multisensory stimulation that uses both right and left hemispheres of the brain is most effective in engaging children as they grow and is best employed by healthcare providers as well as parents and educators.

Role and Perspective of the Patient/Participant

1. The patient, especially a pediatric patient, benefits most when material for health and/or education is presented in a multimodal manner.

2. Parent education and involvement in a family-centered approach to healthcare and learning, coordinated with healthcare providers and teachers, best serves the needs of the child.

3. A successful model of a voucher-funded program for combining the education and healthcare of children exists. Research data show increased academic skills, behavioral adjustment, and health functioning for children who participate in this program.

Interconnection: The Global Perspective

1. Children with special needs need special attention.

2. "Upstreaming" allows guided opportunities for each child to learn to function at the highest level possible and cope with challenges. It opens the door for reverse inclusion of children of all ages and ability levels.

3. A successful, cost-effective model for a voucher-funded program for combining the education and healthcare of children with special needs exists. This model may also hold the potential for providing a successful model for access to healthcare for a wider population of both children and adults.

REFERENCES

Achilles, C. M. (2003, February 24). *How class size makes a difference: What the research says: The impact of class-size reduction.* Paper presented at the SERVE Research and Policy Symposium on Class-Size Reduction and Beyond, Raleigh, NC.

Achilles, C. M., Egelson, P., & Finn, J. D. (1998, November 5–7). *Teaching in small classes: What is the difference?* Paper presented at the Annual Meeting of the Mid-South Educational Research Association, New York.

Achilles, C. M., & Finn, J. D. (2002, February 14–17). *Making sense of continuing and renewed class-size findings and interest.* Paper presented at the Annual Meeting of the American Association of School Administrators, San Diego, CA.

Barnes, N. S., Brinster, P. A., & Fahey, P. (2005). Exploring tableau vivant: An integrated approach to interpretation. *Gifted Child Today, 28,* 24–37.

Donaghy, S., & Wass, P. J. (1998). Interrater reliability of the functional assessment measure in a brain injury rehabilitation program. *Archives of Physical Medicine Rehabilitation, 79*: 1231–1236.

Doonan, M. (2002). *The Miami Dade County immigrant health access task force/access to public health trust services: Success and challenges*. Retrieved July 16, 2006, from www.hscdade. org/pubs/Access%20to%20Public%20Health-Miami1.pdf

Greene, J. P. (2001a, February). *Florida A-Plus Accountability and School Choice Program*. Retrieved January 29, 2005, from http://ksg.harvard.edu/taubmancenter/pdfs/ working-papers/greene_01_florida.pdf

Greene, J. P. (2001b, Summer). Vouchers in Charlotte. *Education Next*, Article 3389746. Retrieved January 29, 2005, from http://www.hoover.org/publications/ednext/ 3389746.html

Greene, J. P., & Forster, G. (2003). *Vouchers for special education students: An evaluation of Florida's McKay Scholarship Program* (Civic Rep. No. 38). New York: June Center for Civic Innovation, Manhattan Institute for Policy Research.

Greene, J. P., Peterson, P. E., & Du, J. (1997). Effectiveness of school choice: The Milwaukee experiment. *Education and Urban Society*. Retrieved January 29, 2005, from http://www.ksg.harvard.edu/taubmancenter/publications/papers_achieve.html

Hatch, G. M., & Smith, D. R. (2004). Integrating physical education, math, and physics. *Journal of Physical Education, Recreation, and Dance, 75*, 42–58.

Hawley, C. A., Taylor, R., Hellawell, D. J., & Pentland, B. (1999). FIM+FAM in head injury rehabilitation: A psychometric analysis. *Journal of Neurology, Neurosurgery, and Psychiatry 67*, 749–754.

Health & Human Services, Agency for Healthcare Research and Quality. (2004). National healthcare disparities report. Retrieved November 12, 2006, from http://www.ahrq. gov/qual/nhdrmeasures/listmeasure.htm.

Hernandez, D. J. (2004). Demographic change and the life circumstances of immigrant families. *Future of Children, 14*, 17–47.

Klas, M. E. (2006, May 3). Senate moves to keep vouchers. *Miami Herald*, 1B.

Kochbar, C., West, L., & Taymans, J. (1999). *Successful inclusion: Practical strategies for a shared responsibility* (2nd ed.). New York: Prentice Hall.

Kulic, K. R., Horne, A. M., & Dagley, J. C. (2004). A comprehensive review of prevention groups for children and adolescents. *Group Dynamics: Theory, Research, and Practice, 8*, 139–151.

Lovaas, O. I. (1987). Behavioral treatment and normal educational and intellectual functioning in young autistic children. *Journal of Consulting and Clinical Psychology, 55*, 3–9.

Market research. (2006). *Miami Herald*.

Mize, J., & Ladd, G. W. (1990). A cognitive-social learning approach to social skills training with low-status preschool children. *Developmental Psychology, 26*, 388–397.

Nieves, G. (2003, August 21). County's number of uninsured rises. *Miami Herald*, 1B.

Peterson, P. E., Howell, W. G., & Greene, J. P. (1999). *An evaluation of the Cleveland voucher program after two years*. Retrieved January 29, 2005, from http://www.harvard.edu/ taubmancenter/pdfs/working_papers/greene_97_cleveland.pdf

Roberts, M. C., Jacobs, A. K., Puddy, R. W., Nye, J. E., & Vernberg, E. M. (2003). Treating children with serious emotional disturbances in schools and community: The intensive mental program. *Professional Psychology: Research and Practice, 34*, 519–526.

Robinson, T. R., Smith, S. W., Miller, D., & Brownell, M. T. (1999). Cognitive behavior modification of hyperactivity—Impulsivity and aggression: A meta-analysis of school-based studies. *Journal of Educational Psychology, 91*, 195–203.

Rouse, C. E. (1998). Private school vouchers and student achievement. *Quarterly Journal of Economics, 113*, 553–602.

Salyer, B. K., Curran, C., & Thyfault, A. (2002, March 7–9). *What can I use tomorrow? Strategies for accessible math and science curriculum for diverse learners in rural schools.* Paper presented at No Child Left Behind: The Vital Role of Rural Schools, 22nd Annual National Conference of the American Council on Rural Special Education, Reno, NV.

Santa Clara Valley Medical Center (2006). *The Center for Outcome Measurement in Brain Injury.* Retrieved March 30, 2007, from http://www.tbims.org/combi

Schectman, Z., Gilat, I., Fos, L., & Flasher, A. (1996). Brief group therapy with low-achieving elementary school children. *Journal of Counseling Psychology, 43,* 376–382.

Schmidt, R., & Schlottman, A. (2006). *Does school district size matter?* Las Vegas: Nevada Policy Research Institute.

Stout, C. (2001). *Special education inclusion.* Retrieved March 19, 2007, from http://www.weac.org/resource/june96/speced.htm

Stull, W. J. (2004). A game-theoretic model of curriculum integration and school leadership. In *Laboratory for Student Success* (pp. 1–28). Philadelphia: Temple University.

U.S. Census Bureau. (2005–2006). *School District Review Program.* Retrieved July 16, 2006, from http://www.census.gov/geo/www/schdist/sch_dist.html

U.S. Department of Education. (2000, August 21). *A back to school special report on the baby boom echo: Growing pains.* Retrieved July 16, 2006, from http://www.ed.gov/pubs/bbecho00/part2.html

Wilkinson, G. S. (1993). *WRAT 3.* Wilmington, DE: Jastak.

Chapter Ten

INTEGRATIVE TRAINING OF PROFESSIONALS AND TRANSDISCIPLINARY PUBLIC KNOWLEDGE

Alan P. Pearson, OD, PhD and James Ferguson, PA-C

INTRODUCTION

In today's technological world, knowledge shock is a syndrome common to healthcare student and practitioner alike. Knowledge shock is a stunning state of disorientation, a feeling of burdensome weightiness, eyestrain, and head-aches. It can manifest itself when perusing journals or searching the Internet or library for topical knowledge. Each year, new disciplines and healthcare options enter the scene, further complicating the web of interrelated knowledge, making it much more difficult for the student or practitioner to digest, inte-grate, and apply. The future will only bring more researchers, generating more results, which will need dissemination to more practitioners. Specialization has certainly become one means of managing this complexity of knowledge, but while it helps the individual manage a coherent body of disciplinary knowledge, it also tends to constrict the focus and fortify the boundaries that separate disciplines. Integrative healthcare is not about building boundaries; rather, it is about what is possible when boundaries are blurred. It is about cross-disciplinary collaborative approaches leading to a melding of disciplines and knowledge, resulting in widening the scope of health and humanness. This presents unique challenges in training and practice, as integrative healthcare demands mastery of cross-disciplinary and disciplinary knowledge.

Not only does knowledge complexity affect individuals, but it also impacts the effectiveness of healthcare teams, systems, and institutions as they struggle to adjust protocols to the new standards that are being rewritten almost daily. The manner and frequency in which a group communicates, the terminology used by the participants, and the social dynamics within a group can all impact the effectiveness of the healthcare delivered to patients. This chapter considers knowledge as an embodied concept: knowledge emerges through the full loop of interactions between the environment, the human, and back to the environment. Embodied knowledge can assist individuals, teams, and institutions in the challenge of knowledge management and training. Disciplines and subspecialties are discussed in relation to other disciplines, and various collaborative team approaches are reviewed. The advantages of interdisciplinary collaboration are particularly emphasized as they relate to the goals of integrative healthcare. Transdisciplinary public knowledge is introduced as a means of fostering interdisciplinary collaborative teamwork.

REHUMANIZING THE KNOWLEDGE CONCEPT: PERSONAL AND PUBLIC KNOWLEDGE

With the ubiquitous success of computer technology, today, we apply information technology metaphors, such as the brain as an information processor, to human situations and then become further stunned as we come up against our limited "processing power" and the apparent superior promise of our technology. The future will only bring far-reaching advances in technology and an ever-widening gap between the information processing capacity of humans versus computers. Information processing is what computers do best—it is what they are designed for, by humans. While the metaphor can certainly be applied to understand better the human brain and mind, it does not follow that the brain and mind are simply, or nothing but, information processing devices. This chapter rehumanizes the idea of knowledge by bringing it back into humans from the disembodied information processing devices of our computer metaphors. This offers advantages for the individual student or practitioner in dealing with the symptoms of knowledge shock. It offers advantages to collaborative teams as it emphasizes the challenges of human-to-human interaction as opposed to human-computer interaction. It offers advantages to institutions and policy makers as it highlights human experience and interrelations as being important to the health and well-being of humans.

EMBODIED KNOWLEDGE, PERSONAL AND PUBLIC

The idea of knowledge presented here recognizes it as an embodied phenomenon. In contrast to disembodied views of knowledge that see knowledge as a stuff that can be extracted, managed, and processed quite separately from the human body, the embodied view of knowledge claims that knowledge is distributed throughout the body's structure and relationships with the environment (Hayles, 1999; Lakoff & Johnson, 1999). Knowledge is not limited

to the inside of the body either, but emerges through the full loop of interactions between the environment, the human, and back to the environment
(Bateson, 1972; Maturana & Varela, 1987). In this embodied view, knowledge is seen as a property of a system rather than a place, part, or product of
a system. Knowledge is more about the nature of the relationships between
the system (in this case, the human) and the environment than a stuff (such
as information) that can flow between various modules, whether within the
system or without.

Personal Knowledge

In the context of an individual person, this view of knowledge is personal.
The person has knowledge in terms of his relationships with objects at many
different levels. The relationships could be described from various frames of
reference such as physically, biologically, neurologically, perceptually, cognitively, socially, or spiritually (Pearson, 2005), but in the end, the human frame
of reference takes in all these simultaneously. Embodied personal knowledge
is a holistic concept.

Since different people have different life experiences, they have different
relationships with objects, and their personal knowledge is also different. No
two people have had the same history of relationships. All people may have
common experiences, such as the feel of water, but however similar, they are
still not exact in all ways. Personal knowledge defines the individual. In this
view of personal knowledge, as a fully embodied property, it is contradictory
to say that two people can have the same knowledge, just as two people cannot
share the same body. Since no two people are equal in all ways, the knowledge
each has is completely personal.

Personal knowledge is primarily developed through direct personal experience. For example, a healthcare provider in training reads a standard medical
textbook, such as Barbara Bates's *Guide to Physical Examinations and History
Taking* (Bickley & Szilagyi, 2005), on how to elicit a history and perform a
physical exam to evaluate a patient's chief complaint. The student internalizes
the information learned from the medical text based on his previous experience and learning style. He refines that information based on an instructor's
training and recommendations and on his own interpretation of what has
been conveyed by the instructor. But even after all this, unless the student clinician has direct personal experience, he will not truly know how to perform
a physical examination or take a history. A critical part of the learning experience is experiential learning through actual patient encounters.

The manner in which a student acquires personal knowledge through
experiential learning is different for every student. A variety of influences
come into play that make experiential learning unique to each student. These

influences might include cultural norms, spiritual traditions, individual learning styles, preconceived ideas about what the student is learning, the student's bias, biases of an instructor or a text author, the philosophy of the program in which the student is studying, and so on.

Another example of how knowledge is primarily developed through direct personal experience is in the learning of specific clinical skills. Community health aide/practitioners (CHA/Ps) are healthcare providers that work in remote Native villages in Alaska. CHA/Ps serve as the backbone of rural healthcare in the state, providing primary healthcare to Alaska Natives in villages where there are no physicians, physician's assistants (PAs), or nurse practitioners (NPs). As part of their skill set, CHA/Ps are responsible for doing blood draws, establishing intravenous lines, and administering injectable immunizations and other medications. Skills such as these are best taught through actual hands-on training. Some have tried to provide this training using lifelike rubber models, but CHA/P students have often stated that they learn best by practicing these clinical skills on each other in a skills lab.

One method that demonstrates this to be true and has worked quite well has been the "show one, do one" method. Through use of this method, an instructor explains the methodology of the skill to be mastered to the students in a small-group format (usually three or less students). The instructor then demonstrates the procedure in a step-by-step fashion on one of the students in front of the group. The students then repeat the procedure on a fellow student in front of the group and the instructor, one at a time. In this manner, the CHA/P students have verbally been instructed on how to do the procedure, have seen a step-by-step demonstration of the procedure by the instructor, have performed the skill themselves under the direction of the instructor, and finally, have seen other students perform the procedure with ongoing instruction by the instructor and, at times, by the students themselves during the skills session. This further reinforces the learning experience.

The above anecdote serves as a good example of how knowledge is not limited to the inside of the body, but emerges through the full loop of interactions between the environment, the human, and back to the environment. The CHA/P students learn a new skill with which they have had no previous experience through interaction with their environment (the hands-on skills lab), process their new knowledge using all their unique individual learning styles, and then apply their new skill in their new working environment—the patient.

Public Knowledge

By itself, personal knowledge does not take into consideration interactions between people or the cultural and historical context of the artifacts, symbols, or tools that may mediate such interactions. Personal knowledge is within an individual person in terms of that person's relationships with the objects of his environment. These objects may or may not be other people. Nonetheless, human interrelationships have significant implications for the development of personal knowledge. As C. Wright Mills (1963) suggested, between multiple people, we begin to perceive a "secondhand world" of patterns, designs, values, symbols, language, and communications that seem to mediate relationships between people. The significance of a social world is that meaning can be derived from social interaction, which results in development of personal knowledge without the need for direct personal experience.

Personal knowledge development is made possible using symbols such as language and writing. The wonder of symbols occurs when two or more people coordinate their symbolic benchmarks. Now one person can have the direct experience, while another person, through symbolic communication, can benefit from the experience and behave as if he had the direct experience also. Social interaction tends to coordinate our symbolic systems, therefore enabling multiple people to derive similar meanings toward objects in the world, which then provides great benefits to our personal knowledge development as we mutually benefit from shared experience.

This social perspective involving symbolic interaction is called *public knowledge*. Whereas personal knowledge is all about relationships between the person and environment, public knowledge is specifically about symbolically mediated relationships between multiple people and the environment. Public knowledge is a collaborative effort to mutually enhance the personal knowledge of the participants. Like personal knowledge, public knowledge cannot be located at any singular point. Public knowledge is not the media, a book, a sculpture, a speech, or anything else physically or abstractly present between people. It links people together such that the dynamics of the multiperson system influence and change the personal knowledge of all participant people. Public knowledge is embodied within the social system of symbolic interaction between multiple people. These social systems impact the development of personal knowledge so significantly that it is very difficult to isolate any perception or behavior of an individual person that is without some public knowledge impact. An example will help to elucidate this distinction between public and private knowledge.

Imagine three fishermen: John, Tom, and Ralph. John and Tom went fishing today. Ralph did not. In the evening, Ralph visits the home of John and is told by John that he did not catch any fish at the north fishing hole. Ralph then visits Tom. Tom tells Ralph that he caught five fish at the south fishing hole. The next day, John, Tom, and Ralph all show up at the south fishing hole.

Both John and Tom had the personal knowledge of fishing that day; Ralph did not. It is reasonable to assume that John went to the south fishing hole the next day because of his personal knowledge of not catching any fish at the north fishing hole the previous day. Likewise, it is reasonable to assume that Tom went to the south fishing hole the next day because of his personal knowledge from successful fishing the previous day. John and Tom both had a personal knowledge they could draw on to make a decision as to which fishing hole they would visit the next day. Ralph, on the other hand, had no such personal knowledge. Why did Ralph go to the south fishing hole?

Both John and Tom communicated to Ralph their personal knowledge. They translated their personal knowledge into public knowledge. Ralph was the recipient of the public knowledge proposals of John and Tom. Ralph then benefited from the personal knowledge of John and Tom by modifying his own personal knowledge as if he had actually been fishing the day before. With the benefit of this public knowledge, Ralph ended up at the same fishing hole, without having to go out and fish at each fishing hole himself.

We can look at the CHA/P model in Alaska to further elucidate this distinction between personal and public knowledge. CHA/P A is a local woman born and raised in an Alaska village along the Bering Sea coast, where harvesting sea mammals for food is part of the subsistence lifestyle of her people. She knows that villagers who work with sea mammals sometimes get a bacterial infection in their fingers known to local villagers as "seal finger." Seal finger is caused by a specific bacteria and requires a specific antibiotic—tetracycline—for its treatment. This is common knowledge among the villagers. CHA/P B is new to the village, having recently moved from a village in the Alaska interior, where working with sea mammals is not part of the subsistence lifestyle. CHA/P B is not aware of seal finger, although her CHA/P training has taught her that finger infections are a common complaint in clinic.

This scenario demonstrates that while both CHA/Ps have a base of public knowledge based on their common medical training, CHA/P A has the benefit of personal knowledge common to the people of her village, and when patients present with finger infections, it is automatic for her to ask whether the patient has been working with sea mammals. Public knowledge comes into play when CHA/P A communicates with CHA/P B concerning the relationship between finger infections and sea mammals. If CHA/P B then begins to ask her patients with finger infections about sea mammal contact, she has learned and integrated new knowledge based on other people's personal experiences.

DISCIPLINE

The embodied concept of knowledge and the distinction between personal and public knowledge are important constructs in the context of this chapter. Personal knowledge develops through active experience, and every student or practitioner in healthcare brings years of life experiences into his career. Throughout life, everyone has participated in countless social groups, such as family, friends, school, religion, and town, to name just a few. Public knowledge has shaped the development of an individual's personal knowledge through participation in such groups. When a person chooses a career path, he enters an educational system and further develops his personal knowledge through participation in the public knowledge of a discipline. In practice, the person may join a collaborative team, working on complex problem situations found in integrative healthcare, and this team itself embodies public knowledge. Participation in such a collaborative team enhances the personal knowledge of all the participants, improving their abilities to effectively serve the needs of their patients.

In the next section, five forms of public knowledge will be introduced. Before this is done, it is important to bring to mind some of the common conceptualizations of discipline, the common root of the five forms. Three conceptualizations are highlighted here, such as that of a learner or disciple being educated within a branch of knowledge (Collen, 2002; Gibbons et al., 1994; Ziman, 2000), a system of rules or standards to be followed by educated participants (Collen, 2003), or a body of knowledge generated by a group of similarly educated participants (Ziman, 1968). Taken together, these conceptualizations can be seen as perspectives highlighting specific functions of the overall discipline system. These perspectives will now be discussed relative to the ideas of personal and public knowledge.

A discipline is composed of people interacting symbolically. Public knowledge links these people together into a coherent discipline. Some people are entering the discipline, while others are leaving. The public knowledge that holds the discipline together exists between people, but is not independent of people. So as people enter, leave, and move within a discipline, the public knowledge of the discipline changes dynamically. More importantly, what distinguishes a discipline from a whimsical group of people are constraints on people entering and moving within the discipline. In this way, the public knowledge of the discipline becomes more than just a random conglomeration of public knowledge linkages between people indistinguishable from any other unorganized group. The constraints, not always explicit, define the discipline since they maintain and stabilize the public knowledge linkages between participants within the discipline.

If people leave a discipline (usually by way of retirement or death), then new people must be recruited to replace them. An educational system is necessary to pass to these new recruits the system of constraints and public knowledge that define the discipline. New recruit training accounts for the learner, disciple, or training characteristic common to many definitions of discipline. Since people that come into a discipline are not blank slates, but rather bring their own personal knowledge, private agendas, variable learning abilities, and public knowledge linkages with other groups and disciplines, the training effect is not perfect. The public knowledge of the discipline will dynamically change as a result of the changeover in discipline membership.

Another source for dynamic change in the public knowledge of the discipline is from the activities of the participants. To promote growth and adaptation, participants within a discipline must generate new public knowledge that is worthy of acceptance by the larger group. The constraints of the discipline define how participants go about generating new public knowledge proposals and provide the criteria for testing and assimilating new public knowledge. The constraints account for the notion of discipline related to a system of rules that are followed by the educated participants.

The third notion of discipline as a body of knowledge reflects the embodied knowledge characteristics of a discipline. A discipline can be viewed as a whole, like an individual or an organism. From this perspective the knowledge of the discipline is embodied within the relationships between the participants in the discipline. A discipline's knowledge dynamically changes as a result of the direct experiences of the discipline as a whole. The discipline is also involved in public knowledge relationships with other disciplines. Public knowledge relationships between disciplines allow the development of knowledge within the discipline without the necessity of the direct experience itself.

Monodisciplinary Public Knowledge

Monodisciplinary public knowledge does not refer to within-discipline knowledge, but rather to the dynamics of knowledge sharing relationships between disciplines. Whereas the higher levels of public knowledge result from the encouragement of sharing knowledge across disciplines, monodisciplinarity is more oriented toward shielding or protecting the discipline from these relationships. While monodisciplinary tendencies are present in all disciplines, the description of monodisciplinarity presented here represents the radical and rare perspective when a discipline views itself as independent and self-sufficient, without any need for interaction with other disciplines.

In monodisciplinarity, the characteristic constraint is that of exclusion of public knowledge links between it and other disciplines. Monodisciplinarity is equivalent to a discipline acting individually and isolated from other disciplines. Isolation can occur through ignorance, neglect, or active exclusion of relationships with other disciplines. When it occurs, knowledge becomes fragmented, separated, and specialized. There may be an attempt within a monodisciplinary approach to achieve objectivity or apodictic truth in the form of a system of knowledge that is pure and uncontaminated by outside influence. For example, a service-oriented discipline may offer a panacea without recognition of any complexity within the problem situation that may require services from other disciplines.

Monodisciplinarity, through ignorance and neglect, may occur when a highly specialized branch of knowledge is pursued without any apparent need to recognize or interact with neighboring disciplines. Monodisciplinarity through active exclusion may occur when neighboring disciplines are considered illegitimate and worthy of elimination since they follow an inferior system of rules and conduct or are ultimately reducible to the pure symbolic system of the true monodiscipline. Education within a monodiscipline is highly specialized and specific. It may involve unlearning patterns of behavior and belief structures that might be considered contaminating influences if they are allowed into the discipline.

Figure 1 represents the monodisciplinary approach in relation to a group of professional disciplines. Each of the professionals is situated within his own house, as if each were in private practice and spread across a city in separate offices. No lines of communication exist between the professionals. Each professional provides diagnosis and treatment services utilizing the disciplinary public knowledge within his respective discipline but does not actively seek to share knowledge across disciplinary boundaries or coordinate diagnostic and treatment plans. No other professionals are recognized as necessary for the purpose of providing in-house services.

This description is an extreme example for illustrative purposes. Pure monodisciplinarity is rarely found; on the other hand, monodisciplinary tendencies

Figure 1
Monodisciplinary public knowledge is represented as the lack of knowledge sharing across disciplinary boundaries; in this case, each professional operates in-house without any interaction between houses (no lines connecting houses)

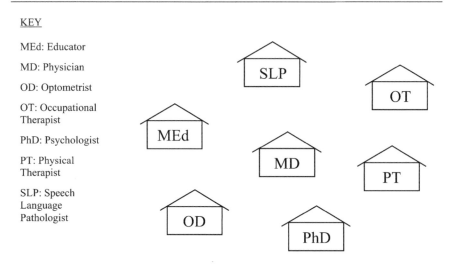

KEY

MEd: Educator

MD: Physician

OD: Optometrist

OT: Occupational Therapist

PhD: Psychologist

PT: Physical Therapist

SLP: Speech Language Pathologist

are at work in all disciplines and serve to consolidate and distinguish the discipline from its surrounding environment. Monodisciplinary public knowledge is represented by the lack of sharing between disciplines, and this requires each discipline to discover knowledge on its own, without any benefit from the experience of other disciplines.

Multidisciplinary Public Knowledge

Multidisciplinarity shares the same constraints as monodisciplinarity, with the exception that other disciplines are not ignored, neglected, or actively excluded. As each discipline recognizes its own limitations, the idea of collaboration emerges, and neighboring disciplines are recognized and given legitimacy. Now public knowledge links are allowed to develop between disciplines as well as within. These links represent multidisciplinary public knowledge.

The key characteristic of these links is that they are informal and unorganized. They represent the inevitable relationships and knowledge sharing that take place when multiple disciplines are brought together in close quarters. Monodisciplinary public knowledge will take form when a discipline is socially isolated; however, when the same discipline is located within the vicinity of other disciplines, informal interactions are inevitable. If the discipline defends itself from these interactions through active avoidance, then it is avoiding participation in multidisciplinary public knowledge. Multidisciplinary public knowledge increases when disciplines no longer avoid, but actually welcome and encourage the informal relationships between disciplines. It flourishes within an institution that brings together similar disciplines under the same roof such as a college of science or university. The various disciplines share a common management, but communications are left informal so that no lines of communication exist that would integrate their research interests. Multidisciplinary public knowledge is formed in places such as the university café or sidewalks, rather than in the laboratory.

In Figure 2, the group of professionals are brought together in a single institution. This institution could be a school or clinic. Inside the institution, each professional works within a separate office. Multidisciplinary public knowledge is represented by the lines that connect the various professionals. The dashed lines represent the informal nature of the sharing of knowledge, much of which occurs in between the professional offices such as in the hallways or common rooms.

Multidisciplinary public knowledge is not systematically taught. People in training for a specific discipline participate in multidisciplinary public knowledge to the extent that their educational environment is adjacent to and informally interacting with other disciplines. It is a street smarts that is acquired by living in the neighborhood of other disciplines. Each discipline

Figure 2
Multidisciplinary public knowledge is represented as disciplines situated inside a single institution and sharing knowledge between disciplines informally

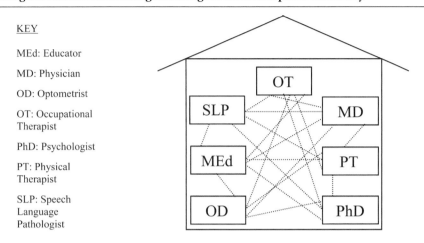

KEY

MEd: Educator

MD: Physician

OD: Optometrist

OT: Occupational Therapist

PhD: Psychologist

PT: Physical Therapist

SLP: Speech Language Pathologist

is allowed to develop its own system of disciplinary public knowledge, and people are expected to be loyal to their disciplines and avoid trespassing on neighboring disciplines. Highly specialized languages and cultures come to characterize disciplines, making it difficult to communicate across disciplinary boundaries, despite close proximity to other disciplines. In multidisciplinarity, there is no method of creating formal public knowledge links between disciplines.

Interdisciplinary Public Knowledge

Interdisciplinarity brings into multidisciplinarity formal lines of communication. Problems that are relevant to multiple disciplines are recognized, and disciplines begin to collaborate in their knowledge-gathering endeavors. Through these intercommunications comes a realization that different approaches have value. Interdisciplinarity begins to recognize the need for such differences in approach and actively seeks the establishment of collaborative relationships. Disciplines are seen as less isolated and more interdependent or open.

Recognizing the limitations of multidisciplinarity, in which the sharing of knowledge across disciplines is informal and unorganized, interdisciplinarity involves a concerted effort at the creation of public knowledge that spans across disciplines, linking them firmly together. Interdisciplinarity may be accomplished by the organizational principles of common goals that guide the construction of the interdisciplinary linkages. Interdisciplinarity results in the creation of many hybrid disciplines and collaborative teams. New knowledge

Figure 3
Interdisciplinary public knowledge is represented as a system of knowledge arrived at through a collaborative effort and the sharing of knowledge between disciplines

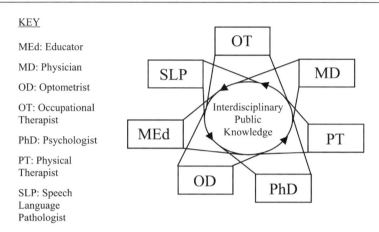

KEY

MEd: Educator

MD: Physician

OD: Optometrist

OT: Occupational Therapist

PhD: Psychologist

PT: Physical Therapist

SLP: Speech Language Pathologist

production results from these collaborative efforts. Interdisciplinary public knowledge is about the sharing of knowledge that takes place when efforts overlap. In Figure 3, the various professionals come together and collaborate for a solution to a problem situation. The knowledge and expertise of each professional overlaps around the common goal, and a system of interdisciplinary public knowledge emerges from this sharing.

Transdisciplinary Public Knowledge

Transdisciplinary public knowledge (TPK) functions as a discipline itself. Participants in the TPK discipline can produce new disciplinary knowledge through the same variety of methods commonly used in other disciplines. Experiments, observations, surveys, interviews, design, or collaboration are only some of the means by which new knowledge can be contributed to the TPK discipline. Knowledge production in TPK can come from individual or collective efforts. Teams utilizing multidisciplinary, interdisciplinary, or transdisciplinary collaboration can contribute to TPK.

Transdisciplinarity has been described as a common language that transcends the borders separating disciplines (Collen, 2003; Koizumi, 2001). The discipline of TPK is specifically about the common language and knowledge that tie a group of disciplines together in a mutual goal. In this way, the TPK discipline transcends the borders separating the various disciplines of the group since it is not about the knowledge of any particular discipline, but rather the knowledge that unites them. Language facilitates the sharing of knowledge between people. Likewise, TPK facilitates the sharing of knowledge between disciplines. Just as public knowledge links individuals together within a discipline, TPK links together multiple disciplines (Figure 4).

TPK emerges from people active within various disciplines. These individuals make a conscious decision to contribute to TPK through individual or collective effort. Through the effort of these people, a system of TPK develops (Figure 5A). TPK then influences and organizes disciplines and collaborative teamwork (Figure 5B). Hideaki Koizumi (2001) defines transdisciplinarity in just such a three-dimensional manner. Transdisciplinarity is the emergence of a new field rising vertically above the flat plane of overlapping disciplines and interdisciplines. It is the organizational influences or common language characteristic of TPK that makes it useful to collaborative teams. Knowledge from experience can be transferred from one collaborative team to another, thus saving the recipient team from having to have the experience itself. This sharing of knowledge allows teams to reach functional and effective outcomes more easily in less time and with less expense.

As a discipline, TPK has the characteristics of being teachable, having a system of rules whereby new knowledge is created, and being a body of such created knowledge. It requires a core group of participants who are literate in both their disciplinary public knowledge and the TPK that unites their disciplines with other similarly focused disciplines. Participants may perform research within their specific disciplines, benefiting from the guidance contributed to the process from their TPK participation. They also perform research that results in new proposals to the TPK related to the field. Participants in the TPK discipline might then adopt the results of such research, thus changing and developing the TPK discipline.

TPK has educational implications. Since it can be described and treated as a discipline in itself, it suggests that new individuals be educated in the

Figure 4
Transdisciplinary public knowledge (TPK) links together multiple disciplines in the same way that public knowledge links together the personal knowledge of multiple people

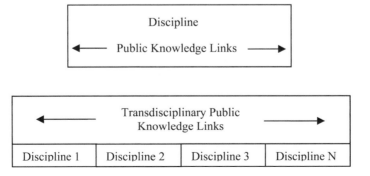

Figure 5
(*A*) TPK is created when contributions are made from individuals, disciplines, or teams and accepted by the members of the TPK transdiscipline. (*B*) Once a system of TPK is developed, it can then influence and organize disciplines and collaborative teamwork

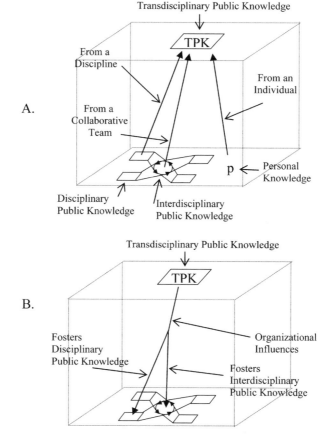

transdisciplinary field as well as their own disciplines. In this way, all the participating disciplines learn the common language that allows them to communicate effectively and mutually benefit each other through collaborative team endeavors. New technological applications may also spring from the development of TPK. Such knowledge may provide the basis for integrating knowledge from a variety of disciplines in ways that could not be conceived from the perspective of a single discipline alone.

Considering collaborative teamwork, interdisciplinary and transdisciplinary teams do not necessarily involve the concept of TPK as it has been defined here. Most often, individual professionals come to the collaborative team without a history of being educated in the common language of a transdisciplinary field. The team may develop a language of its own that facilitates communications among members, but it is specific to the team. The coherent system of public knowledge the team creates in such a case is interdisciplinary public knowledge, not TPK. Only when the team, or members of the team, decide to formally propose their team's interdisciplinary public knowledge to the TPK discipline, and the proposal is accepted by the wider group of TPK participants, does the knowledge actually become TPK.

Metadisciplinary Public Knowledge

Collen (2002) describes metadisciplinarity as a dissolving of disciplinary boundaries and an interwoven collaborative and collective pursuit of knowledge. The extent of the integration becomes such that there emerges a superordinate monodiscipline able to deal effectively with greater complexity. The hierarchy of disciplinary public knowledge developed in this chapter suggests a similar concept of metadisciplinarity. Just as TPK becomes a superordinate monodiscipline useful to a field of disciplines, metadisciplinary public knowledge also represents a monodiscipline, but superordinate to a much wider group of disciplines, including the TPK disciplines. Metadisciplinary public knowledge is most general and abstract and can be applied in the guidance of most domains of transdisciplinary, disciplinary, and personal knowledge. A good example of a research endeavor attempting to generate metadisciplinary public knowledge is the field of general systems theory (Hammond, 2003). The principles developed from such a science of systems can be applied to any theory or discipline that describes the objects of its study as systems. The principles may have application in fields of study as diverse as physics and anthropology. General systems principles are frequently applied to educational and health-related issues and theory. Another example of a metadiscipline is the domain of ethics. Ethics, as a metadiscipline, has impact on human behavior and interaction at all subordinate disciplines.

In Figure 6, a schematic of the hierarchy of disciplinary public knowledge is presented. The informal public knowledge relationships between individuals are organized into disciplines by disciplinary public knowledge. From the perspective of disciplinary public knowledge, informal public knowledge begins to blur. When disciplines collaborate, disciplinary public knowledge begins to blur as interdisciplinary public knowledge begins to organize the subordinate forms of public knowledge. In a like manner, TPK and metadisciplinary public knowledge organize their respective subordinate forms of public knowledge, and borders continue to blur.

The concept of metadisciplinary public knowledge suggests that disciplinary education may involve a curriculum involving at least three levels of public knowledge: disciplinary, transdisciplinary, and metadisciplinary.

Figure 6
Relationships and hierarchies between the various domains of public knowledge
are shown. Superordinate levels encompass subordinates, and subordinate level
boundaries begin to blur. PK, personal knowledge; DPK, disciplinary public
knowledge; IPK, interdisciplinary public knowledge; TPK, transdisciplinary public
knowledge; MPK, metadisciplinary public knowledge

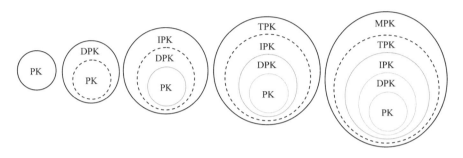

TRANSDISCIPLINARY PUBLIC KNOWLEDGE
AND COLLABORATIVE TEAMWORK

Traditionally, professionals are trained to diagnose and treat problems that
are within a certain scope of practice. When a problem situation arises that
is outside his scope of practice, the professional's responsibility is to refer the
individual to another appropriate professional. Referral is very common in
medicine. For example, if an internist were treating a patient for a condition that required prednisone, and as a result, the patient developed cataracts
(a side effect of prednisone use), the patient would then be referred to an oph-
thalmologist for assessment and surgical removal of the cataracts. The internist would not attempt to remove the cataracts himself. The situation is much
different when considering diagnosis, treatment, and lifestyle coaching in
integrative healthcare. The situations are complex and simultaneously involve
issues relevant to a variety of professionals. One professional's therapy may
not be implemented effectively without taking into consideration the issues,
approaches, and therapy of other professionals also involved with the patient.
This fact has prompted much development and acceptance of a variety of team
approaches (Woodruff & McGonigel, 1988).

TEAM APPROACHES

Different approaches have been explored toward meeting team requirements. Usually, a group of professionals of varied disciplines are recruited
or employed by an institution, such as a school or clinic, for the purpose of
assessment and treatment. Three characteristic team approaches have been
described for organizing the services of varied professionals. These are the

multidisciplinary team, the interdisciplinary team, and the transdisciplinary team (Garner, 1994b; Gilles & Clark, 2001; McGonigel et al., 1994; Orelove & Sobsey, 1996; Rainforth & York-Barr, 1997; Ryndak, 1996; United Cerebral Palsy Associations of America [UCPAA], 1976; Woodruff & McGonigel, 1988). This characterization is an example of the hierarchical organization of descriptive terms, with an emphasis on the collaborative nature of the teamwork taking place. Each of these will be briefly reviewed and then discussed relative to a hierarchy of public knowledge that emphasizes knowledge sharing.

Multidisciplinary teams involve professionals that work independently from each other. The approach is most similar to the medical model of service delivery, and since many professionals were trained in this model, it was most often the first approach tried when teams were first forming. Members of a multidisciplinary team may share the same space and utilize some of the same tools, but they often function independently from one another. Each team member performs a separate assessment. Team members develop separate treatment plans relevant to their particular disciplines and presume that only they are capable of providing the service. Team members have only informal lines of communication among themselves and, while recognizing the importance of contributions from other disciplines, often do not cross disciplinary boundaries within their professional continuing education and research.

The multidisciplinary team approach has been criticized for not fostering services that reflect a holistic view (Linder, 1983). Communication among the professionals is considered poor; therefore, in the case of a child, a parent often must consolidate the information from the various professionals and take on a case management role (Woodruff & McGonigel, 1988). With individualized assessment and poor communication, team members often find themselves recommending opposing therapeutic interventions (Orelove & Sobsey, 1996). When each team member suggests his own unique treatment, plans can easily become complicated and expensive to implement.

Interdisciplinary teams address the communications difficulties inherent in the multidisciplinary model. For the most part, interdisciplinary teams still involve individual assessments by the various disciplines, but formal channels of communication are structured for the purpose of sharing assessment results and discussing treatment options and priorities. Even though some of the communication and isolation issues are dealt with, significant problems still exist. Professional turf battles appear to be a major problem (Woodruff & McGonigel, 1988). These are usually brought on by a lack of interdisciplinary understanding. Team members may not understand the expertise of other team members, or terminology may carry different meanings between disciplines. The interdisciplinary team approach still relies on direct hands-on therapy by the therapist, which can become an issue when therapists are constrained for time or monetary resources are low (Ore-love & Sobsey, 1996).

The transdisciplinary team model was originally designed to serve high-risk infants (UCPAA, 1976) but has since been applied in other settings involving special needs and inclusive practices (Gilles & Clark, 2001; Orelove & Sobsey, 1996) and healthcare. The model attempts to transcend traditional disciplinary boundaries for the purpose of fostering greater communication, understanding, cooperation, and coordination of treatment approaches by therapists. In the transdisciplinary model, the status of the patient or family as a member of the team is heightened over the multidisciplinary and interdisciplinary models (Woodruff & McGonigel, 1988). Patients or families are viewed as having a great impact on the outcome of the treatment approach and therefore need complete participation in setting goals and providing therapy.

Usually, a team member is designated as the primary service provider. In this role the team member is responsible for the primary intake, arranging the evaluation, coordinating the overall treatment plan, and providing a significant portion of the therapy. These responsibilities may involve the primary service provider in therapeutic roles that cross over into other disciplines. The patient intake is only done once by the primary service provider, rather than multiple times by each individual discipline.

Following assessment, the team formulates a treatment plan. The treatment plan involves all team members, including the patient or family, and integrates suggestions from everyone. The program implementation is usually carried out by the patient, family, or primary service provider. If specific therapeutic activities are needed, then the appropriate professional may instruct the primary service provider on proper techniques. Sometimes this is not possible, and only the professional can provide the direct therapy. In such cases the professional might be assigned a role support function that is more traditional in format. The same basic pattern of arena assessment and team planning is utilized for all reassessments and progress checks (Wolery & Dyk, 1984).

In application, the transdisciplinary team model has generated controversy and confusion, usually centered around issues related to clarification of roles, logistics, practicality, accountability, and liability (Landerholm, 1990; Orelove, 1994; York et al., 1990). Because of the extensive preparation, training, and experience needed to develop a transdisciplinary team as well as the expense and logistics of getting all team members together, the ideal of a transdisciplinary team is rarely practiced as described above. More often, professionals strive to implement key aspects of the model such as involving patients or families as equal team members or role releasing therapeutic approaches between professionals (Albano, 1983; Landerholm, 1990; Magrum & Tigges, 1982; Reed, 1993). Recently, there is a trend toward using the more generic description of so-called collaborative teamwork to describe teams that may implement aspects from the multi-, inter-, and transdisciplinary models but do not situate themselves exclusively within one model (Snell & Janney, 2000; Gilles & Clark, 2001).

PUBLIC KNOWLEDGE UTILIZATION WITHIN TEAMS

The hierarchy of disciplinary public knowledge can now be applied to the collaborative teamwork in use by professionals. Figure 7 presents a field of professional disciplines. Each of the forms of disciplinary public knowledge is highlighted. As an example, speech language pathology (SLP) is a professional

Figure 7
The hierarchy of disciplinary public knowledge is represented. Disciplinary public knowledge is within each box, multidisciplinary public knowledge is shown as informal links between boxes, interdisciplinary public knowledge is the result of a collaborative effort, and TPK has influence on all disciplines and collaborative processes

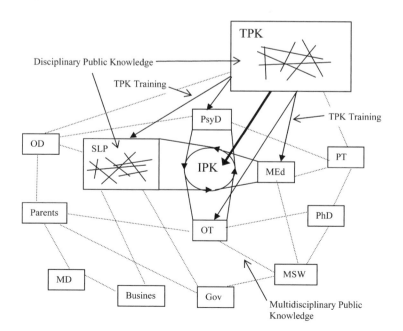

KEY

Gov: Government
IPK: Interdisciplinary Public Knowledge
MEd: Educator
MD: Physician
MSW: Social Worker
OD: Optometrist

OT: Occupational Therapist
PhD: Researcher
PsyD: Psychologist
PT: Physical Therapist
SLP: Speech Language Pathologist
TPK: Transdisciplinary Public Knowledge

discipline actively involved in developmental contexts. As such, SLP develops a disciplinary system of public knowledge involving the individual SLPs' personal knowledge and the links connecting together these participants in the discipline. This disciplinary public knowledge is represented in Figure 7 as the web of relationships internal to the SLP discipline. All the other disciplines represented within the field also have their own disciplinary public knowledge web.

SLP interacts with other professional disciplines informally and develops public knowledge links between members of the discipline and surrounding disciplines involved in the field. These relationships are informal in that there are no intentional goals to collaborate as a team to research and develop a public knowledge about common interests and concerns. These informal relationships between disciplines become multidisciplinary public knowledge and are represented in Figure 7 as the web of dotted lines between the various disciplines.

The SLP, PsyD, MEd, and OT decide to collaborate as a team on a specific problem situation, the outcome of which is a useful system of interdisciplinary public knowledge. While each of these professionals has not made formal contributions to the field's TPK, the professionals have been trained in the TPK discipline. This training results in benefits that foster the collaborative efforts of the team. The team reaches an effective solution to the problem situation more quickly.

STAGES OF COLLABORATIVE TEAM BUILDING

The benefits of TPK can be further developed by consideration of some of the stages involved in development of an effective team (at this point, references to the transdisciplinary team refer to a collaborative process leading to interdisciplinary public knowledge, not to be confused with TPK, which refers to a distinct discipline that guides and organizes such collaborative teams). The development of a transdisciplinary team requires what the United Cerebral Palsy National Collaborative Infant Project (UCPAA, 1976) calls *role release*. The team approach becomes transdisciplinary when the professionals give up, or release, their direct intervention with the clients. Role release is accomplished by training team members other than the specialists among the team to provide the therapy. There are five processes that the professionals must address to have the proper support for role release: role extension, role enrichment, role expansion, role exchange, and role support (Lyon & Lyon, 1980; Woodruff & McGonigel, 1988).

Role extension represents the usual continuing education within a discipline. It is important for professionals to keep up with current knowledge in their fields. Role enrichment follows role extension. Once the professional is well versed within his own discipline, he is ready to learn about other disciplines. Role enrichment refers to the cross-discipline education that is necessary to support a cooperative team approach. Role expansion continues this process when the various professionals start working together as a team and learn more specific information about each other's disciplines through interaction and discussion. Once knowledge has been shared between the various team members, the professionals move toward role exchange. At this point the professionals may perform assessment and therapeutic techniques that cross over into another team member's discipline. Role exchange is facilitated by team members working side by side. Finally, the professionals exhibit role release, where there is enough trust between professionals that assessment and therapeutic needs can be addressed by any team member. This accomplishment does not mean that the team is then broken up and the professionals work independently with clients outside of their particular scopes of practice, but rather that in the transdisciplinary team, roles are not isolated or segmented, but all team members can share roles, more or less. Sometimes, however, there are assessment or therapy techniques that require extensive training or experience and cannot be easily released to other team members. In these cases the qualified professional exhibits a role support function to the team, performing the specific assessment or therapy directly.

When any group of individuals comes together in a team for the purpose of collaborating to solve a problem situation, there are characteristic stages of team development that typically occur prior to reaching full effectiveness. Performance differences among teams in similar organizations can usually be attributed to differences in the teams' stage of development (Garner, 1994a). Tuckman (1965) describes team development according to a four-stage model: forming, storming, norming, and performing. Forming involves the coming together of team members and the establishment of a sense of purpose and identity as a team. Storming usually involves conflict as the team begins to search for values and norms. Norming is a transition stage as the group discovers and implements shared values and norms. Performing is characterized by less attention being paid to internal team issues such that the effort of the team is directed more fully toward solving the problem situation that brought together the team in the first place.

TRANSDISCIPLINARY PUBLIC KNOWLEDGE ACCELERATION OF THE TEAM BUILDING PROCESS

There is considerable direct experience that is involved currently in the process of building a collaborative team. Not only do team members need direct experience to progress through the stages leading to role release, they also directly experience the social dynamics of team development leading to the performing stage. If a team member were to exit a team, the new member does not have the benefit of direct experience and may hinder the function of the team for a time as his personal knowledge develops, through direct experience, to a functional level. The whole team may be pulled down to a lower stage while the new member catches up. Furthermore, when a problem situation arises that is best dealt with through the utilization of a collaborative team, it may take considerable time to form and develop the team to a level of functionality appropriate to the problem situation.

Public knowledge allows an individual person to benefit from the direct experience of another. While it is unlikely that all of the direct experience involved in the establishment and orchestration of a transdisciplinary team could be transferred from one individual to another, it is likely that significant aspects can be. By utilizing public knowledge to substitute for some of the direct experiences involved in team building, it may be possible to build teams to highly effective levels much more quickly and economically.

TPK is about public knowledge that will assist the formation and maintenance of teams and collaborative networks. Through TPK, individuals new to a collaborative team become fully functional much more rapidly than they could if they had to acquire personal knowledge through direct experience alone. Because individuals who participate in TPK may benefit from the experiences of others as if they had had the experience themselves, they enter the team building process with a head start.

A key characteristic of a transdisciplinary team is role release. The sequence of stages leading to role release were outlined previously as role extension, role enrichment, role expansion, and role exchange, leading then to role release. Role extension involves the professional involving himself in the public knowledge specific to his discipline. Role extension is primarily attention being paid to disciplinary public knowledge. Role enrichment is a familiarization with peripheral disciplines and learning a bit of their language and techniques. Role enrichment might involve multidisciplinary or interdisciplinary public knowledge. Role expansion and role exchange involve greater degrees of interaction with the public knowledge of another discipline as well as considerable direct experience from the side-by-side interaction between professionals. Role expansion and exchange recognize that a professional discipline involved with human learning and development cannot be mastered entirely through public knowledge, but also requires some direct experience. Before a team can reach the level of role release, the team members must become familiar with the public knowledge of the other disciplines and also attain personal knowledge through direct experience in the process of role exchange. TPK is not about any particular discipline, but is a general knowledge that will help to facilitate the team building process toward role release. TPK accelerates the processes of role enrichment, role expansion, and role exchange, leading to role release.

BUILDING TRANSDISCIPLINARY PUBLIC KNOWLEDGE

While the concept of TPK is new, there exists considerable literature related to collaborative teams in a variety of contexts. Much of this literature has been reviewed in previous sections. Books, journal articles, conferences, and other presentations of the results of research and experience in collaborative teaming have been published. Collectively, these presentations and the activities of the individuals who authored them indicate that TPK disciplines are emerging.

As stated previously, TPK does not depend on any particular research methodology for its production. As a discipline, it is free to explore any means of research. While TPK is generally applied to fostering collaborative teamwork, and the experiences of teams will likely be a rich source of TPK contributions, there is no requirement that TPK be generated only through collaborative efforts. Individual researchers can equally generate proposals of TPK, as can collaborative teams.

One of the most utilized means of sharing public knowledge within a discipline is through the use of text. Textbooks, used by most new students entering a discipline, provide a general overview of the discipline's fundamentals or consensus views. They provide the language training and concept development the student will need to become an active practitioner or contributor within a discipline. Journal articles, editorials, conference proceedings, and other uses of text bring personal knowledge into the sphere of the discipline's public knowledge. Individuals make contributions to the public knowledge of the discipline, but these contributions have not reached the level of consensus common in textbooks. Also, participants in a discipline informally interact using text such as e-mail communication.

In a similar manner, text could be used as a medium in the establishment of TPK within a field of multiple disciplines. Students could interact with texts representing TPK consensus in the field. In this way the process of developing the language and skills of collaborative teamwork could be accelerated. TPK consensus would emerge from the efforts of researchers actively contributing to the field the results of their investigations or ideas. Participants in this TPK generation and distribution system would test its utility in their day-to-day professional practice when called on to collaborate with other professionals.

As further strides are made in the area of interdisciplinary collaboration, opportunities for cross-disciplinary training need to be developed, systematized, and actively promoted throughout the spectrum of healthcare professions. We can see current evidence of such cross-disciplinary training in a number of healthcare professions, but more needs to be done. Physicians are beginning to receive more structured training in alternative-complementary medical concepts, public health, hospital administration, medical-legal training, and more. Nurses are also gaining valuable training in areas such as public health, administration, and advanced clinical practitioner training, to name but a few. Within the field of early intervention, healthcare professionals, such as occupational, physical, and speech therapists, have been involved in cross-disciplinary training with child educators for a number of years now.

Efforts to publish texts like this text on humanizing healthcare will serve to educate professionals in all fields about the importance of cross-disciplinary training in healthcare and can lay the groundwork for further research.

TRAINING IMPLICATIONS

Any discussion of embodied knowledge warrants comments concerning the application and implications of the ideas presented above to various individuals and groups involved in training and education in integrative healthcare.

The Trainee

Students bring into their academic arena a vast personal knowledge developed over years of personal experiences and interaction with public knowledge. Students do not start as blank slates. The existing personal knowledge of the student will shape how the student sees, hears, and otherwise interacts with new direct experiences and public knowledge. Learning is a dynamic that begins where the student is at the moment, with new patterns of behavior emerging through the learning process. Learning is not simply the absorption or acquisition of new knowledge such as the writing of new information in the memory of the brain, as our common computer metaphors would suggest. The embodied view of knowledge emphasizes the importance of the relationships that develop between the student, teacher, and symbolic mediators such as texts. By participation in the public knowledge relationships organized and structured by an institution and teacher, the student will develop his personal knowledge in ways that do not require direct personal experience. In this way the student can take an accelerated learning track and achieve functional competence in the field much faster than would be possible if direct personal experience were the only way to learn.

On the other hand, there are considerable skills, especially in a field such as healthcare, that necessitate direct experience. Examples of such skills include learning how to elicit a medical or social history and perform complete as well as problem-specific examinations: learning how to do blood draws and start intravenous lines; learning the fine art of suturing and casting; learning basic and advanced life support skills; learning how to give immunizations and other injectable medications; and so on.

It is easy to talk about how professionals might formally interrelate as an interdisciplinary team, but there are considerable relationship skills that are critically important in the success of such a team that cannot be learned simply through public knowledge. Students should have participatory experiences to develop teamwork skills prior to entering practice situations. Not only will this enable more effective teamwork in practice, but it will also remind students of the possibilities and benefits of relating with other professionals in an interdisciplinary manner.

The CHA/P program in Alaska offers an excellent example of developing this interdisciplinary model and the inherent challenges that present themselves. The majority of CHA/P trainees and graduates are Native Alaskans representing a variety of tribes each with unique cultures, language subtleties, and experiences interacting with the non-Native cultures that coexist in their areas. The CHA/Ps are the first responders to medical emergencies in their villages. They are called on not only to utilize their personal knowledge and experience in responding to these emergencies, but they also must tap into the knowledge and experience of others in their villages and in the region. These other resources include other villagers who might have medical training in basic first aid, firefighters who have experience dealing with smoke inhalation, or others in the village with experience in cold water injuries, gunshot wounds, and other trauma, all of which are very common in Alaska. There may be a traditional healer in the village who offers advice or guidance to the CHA/P that must be given consideration along with the CHA/P's Western medical training when making important health decisions.

The CHA/Ps have ample opportunity for participatory experiences through interaction with traditional healers as well as with advanced Western medical providers in their region and around the state. These include physicians, PAs, NPs, and other veteran CHA/Ps. On a daily basis, CHA/Ps report complicated patients outside the scope of their practice to physicians in their regional health center via telephone. CHA/Ps interact with PAs, NPs, nurses, and paramedics on a regular basis. A CHA/P might receive a call to consult about a patient in the village from a specialist at the Alaska Native Medical Center in Anchorage. These interactions provide opportunities for developing mutual respect between members of a very diverse interdisciplinary team. Other medical resources with whom CHA/Ps have regular interaction include emergency medical technicians (EMTs), dentists, optometrists, mental health professionals, social workers, and public health specialists. Making such a multidisciplinary team work effectively is a challenge.

There are other aspects of effective teamwork that may indeed be learned through participation with public knowledge. This is the case for transdisciplinary public knowledge. If students are also taught the language and understanding developed by the field's TPK, in certain aspects they will come to the interdisciplinary team process with advanced skills based on the accumulated experience of those who have tried various approaches in the past and discovered certain best practices.

An example to illustrate this point is seen in the PA profession. A PA's education is composed of the medical field's language and understanding, which is this field's TPK. The same can be said of physicians and NPs and, to a degree, of CHA/Ps in Alaska. A rigorous medical education is based on the latest best practices, and this is an evolving body of knowledge that changes daily. Through study of an evolving body of best practice knowledge, one is able to bring the latest information to the interdisciplinary team for consideration in the care of patients. PAs come to the interdisciplinary team process already with advanced skills based on the accumulated experience of those who have tried various approaches in the past and discovered certain best practices. For a PA to be accepted into PA training, he must have some previous hands-on medical experience. He has gathered a foundation of skills and knowledge prior to his PA training, and this only serves to enhance his contributions to the interdisciplinary team.

The Trainer

The teacher or trainer represents the primary human relationship that modulates the student's interactions with public knowledge toward a goal of demonstrating personal knowledge competence in the field. The trainer must have insight and respect for the existing personal knowledge of the student; otherwise, it is difficult to guide the student through a sequence of direct experience and public knowledge encounters as appropriate stepping stones toward mastery of a subject or skill.

A teacher will function as a guide or coach for learning by doing experiences. In this way the teacher sets up situations for students to directly experience, and through such direct experience, the students' personal knowledge is developed. Earlier examples have been shared that emphasize this point using the CHA/P program in Alaska as a model. Using the "show one, do one" method has been found to be a successful training method for developing a CHA/P's personal knowledge. Having a trainer/teacher set up controlled learning experiences for the trainees provides them a safe opportunity to learn critically important skills such as eliciting a medical history, performing a physical exam, doing blood draws, and inserting intravenous devices, giving injections by practicing these skills on their colleagues.

A teacher also functions as a guide or coach for immersion in public knowledge relevant to the discipline, transdiscipline, or metadiscipline. Through a lecture, reading, discussion group, or any other variety of symbolic interaction utilized in educational contexts, the teacher will ensure that the student encounters and is influenced by relevant public knowledge. The teacher cannot be ensured that such interaction will have the same results for all students, only that the interaction should move the student toward the educational objectives. For example, the most relevant public knowledge for a CHA/P to be exposed to is the community health aide manual (CHAM). The CHAM serves as the CHA/P's standard of care. It must be used with every patient encounter. It is a detailed, step-by-step manual to assist the CHA/P in his patient encounters. Their medical standing orders are based on their demonstration of thorough understanding of how to use this manual. During their training, every facet of their experience involves how to use the CHAM or where to find information in their CHAM. Through lectures, homework assignments, medical standing orders exams, skills labs, group and individual discussions, and experiential learning in the clinic setting, the CHA/P trainee is immersed in the CHAM, thus ensuring an intense and ongoing encounter with the source of a CHA/P's relevant public knowledge.

In Practice: The Patient-Healer Relationship

When a macrophage gobbles up nasty bacteria, thus preventing a deadly infection, we stand back in amazement and applaud at the embodied knowledge within the person. Certainly without this disease-fighting knowledge, a body would find it tough to grow into a system composed of trillions of cells in intimate relationship. Embodied knowledge is not always explicit and conscious; in fact, most personal knowledge—the integration of experience and expression with the environment—is implicit and unconscious. This is an important point to remember for the practitioner working with a patient. The patient already has a vast amount of personal experience, not only developed through real-life experiences, but also developed through the evolution of the species having to deal with health and survival for millions of years. The healer cannot hope to understand all the personal knowledge within the patient, and this demands a certain humility and respect for the natural processes that are at work.

The healer's relationship to the patient is much like the teacher's to the student. It is a public knowledge–modulating relationship. The healer can guide and coach the patient toward direct experiences that should move the patient toward health. The healer can guide and coach the patient toward interaction with public knowledge such that the patient adopts patterns of behavior that have shown through experience to help positively the healing outcome of the situation.

In the role of a teacher or health guide to the patient, the best the provider can hope for is to use the provider's personal knowledge, the wealth of public knowledge available in the disciplines, and the wisdom of the interdisciplinary team to educate and help the patient help himself. The personal knowledge and experience of the patient and his culture are also critical components to consider. Healthcare providers cannot force a patient to do anything that he does not want to do for himself.

The effects of this one point are clearly demonstrated when we consider the serious problem that exists today with drug-resistant bacteria. Part of the problem is due to the wanton prescribing of antibiotics by providers for diseases where antibiotics are of no value (e.g., the treating of viral illnesses with antibiotics). Another part of the problem is the misuse of antibiotics by the patient—not taking the full course of the antibiotic or not taking it as directed. This is especially problematic when the patient is a child and the parent has the responsibility to administer the antibiotic to the child according to the healthcare provider's direction. Even with education from the provider about the benefits of the antibiotic and how to take the medication properly, patients often do not adhere to the directions. The end result is a drug-resistant bacteria conundrum with which medical science is barely keeping up.

The nature of the relationship between the healer and the patient is more along the lines of sharing rather than prediction and control. The patient is not submitting himself to the control of the healer; rather, the healer, through a public knowledge relationship, is sharing with the patient knowledge that leads to health. The sharing is not always verbal, but could be physical, biological, cognitive, or spiritual—or a combination of these.

In Practice: Interdisciplinary Relationships

In practice, professionals will find themselves in a variety of settings, some of which will be more conducive to the establishment of informal and formal relationships with other professionals, and others that will not. Previously, monodisciplinary public knowledge was discussed as necessary for defining the scope and borders between disciplines, but when carried too far, it can lead to the extinguishing or lack of important relationships between professionals. Multidisciplinary public knowledge was presented as the informal relationships that form between professionals when working close together. Interdisciplinary public knowledge relationships form when the process of relationship building becomes formalized, directed, and actively pursued. With these forms of public knowledge in mind, some principles compatible with the goals of a more integrative healthcare become apparent.

Active exclusion, negation, and denial of other professionals and their practices is a monodisciplinary tendency that works against cross-disciplinary integration of knowledge, which is a key feature of integrative healthcare. This does not mean that rigorous and critical inquiry should not have its place in the research and application of healthcare practices, only that recognizing the diversity of disciplines and approaches can bear considerable fruit in the development of healing insights when explored in an interdisciplinary fashion, and monodisciplinarity tends to work against the recognition of these possibilities.

Professionals have daily opportunities to interact with other professionals in a multidisciplinary fashion these days that does not always require the professionals to meet face-to-face. Communication technology, such as telephones, mail, and e-mail, will bring professionals together as they deal with mutual cases. Professionals who are supportive of the goals of integrative healthcare should look for opportunities to communicate with other professionals of diverse disciplines. Simply asking patients during the case history what other professionals they are currently or have recently worked with will open up communicative opportunities such as sharing testing results and assuring that treatment approaches are not conflicting. Such communication can not only develop each professional's cross-disciplinary knowledge, but also has the potential for developing better interprofessional referral networks that bring patients in contact with a wider array of services from which they may benefit.

When professionals recognize the mutually beneficial multidisciplinary public knowledge that is emerging through informal means, groups may be formed to formalize and pursue deliberately the development of interdisciplinary public knowledge relevant to mutually important problem situations. These problem situations might be concrete individual patient cases or could be more abstract issues and procedures that impact collaborative healthcare in general. An example of formalizing and pursuing deliberately the development of interdisciplinary public knowledge relevant to mutually important problem situations can be seen in the field of telemedicine. There has been an explosion in telemedicine technology in the past 10 years that has served to link health professionals, researchers, specialists, and others together. In the Norton Sound region of northwest Alaska, for example, this technology was introduced in the mid-1990s. The technology was tested in a few of the larger villages in the region. Today, all 15 villages have telemedicine technology, making it possible for CHA/Ps to consult with advanced healthcare providers throughout the state and establishing a beginning network for true transdisciplinary public knowledge and training to take place.

TOOL KIT FOR CHANGE

Role and Perspective of the Healthcare Professional

1. Training of the healthcare provider includes educating the provider about the differences in personal and public knowledge that are embodied in the experiential/

expressive relationship between the person and the environment and in relationships between people.
2. The healthcare provider must be willing to learn the language of other disciplines to best meet the needs of the patient.
3. The healthcare provider must be willing to participate nondefensively and nonaggressively in personal, experiential learning opportunities to work with others on well-functioning teams for the best interest of the patient.

Role and Perspective of the Patient/Participant

1. The patient must be willing to establish multiple relationships to form a healing network to address his health concerns.
2. The patient must request, tirelessly at times, that multiple team members communicate with each other and with the patient about health choices.
3. The patient must request that information be shared in as clear a layman's language as possible so that the patient can participate in his own care and make healthcare decisions.

Interconnection: The Global Perspective

1. As the flow of information increases with the progress of technology, attention to group communication, terminology, and dynamics among healthcare disciplines becomes increasingly important—but also time consuming and difficult.
2. Specific training models for addressing this communication dilemma are essential.
3. Models for making healthcare knowledge more available across the boundaries of different professions currently exist. They use both computer-based analysis and face-to-face training, which can stimulate the evolution of quality integrative healthcare.

REFERENCES

Albano, M. (1983). *Transdisciplinary teaming in special education: A case study.* Urbana-Champaign: University of Illinois.
Bateson, G. (1972). *Steps to an ecology of mind.* New York: Ballantine Books.
Bickley, L. S. & Szilagyi, P. G. (2005). *Bates' Guide to Physical Examination and History Taking. 9th edition.* New York: Lippincott Williams & Wilkins.
Collen, A. (2002). Disciplinarity in the pursuit of knowledge. In G. Minati and E. Pessa (Eds.), *Emergence in complex cognitive, social, and biological systems* (pp. 285–296). New York: Kluwer Academic / Plenum.
Collen, A. (2003). *Systemic change through praxis and inquiry.* New Brunswick, NJ: Transaction.
Garner, H. G. (1994a). Critical issues in teamwork. In H. G. Garner and F. P. Orelove (Eds.), *Teamwork in human services* (pp. 1–18). Boston: Butterworth-Heinemann.
Garner, H. G. (1994b). Multidisciplinary versus interdisciplinary teamwork. In H. G. Garner and F. P. Orelove (Eds.), *Teamwork in human services* (pp. 19–36). Boston: Butterworth-Heinemann.
Gibbons, M., Limoges, C., Nowotny, H., Schwartzman, S., Scott, P., & Trow, M. (1994). *New production of knowledge: Dynamics of science and research in contemporary societies.* London: Sage.

Gilles, D., & Clark, D. (2001). Collaborative teaming in the assessment process. In S. Alper, D. L. Ryndak, & C. N. Schloss (Eds.), *Alternative assessment of students with disabilities in inclusive settings* (pp. 75–87). Boston: Allyn and Bacon.

Hammond, D. (2003). *The science of synthesis.* Boulder: University Press of Colorado.

Hayles, N. K. (1999). *How we became posthuman.* Chicago: University of Chicago Press.

Koizumi, H. (2001). Trans-disciplinarity. *Neuroendocrinology Letters, 22,* 219–221.

Lakoff, G., & Johnson, M. (1999). *Philosophy in the flesh: The embodied mind and its challenge to Western thought.* New York: Basic Books.

Landerholm, E. (1990). The transdisciplinary team approach. *Teaching Exceptional Children, 22,* 66–70.

Linder, T. (1983). *Early childhood special education: Program development and administration.* Baltimore: Paul H. Brookes.

Lyon, S., & Lyon, G. (1980). Team functioning and staff development: A role release approach to providing integrated educational services for severely handicapped students. *Journ-al of the Association for the Severely Handicapped, 5,* 250–263.

Magrum, W. M., & Tigges, K. N. (1982). A transdisciplinary mobile intervention program for rural areas. *American Journal of Occupational Therapy, 36,* 90–94.

Maturana, H. R., & Varela, F. J. (1987). *The tree of knowledge.* Boston: New Science Library Shambhala.

McGonigel, M. J., Woodruff, G., et al. (1994). The transdisciplinary team: A model for family-centered early intervention. In L. J. Johnson, R. J. Gallagher, M. J. LaMontagne, and J. B. Jordan (Eds.), *Meeting early intervention challenges: Issues from birth to three* (pp. 95–131). Baltimore: Brookes.

Mills, C. W. (1963). *Power, politics, and people: The collected essays of C. Wright Mills.* New York: Ballantine.

Orelove, F. P. (1994). Transdisciplinary teamwork. In H. G. Garner and F. P. Orelove (Eds.), *Teamwork in human services* (pp. 37–59). Boston: Butterworth-Heinemann.

Orelove, F. P., & Sobsey, D. (1996). Designing transdisciplinary services. In F. P. Orelove and D. Sobsey (Eds.), *Educating children with multiple disabilities: A transdisciplinary approach* (pp. 1–33). Baltimore: Paul H. Brookes.

Pearson, A. P. (2005). *Transdisciplinary public knowledge for collaborative teamwork in the education of children with disabilities.* Doctoral dissertaion, Saybrook Graduate School and Research Institute, San Francisco, CA. UMI Dissertation Services, Proquest. Microform 3160023.

Rainforth, B., & York-Barr, J. (1997). *Collaborative teams for students with severe disabilities.* Baltimore: Paul H. Brookes.

Reed, M. L. (1993). The revised arena format (RAF): Adaptations of transdisciplinary evaluation procedures for young preschool children. *Education and Treatment of Children, 16,* 198–205.

Ryndak, D. L. (1996). Educational teams and collaborative teamwork in inclusive settings. In D. L. Ryndak and S. Alper (Eds.), *Curriculum content for students with moderate and severe disabilities in inclusive settings* (pp. 77–96). Needham Heights, MA: Allyn and Bacon.

Snell, M. E., & Janney, R. (2000). *Collaborative teaming.* Baltimore: Paul H. Brookes.

Tuckman, B. W. (1965). Developmental sequences in small groups. *Psychological Bulletin, 63,* 384–399.

United Cerebral Palsy Associations of America. (1976). *Staff development handbook: A resource for the transdisciplinary process.* New York: Author.

Wolery, M., & Dyk, L. (1984). Arena assessment: Description and preliminary social validity data. *Journal of the Association for the Severely Handicapped, 9,* 231–235.

Woodruff, G., & McGonigel, M. J. (1988). Early intervention team approaches: The transdisciplinary model. In J. B. Jordan (Ed.), *Early childhood special education: Birth to three* (pp. 163–181). Reston, VA: ERIC Clearinghouse.

York, J., Rainforth, B., & Giangreco, M. F. (1990). Transdisciplinary teamwork and integrated therapy: Clarifying the misconceptions. *Pediatric Physical Therapy, 2,* 73–79.

Ziman, J. M. (1968). *Public knowledge: The social dimension of science.* New York: Cambridge University Press.

Ziman, J. M. (2000). *Real science: What it is, and what it means.* New York: Cambridge University Press.

Chapter Eleven

THE INTERNATIONAL CLASSIFICATION OF FUNCTIONING: FACILITATING INTEGRATIVE HEALTHCARE

Gerry E. Hendershot, PhD and Don Lollar, EdD

ORIGIN AND DEVELOPMENT OF CLASSIFICATION OF FUNCTIONING AND HEALTH

Integrative healthcare combines two terms into a description of an orientation toward taking care of the health of individuals in a society. *Integration* is a term most associated with social relations. The word describes a quality of coming together, usually of distinct, if not disparate, elements. The opposing term is *segregation,* implying elements that are separate and kept apart. When applied to healthcare, integration becomes *integrative,* which implies an effort to combine several things. First, *integrative* implies seeing the whole person, not just the physical component. Involving the whole person means being concerned for the emotional, behavioral, social, and even spiritual dimensions of the person. Integrative healthcare also adds the element of prevention to treatment. Indeed, prevention becomes a hallmark of integrative healthcare, emphasizing the promotion and maintenance of health beyond the treatment of illness. Attention to the positive end of the health-illness spectrum is allowed, even encouraged, by integrative healthcare. *Healthcare* suggests an emphasis on health. This, however, is usually not the case since the focus of health-related visits is usually to alleviate illness and disease, not the promotion of health. The vision is to address healthcare—caring for and promoting the health of the population—beyond treatment of disease.

With integration of the varied dimensions of well-being within the person and both prevention and treatment, however, come substantial challenges to the science base that undergirds our systems addressing medical care. Medical interventions focusing on improved treatments for injuries, illness, disorders, and diseases have been founded on a strong scientific process. That process is based on breaking the problem into its component parts and finding answers at the most basic of levels, whether cellular or systemic. It focuses on etiology of the problem and diagnostic categories under the auspices of the World Health Organization (WHO) that are used to identify so-called health concerns. Healthcare research most frequently is based on medical conditions that are framed by the same diagnostic system used throughout the world—the International Statistical Classification of Diseases and Related Health Problems (World Health Organization [WHO], 1992–1994).

Integrative healthcare confounds this paradigm by extending beyond the medical, addressing additional factors contributing to health and focusing on outcomes beyond those that are medically based, including the individual's functioning in society. That said, scientific analysis can be a part of healthcare that looks at the whole person and cumulatively analyses factors beyond the medical dimension. The WHO began to consider these broader issues of health in the 1970s. At that time, there emerged an emphasis on the consequences of disease, from which developed a novel conceptual framework. The International Classification of Impairment, Disability, and Handicap (ICIDH), the product of the novel conceptual framework, was presented by WHO with provisional status in 1980. This model described the planes of experience affected by diagnoses—the body, the person's activities, and the individual's interaction with his environment. It asserted that there are experiences beyond the medical condition that can and should be conceptualized, measured, and classified. This new framework in itself was a major advance. The ICIDH was never officially approved by WHO as a classification system for global use but set the foundation for what was to come.

In the early 1990s, WHO began a process for revising the ICIDH. With the assistance of collaborating centers representing all regions of the world and over almost a decade, the World Health Assembly officially approved the International Classification of Functioning, Disability, and Health (ICF) in 2001 (WHO, 2001). In the title alone, one begins to see the difference in language between the older and newer conceptual frames. Negative terms like *impairment* and *handicap* are replaced with neutral *(functioning)* or positive *(health)* terms. Neutral terms were only one of the basic conceptual changes that allow use of the ICF for integrative healthcare purposes.

The ICF "defines components of health and some health-related components of well-being (such as education and labour)" (WHO, 2001, p. 3). The characteristics and concepts embedded in the ICF are particularly relevant for integrative healthcare, including the following.

Universality: The classification is about all people, but it does not classify people. Rather, it describes experiences or health states.

Scope: The experiences covered include body functions, personal activities, societal participation, and environmental factors influencing the person's body, activities, and participation. Inclusion of environmental factors is, perhaps, the most extraordinary conceptual improvement. The interaction between the individual and his environment often enhances or deters participation in and satisfaction with life. The opportunity to identify environmental facilitators and barriers and assign ranks to the degree of help or hindrance to each is a powerful quantitative tool.

Reciprocity: The concepts of the model, presented in Figure 1, are interactive, not linear. Linearity assumes that a medical condition/diagnosis leads to impairments of the body, which lead to personal limitations and then to societal restrictions— for example, cerebral palsy leads to neuromuscular deficits that lead to mobility problems and, finally, to being unable to work. Reciprocity suggests that living is not that simple. It is possible, for example, that one can be physically able to work but have substantial mobility or communication limitations. Likewise, an individual may have a body impairment, such as scoliosis, but without limitations of activity. That same individual, however, may not be able to work due to the stigma of his appearance creating misunderstanding in a work setting. Also, the environmental factors, for example, a schoolteacher, may facilitate or hinder the academic and social function of a child with a diagnosis of attention-deficit/ hyperactivity disorder. Whether or not an individual has access to eyeglasses through a healthcare system may determine whether a visual impairment actually limits the person's ability to read or drive. *Integration*, again, is the operative word—the interaction of the environment and the individual.

Conceptual model: The ICF attempts to bridge the gap between a traditional medical model of functioning, disability, and health and the emergent social model that has developed in the past 35 years. In addition, the ICF conceptual model provides a base for integrative healthcare. The traditional medical model places the problem

Figure 1. Interaction of concepts: ICF 2001.

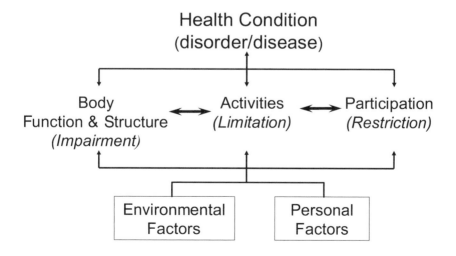

within the person, requiring medical interventions by medical care professionals to cure the problem. The social model posits that the source of the problem is in the society, associated with negative perceptions of disability and environmental barriers, resulting in the outcome of poor participation in community and society. Intervention, therefore, should be at the level of society, addressing physical, attitudinal, and systemic barriers. The ICF proposes the integration of the medical and social models into a biopsychosocial approach that acknowledges the strength of both perspectives and will encourage full health and well-being.

INTERNATIONAL CLASSIFICATION OF FUNCTIONING (ICF) CLASSIFICATION, CODES, AND QUALIFIERS

The ICF operationalizes the concepts through a classification of the components—body functions, activities and participation, and environmental factors. Figure 1 provides the model portraying the components and their relationship to one another. Particularly relevant for integrative healthcare is the ubiquitous role of the environment on body, personal activity, and societal functioning.

Body functions and *body structures* include the physiological functions, including mental, and the anatomical parts of the body. *Impairments* describe problems in body function or structure as a significant deviation or loss (WHO, 2001, p. 12). *Activity* is the execution of a task or action by an individual. *Activity limitations* are problems an individual may have in carrying out a task (WHO, 2001, p. 14). *Participation* is involvement in a life situation, while *participation restrictions* are difficulties a person may experience in a life situation (WHO, 2001, p. 14). *Environmental factors* are the physical, social, and attitudinal settings in which people conduct their lives (WHO, 2001, p. 16).

Central to the ICF coding system is the use of universal qualifiers. This distinguishes the classification from the International Classification of Diseases (ICD). Qualifiers are used across the dimensions (body function and structure, activities and participation, and environment) and use generic numeric codes after the decimal point to characterize severity of difficulty from none (0), to mild, to moderate, to severe, to complete (4). In addition, the qualifiers for activities/participation add two conceptual elements—*capacity,* defined as an individual's ability to execute a task or action within a standardized environment, and *performance,* defined as what an individual does in his current environment. For integrative healthcare, the ICF codes that are most relevant focus on the possibility of coding environmental factors positively or negatively; that is, the ICF allows the description of environmental elements such as attitudes of professionals or the medical or educational systems as either facilitators or barriers to functioning at the personal or societal level. Also, the difference seen between capacity and performance represents the gap between what is and what might be. Emphasis on narrowing the gap is possible using the ICF conceptual and coding system. For instance, a person with a mobility limitation may not be able to use public transportation because of current barriers to wheelchair access to buses and vans, a limitation in *performance;* however, with the addition of wheelchair-accessible buses and vans to the vehicle fleet, the person would have the *capacity* to use public transportation.

RECENT APPLICATIONS OF THE ICF: IS IT LIVING UP TO ITS PROMISE?

The introduction to the ICF (WHO, 2001) says, "The ICF is a multipurpose classification designed to serve various disciplines and different sectors" (p. 5). It goes on to specify that its aim is "to permit comparison of data across countries, health care disciplines, services and time" (p. 5). *Time* is here regarded as including not only historical time, but also life cycle stages from infancy through old age.

These multicultural, multidisciplinary, multi-life-cycle stages aims of the ICF conceptual framework and classification could play an extremely important role in the integration of healthcare. Most care providers are trained and experienced to work with particular cultural groups, particular disciplinary approaches, and particular life cycle stages. Working in integrated care settings requires that they interact with other providers and patients with different particularities, and this can result in communication difficulties and barriers to integration. The promise of the ICF is to provide a common language about function that overcomes communication difficulties and facilitates integration of care.

But is the ICF fulfilling its promises of a multicultural, multidisciplinary, and across-the-life-cycle language for communication about function? Perhaps it is premature and unfair to ask that question so soon after the ICF arrived on the scene—at the time of this writing, it has been only five years since the ICF was approved for use by the World Health Assembly (whereas the ICD has been in use for over 100 years). Although it may be too soon for a definitive evaluation, we believe that there has been enough experience with the ICF to date to begin to formulate a judgment about its probable future as a language for integrated care. Therefore, in this section, we will briefly review some published reports of ICF applications in research and practice with respect to their coverage of cultures, disciplines, and life cycle stages.

As a source of information on applications of the ICD, we searched PubMed, the computer database of the National Institutes of Health for English publications, on the "International Classification of Functioning, Disability, and Health" in the years 2001 through early 2006. About 75 publications were identified. As a database for the present study, the identified articles have some shortcomings. First, we did not do an exhaustive search—if we had used additional search terms, we probably would have found additional publications. Second, PubMed focuses on health research; therefore its coverage of applications that are not, or only marginal to, health research is not complete, and applications that are not clearly scientific research might not be included. We make no claim, therefore, that this evaluation is itself scientific, but we believe it is sufficient to give clear indications of the directions ICF applications were headed in the first five years after its approval.

Cross-Cultural Applications

An important part of the WHO process for developing the ICF was cross-cultural applicability research (Trotter et al., 2001). By testing drafts of the ICF in different cultural contexts around the world, cultural variations in language and meaning were identified and, insofar as possible, eliminated or reduced. The version of the ICF approved by the World Health Assembly was in the English language, but following its approval, it was translated into the other official WHO languages: French, Spanish, Arabic, Chinese, and Russian. Searchable versions of the ICF are available on the ICF Web site (http://www.who.int/icf) in all the official WHO languages, plus Swedish and German. In addition, the ICF has been translated into many other languages in all major geographic areas of the world.

The linguistic ubiquity of the ICF is paralleled by the national origins of the ICF researchers who authored our list of publications from 2001 to 2006. Using as the nationality indicator the locations of the institutions with which lead authors were affiliated, 19 nations are represented, as follows:

Austria
Canada
Czech Republic
Egypt
France
Germany
India
Ireland
Italy
Japan
Netherlands
New Zealand
Norway
South Africa
Spain
Sweden
Switzerland
United Kingdom
United States of America.

With a few exceptions, these are modern, industrially developed nations. While this probably reflects accurately the recent cultural distribution of *health-related* ICF *research*, it fails to capture the many nonresearch applications of the ICF currently under way in economically developing nations (Mbogoni, 2003). Thus the cultural diversity suggested by the national origins of the authors of research publications, although impressive in itself, understates the considerably greater cultural diversity of ICF applications worldwide.

Interdisciplinary Applications

It is a central concept of the ICF that level of function has no necessary relationship to medical diagnosis. Different diagnostic conditions may be associated with the same type and level of function, and similar diagnostic conditions may be associated with different types and levels of function. For that reason the labels and definitions of functional categories rarely mention traditional diagnostic categories. There are some exceptions in the impairments section of the ICF, which covers body structures and body functions; even in those cases, however, the diagnostic categories are not used etiologically, but with respect to variation in structure and function.

A promise of the ICF is that by using nonetiological language, the traditional boundaries among healthcare specialties will be more easily traversed. By focusing on function—walking, for example—specialists in stroke or spinal cord injury or postpolio can communicate more effectively among themselves, with caregivers, and with patients.

As an indicator of the cross-disciplinary application of the ICF, we looked at the medical diagnoses covered in the 2001–2006 ICF publications we identified. Many of the publications were not condition-specific; rather, they were setting-specific, as in studies of patients in post-acute-care facilities. Among the publications that did identify one or more diagnoses, the following diagnoses were mentioned:

brain injury
cerebral palsy
chronic obstructive pulmonary disease
chronic widespread pain
clubfoot
depression
diabetes mellitus
distal radius fracture
epilepsy
hearing loss
idiopathic intracranial hypertension
ischemic heart disease
low back pain

muskuloskeletal conditions
neurodegenerative disease
neurodevelopmental disorder
obesity
oral health
osteoathritis
osteoporosis
rheumatoid arthritis
soft tissue sarcoma
spinal cord injury
stuttering.

These diagnostic categories differ widely in their scope from general (e.g., oral health or muskuloskeletal conditions) to specific (e.g., clubfoot or distal radius fracture). Taken as a group, however, the categories cover a wide range of conditions arising from a variety of causes, both acute and chronic, and affecting persons of both sexes and all ages. We take this as evidence that even in its relative infancy, the ICF already has become multidisciplinary in the sense that researchers interested in a variety of medical conditions, representing a wide range of disciplines, are using it in their work.

As a more direct assessment of that assertion, we attempted to identify the specialized professions of the researchers, but this usually was not possible because institutional affiliations, the best evidence available, did not often permit identification of a particular discipline. To the extent that disciplines of authors were identified, however, there was a notable concentration in the field of rehabilitation. This suggests that whereas many different conditions may be considered by ICF researchers, there may still be a bias toward its use in the rehabilitation sciences.

Before leaving the topic of multidisciplinary applications, we should note the work being done by an international group of researchers based at the ICF Research Branch of the WHO Collaborating Center for the Family of International Classifications at the German Institute of Medical Documentation and Information in Munich (Stucki, Ewert, & Cieza, 2003). Most of the work done by the WHO on the ICF (like most of the work by WHO in general) is done with its so-called collaborating centers, policy and research centers with whom WHO has agreements to collaborate on specific research areas of mutual interest. The Munich group has undertaken to create so-called core sets of ICF categories specific to particular health conditions. Using a mix of qualitative and quantitative techniques—such as focus groups, literature reviews, systematic consultations with specialists (the Delphi method), and clinical trials—they have identified subsets of ICF categories (core sets) that are most useful to specialists treating particular conditions such as osteoarthritis, lupus, obesity, and so on. The existence of core sets for specific conditions, derived using systematic and replicable procedures, is making it easier for specialists to adopt the ICF, extending their emphasis beyond diagnosis to function. Caution should be used, however, in the application of core sets; if they are too narrowly applied to isolated sets of conditions, the commonality of functional outcomes across sets could be overlooked.

Life Span Applications

During the development of the ICF, questions were raised about its applicability to children. Whereas the level of functioning among adults can be considered relative to some explicit or implicit standard that applies to most adults most of the time, that was clearly not the case for children. Children grow and mature over time in a developmental process, and the standards for evaluating their function also change. Evaluating the functions of walking and talking, for instance, is different for children aged 1 year, 5 years, and 10 years. Not only do standards for evaluation change, but the typical activities of children are much different than those of adults, with play and learning occupying a much larger part of their time.

The ICF developers attempted to make it applicable for persons of all ages, but they also recognized that specialized versions of the ICF, adapted to special populations, would be needed, among them an ICF for children and youth. Thus, even before the ICF was approved by the World Health Assembly in 2001, steps were taken to develop an ICF for Children and Youth (ICF-CY). Working under the auspices of the WHO, with funding from the U.S. Centers for Disease Control and Prevention, an international task force of specialists in the functioning, disability, and health of children and youth was formed and began to meet on a regular basis. They drafted and tested additions and modifications to the ICF to make it more applicable to children and youth (Lollar & Simeonsson, 2005). Their guiding principle was to make as little change in the ICF itself as possible; the ICF-CY was not to be an alternative to the ICF, but a specialty version of the ICF.

The effort can be compared with special versions of the ICF's older sibling, the International Classification of Diseases (ICD), also operated under the auspices of WHO. The ICD was originally developed more than 100 years ago as a classification of causes of death; now in its 10th revision, the ICD-10 is still used for that purpose. However, health researchers, health administrators, and health payers needed a system for classifying not just conditions leading to mortality, but also conditions leading to morbidity (illness). The need gave rise to so-called clinical modifications for use in classifying the conditions for which people were hospitalized, known in the United States as ICD-9-CM and ICD-10-CM. The development of these clinical modifications by the United States and other countries is not strictly analogous to the development of the ICF-CY, but both illustrate the general principle that standard classifications can be modified for specialized applications, and such modifications need not undermine the integrity of the original classification. The ICD and ICF are now considered members of a Family of International Classifications, which includes derived classifications as well as related classifications (http://www.who.int/classifications/en/).

The ICF-CY was accepted by WHO in 2006 and will be published in 2007; a preliminary version is available online at the ICF Web site. As an illustration of the kind of modification to the ICF that is incorporated in the ICF-CY, consider the code category d811, "Play, engaging in play." That category (and that alphanumeric code value) is not in the parent ICF. Playing was included as a recreational activity. The Children's Task Force separated play as recreation from the play that children do as their major life activity. Therefore d811 was included in Major Life Activities, with its accompanying developmental sequence; that is, in the ICF-CY, play (d811) is further specified as solitary play (d8110), onlooker play (d8111), parallel play (d8112), and shared cooperative play (d8113).

HOLISTIC ASPECTS OF THE ICF

It was the ambitious goal of the ICF developers to include within its scope *all* human functioning. It was not the goal that all specific functions would be *identified* and *described* by the ICF, but that the classification would be sufficiently broad in its scope and language that any specific human function that might be identified could find a niche within it. An illustration is provided in the previous section: the original ICF did not include a category for play, appropriate for the life activity of children, but that function was easily accommodated in the special version of the ICF-CY.

In this regard, the ICF is certainly holistic, by which we mean simply the understanding of the person as more than the sum of all of his parts. Science, including medical science, has achieved tremendous success over the centuries by deconstructing persons into their constituent parts and understanding each of those parts: the circulatory system, the neural system, and so on. Classification systems have aided and abetted this decomposition process, slicing and dicing human function into smaller and smaller units.

The ICF recognizes the value of having categories for very fine classes of human functioning and implements the received wisdom of science. But it goes forward from there in a more holistic direction by insisting that *all* human functioning should be included within the scope of scientific interest, not just those functions that, for historical reasons, have been of interest to scientists.

BODY, PERSON, AND COMMUNITY

It is commonplace these days in disability and rehabilitation circles to describe disability as "multidimensional" or "multiaxial." Unfortunately, outside of those circles, that language is less common, although it does seem to be making inroads. The predecessor to the ICF, the ICIDH, formulated in the 1970s, was one of the first full conceptualizations of disability to incorporate multidimensional constructs.

The dimensions or components of the ICF were described above: body structures and functions, activities and participation, and environmental factors. To emphasize the holistic nature of the ICF, we would like to recast those components in terms of body, person, and community. All of us have, or are, a body: flesh and bones, aches and pains, strong or weak, sick or well, and so on. We pay more or less attention to ourselves as body, depending on many variables. But we are more than body; we are persons, ourselves, the entity in our mind that reflects on our bodies and, reflexively, on ourselves. Furthermore, we are more than persons in ourselves; we are participants in community, interacting with other persons, learning from them who we are and giving definition to them as persons in relationship to us. We are, collectively, simultaneously, and interactively, body, person, family, and community. To consider humans in that way is to consider them holistically.

The ICF does not explicitly espouse a holistic worldview. We were participants in its development, and we can attest that no such grand ideas were ever part of the debate. Nevertheless, through a fortunate convergence of influences, the outcome of the ICF process was a view of human functioning that is, however unintentionally, holistic in its implications, if not in its public pronouncements. The ICF is so structured as to allow inclusion of any human functioning—body, person, or community—within its system, although to do so will require that specialists in particular realms of functioning develop new ICF categories according to WHO guidelines and under WHO auspices.

HUMAN RIGHTS, RELIGION, AND SPIRITUALITY

To illustrate the holistic breadth of the ICF, we invite attention to two of its categories. Chapter 9 of the Activities and Participation component of the ICF is titled "Community, Social and Civil Life," defined as "the actions and tasks required to engage in organized social life outside the family, in community, social and civic areas of life." Code d940 (the *d* identifies the ICF component Activity and Participation) in Chapter 9 is labeled "Human Rights" and is described as follows:

> Enjoying all nationally and internationally recognized rights that are accorded to people by virtue of their humanity alone, such as human rights as recognized by the United Nations Universal Declaration of Human Rights (1948) and the United Nations Standard Rules for the Equalization of Opportunities for Persons with Disabilities (1993); the right to self-determination or autonomy; and the right to control over one's destiny. (p. 170)

The inclusion of this code in the ICF implies that a complete assessment of human functioning should include an assessment of the human rights accorded to people. It is remarkable that the World *Health* Organization should include in its family of *health* classifications a type of function so far removed from everyday understandings of health.

Similarly, ICF code d930, "Religion and Spirituality," also surprises conventional expectations of health classifications; it is defined as

> engaging in religious or spiritual activities, organizations and practices for self-fulfilment, finding meaning, religious or spiritual value and establishing connection with a divine power, such as is involved in attending a church, temple, mosque or synagogue, praying or chanting for a religious purpose, and spiritual contemplation. (p. 169)

In the current version of the ICF, approved in 2001, the codes for human rights and religion and spirituality are not much more than placeholders. Code d940, "Human Rights," has no specified subcategories, and code d930, "Religion and Spirituality," has only two subcategories: d9300, "Organized Religion," and d9301, "Spirituality." To have much practical value in assessing function, both codes would need to be elaborated. Fortunately, rigorous methods for elaborating codes are available. In fact, one of the coauthors of this chapter has experimentally elaborated the "Organized Religion" code to include the categories d9300, "Prayer"; d9301, "Worship Activities"; d9302, "Religious Education"; and d9303, "Congregational Life and Service" (Hendershot, 2004). The method used to elaborate the religion and spirituality codes could as easily be applied to code d940, "Human Rights."

Although the paucity of detailed codes for human rights and religion and spirituality currently limit their application in assessing function in practical situations, our main point in drawing attention to these codes in the ICF is to emphasize its inherently holistic approach to human functioning. By including these codes within its framework, even in adumbrated form, the ICF signals to its users—health researchers, health policy makers, healthcare providers, and others—that human rights, religion, and spirituality are legitimate health concerns.

LOW, NORMAL, AND ADVANCED

One of the criticisms of the ICIDH, the WHO's predecessor to the ICF, was that it described function in negative terms (WHO, 1980). That bias was evident in its definitions of its key concepts:

> "In the context of health experience, an impairment is any *loss or abnormality* of psychological, physiological, or anatomical structure or function" (p. 27).

"In the context of health experience, a disability is *restriction or lack* (resulting from an impairment) of ability to perform an activity in the manner or within the range considered *normal* for a human being" (p. 28).

"In the context of health experience, a handicap is a *disadvantage* for a given individual, resulting from an impairment or disability, that limits or prevents the fulfilment of a role that is *normal* (depending on age, sex, and social and cultural factors) for that individual" (p. 29).

The ICIDH, reflecting the conventional view of functional assessment, presumed that for every function, there is some so-called normal level of functioning, and that assessing function means measuring deficiency in functioning relative to the norm. The goal of treatment, insofar as it was concerned with functional outcomes, was to remove or correct deficiencies, raising the level of functioning toward that hypothetical normal level. The scores for level of functioning ran from 0 for normal to 6 for "complete inability."

Critics of the ICIDH (and other approaches to functional assessment that shared its bias) noted that level of functioning extends above normal as well as below: there is normal bicycle riding, for instance, and then there is Lance Armstrong's exceptional bicycle riding. Any assessment of overall functioning, holistic functioning, should not be limited to low functioning, nor even normal functioning, but also include advanced functioning. Viewed holistically, a personal profile of level of functioning might show low functioning in some functions, normal functioning in others, and advanced functioning in yet others. A person who is low in mobility function, say, unable to walk unassisted, may have normal intellectual function and may function at an advanced level in interpersonal relationships, having an extensive and active network of friends and relatives.

Although this viewpoint was vigorously advocated by some participants in revision of the ICIDH (that led to the ICF), especially participants with disabilities, it met with limited success. There was significant change in the language used to define the components of the ICF system: body structure, body function, activity, participation, and environment. The language is mostly neutral and descriptive, with no reference to normal and abnormal functioning. In a key respect, however, the idea that functioning can be advanced, not just normal or low, fell by the wayside: the scoring of level of function runs from 0 (no problem) to 4 (complete problem); that is, the scoring assumes that functioning is either normal (no problem) or low (mild to complete problem), with no provision for persons who may be the Lance Armstrongs of their area of functional excellence. Advanced functioning is certainly an area that needs to be addressed by those interested in integrated healthcare.

The low-normal scoring system applies to level of functioning categories in body structure, body function, activity, and participation, the central components of the ICF. However, the ICF also includes a section on environment. Environment is one of two contextual factors the ICF recognizes as affecting function (the other is personal factors, which is not classified in ICF). In the scientific-political process that led to the ICF, many participants, especially persons with disabilities and their advocates, argued that environment (physical and social) was crucial to understanding functioning. In a compromise, it was decided that environment would be recognized as an important contextual factor by including a list of environmental factors.

The categories in the environment section are not detailed, but they do cover a wide range of factors that should permit it to be filled out in future developments. Just as importantly for holistic concerns is the inclusion in the environment section not only of the low-normal levels described above, but a corresponding set of normal-advanced codes, running from 0 (no facilitator) to 4 (complete facilitator); that is, the ICF not only recognizes the importance of environmental factors, it also recognizes that the environment can create both *barriers* to functioning and *facilitators* to functioning. This is a step toward a more holistic ICF, and we can hope for, and work toward, the extension of normal-advanced codes in the main components of the ICF in its next revision.

CONCLUSION

In this chapter we have introduced the reader to the WHO's relatively new International Classification of Functioning, Disability, and Health—the ICF. The ICF provides a conceptual framework for thinking about human functioning, a detailed and comprehensive set of functional categories, and guidelines for assessing functioning in those categories. The international network of disability researchers and advocates who developed and tested the ICF intended that it would be useful across nations, professions, and life cycle stages. Although the ICF was approved for use by the World Health Assembly only five years ago (at the time of this writing), there is evidence in the published literature that it is being used in many nations by researchers interested in many different medical conditions. Also, the use of the ICF has been extended across additional life cycle stages by the creation of a version for children and youth (ICF-CY).

We have suggested that the ICF can be a tool for the greater integration of healthcare because it takes a holistic view of the individual as body, person, and community participant. It incorporates a much wider range of human functioning than is typical in health contexts, and we cited its inclusion of functioning in the areas of human rights and religion to illustrate that inclusiveness. We were also critical of approaches to human functioning, such as the ICF, that focus on the range of function from normal to abnormal, failing to recognize that many persons function at an advanced level in some areas. We noted that one part of the ICF, its list of environmental factors, does allow for so-called above normal situations ("facilitators" in the environmental field), and suggested that that mode of assessment could be extended to the other components of the ICF—body structure and function, activity, and participation—in future revisions of the classification.

The fiscal and administrative structure of healthcare requires that records be kept on patient treatments and outcomes. To be effective, record systems must use standard definitions and information systems, including standard classification systems. The effect of classification systems on the organization and delivery of healthcare services is pervasive but often unrecognized. Classification systems that are indifferent to holistic care (or worse) can create substantial barriers to the integration of healthcare. We have argued here that the ICF is a classification system that treats humans holistically and therefore supports the movement toward integrated healthcare.

TOOL KIT FOR CHANGE

Role and Perspective of the Healthcare Professional

1. Through the use of the ICF, the healthcare provider focuses on healthy function, not on disease alone.
2. The ICF is a tool that the healthcare provider can use to assess function independent of diagnosis.
3. The mind and body are unified for functional assessment in the ICF, eliminating the duality of the mind-body split for the healthcare provider.

Role and Perspective of the Patient/Participant

1. The patient's health is defined not through diagnosis, but through ability to function in activities and participate in the environment.
2. Assessment of the integrity of the physical body structure is viewed separately from the function of the patient, both in clinical settings and in the patient's daily life.
3. With the ICF focus on function as a definition of health, the patient has the opportunity to shift the focus from illness and disease to enhancing a positive focus on coping, which is a more healing aspect of healthcare.

Interconnection: The Global Perspective

1. The ICF provides a valid and reliable language that allows clear communication about health and function between the healthcare provider and the patient, among many different disciplines in healthcare and across professional boundaries outside of healthcare.
2. Use of the ICF allows the healthcare system to define health and quality of life in a reciprocal manner: health affects quality of life, and quality of life affects health.

REFERENCES

Hendershot, G. (2004, June 1–4). *Elaborating ICF codes for specialized applications: The case of "Organized Religion" (D9302)*. Paper presented at the Annual Meeting of the North American Collaborating Center on the International Classification of Functioning, Disability, and Health, Halifax, Nova Scotia, Canada.

Lollar, D., & Simeonsson, R. (2005). Diagnosis to function: Classification for children and youths. *Journal of Developmental Behavior and Pediatrics, 26,* 323–230.

Mbogoni, M. (2003). On the application of the ICIDH and ICF in developing countries: Evidence from the United Nations Disability Statistics Database (DISTAT). *Disability and Rehabilitation, 25,* 644–658.

Stucki, G., Ewert, T., & Cieza, A. (2003). Value and application of the ICF in rehabilitation medicine. *Disability and Rehabilitation, 25,* 628–634.

Trotter, R., Ustun, B., Chatterji, S., Rehm, J., Room, R., & Bichenbach, J. (2001). Cross-cultural applicability research on disablement: Models and methods for the revision of an international classification. *Human Organization, 60,* 13–27.

World Health Organization. (1980). *International classification of impairments, disabilities, and handicaps.* Geneva, Switzerland: Author.

World Health Organization. (1992–1994). *International statistical classification of diseases and related health problems* (10th rev., Vols. 1–3). Geneva, Switzerland: Author.

World Health Organization. (2001). *International classification of functioning, disability, and health.* Geneva, Switzerland: Author.

Chapter Twelve

RISK PREVENTION AND PATIENT PROTECTION IN INTEGRATIVE HEALTHCARE

Steven E. Stark, JD, LHCRM, Mark G. DiCowden, JD, and Alan L. Goldberg, PhD, JD

INTRODUCTION

Recently, the public, government regulators, the medical profession, and other traditional healthcare delivery systems have become increasingly more interested in the efficacy, safety, and usability of integrated models of healthcare delivery and complementary and alternative medicine (CAM). CAM can be defined as a group of medical, healthcare, and healing systems other than those currently included in mainstream healthcare in the United States. CAM includes the worldviews, theories, modalities, products, and practices associated with these systems and their use to treat illness and promote health and well-being (National Institutes of Health, 2002). Integrative medicine, as defined by the National Center for Complementary and Alternative Medicine (NCCAM), which operates under the auspices of the National Institutes of Health (NIH), combines mainstream medical therapies and CAM therapies for which there is some high-quality scientific evidence of safety and effectiveness (National Center for Complementary and Alternative Medicine [NCCAM], 2002). This definition follows the growing availability and use of these types of therapies in both traditional and nontraditional settings.

According to studies reported in the *Journal of the American Medical Association,* for the last 10 years, there have been more visits to CAM practitioners than to primary care physicians (Astin, 1998; Eisenberg et al., 1998). As this interest continues, there has been a concurrent rise in discussions about the sometimes difficult and usually unanswered questions about legal liability, regulatory oversight, scope of practice, liability insurance availability and coverage, payment, and practice standards related to these developing models of care delivery. This chapter will address these issues and the public health and public policy implications of these trends.

PROFESSIONAL MALPRACTICE DEFINED

Professional malpractice is essentially negligent acts of omission or commission on the part of professionals that result in harm to clients or patients. In most circumstances, a professional is defined as a person who has undertaken a course of professional study and is required to be licensed to practice that profession (Wetzel, Eisenberg, & Kaptchuk, 1998). The amount of time that a patient may wait to bring such a claim, called the statute of limitations, varies from state to state but is usually within the range of from 2 years after the event to 7–10 years in the case of fraudulent concealment of the event on the part of the practitioner. Many of these time periods begin to run only after the patient knew or should have known of the negligent event that caused an injury. A number of states also have statutes of repose, which cut off the right to bring a claim a specified number of years after the treatment at issue, regardless of when or even whether the patient became aware of the potential claim for negligence.

Negligence consists of four elements: duty, breach of that duty, injury, and causation. In cases involving healthcare professionals, the standard of care is ordinarily that level of care that a reasonably careful healthcare provider of the same or similar specialty would exercise under the circumstances. In most jurisdictions, the party alleging negligence has the burden to present the testimony of a medical expert establishing the elements of the cause of action. In some circumstances, however, such as cases of obvious mistakes—that is, retained objects such as surgical instruments, sponges, and so on—or misconduct that adversely affects the ability to pursue the claim—that is, loss or destruction of treatment records—the burden shifts to the practitioner to prove that they were not negligent under the circumstances.

The existence of a legal duty is ordinarily a question of law for the court. In a negligence case involving a healthcare practitioner, such a duty is usually assumed based on the special relationship and public expectations of safe practice that are established between a practitioner and his patient or client. In some circumstances, such as in the case of the existence of a duty to prevent suicide or harm to third persons, the law is less clear and varies among the states. In some states, the existence or nonexistence of a legal duty in these more difficult cases is established by the state legislature as part of a state statute. In others, the courts, as part of the court-made common law, decide these issues through the individual cases that come before the courts. All other elements of a negligence claim—breach, causation, and damages—are usually questions of fact for the jury, unless the evidence is so clear that there are no material questions of fact for a jury to decide. If so, the court can decide the issue as a matter of law.

In deciding questions of practitioner negligence, juries are given written or verbal instructions regarding the law they should apply to the case. These instructions also vary from state to state but generally address issues such as credibility of witnesses, the effect of evidence either admitted or excluded, the factual and legal questions to decide, the types of available damages, the process of deliberation, and the form of the verdict. These also will identify the burden of proof that must be met. In most states, the burden of proof standard is a "preponderance of evidence," which means that the result is more probable than not (50% or higher). This is a much lower burden than the criminal standard of "beyond a reasonable doubt." A few states have adopted a slightly elevated burden of proof, such as a standard of proof requiring a finding of "gross negligence" or other heightened levels of review, such as a standard of proof that requires "clear and convincing evidence." Regardless of the applicable standard, if the jury concludes that the patient has proven each of the elements of negligence, then they will enter a verdict against the practitioner.

SCOPE OF PRACTICE

Although the bases for potential harm to patients and for professional liability or discipline of providers are numerous and varied, these potential consequences implicate primarily the issues of scope of practice and clinical activities beyond the scope of licensure and qualification. Most, if not all, other issues, and the most reliable methods to resolve them, should flow from that initial inquiry.

Each state has different laws related to licensure and scope of practice for allied healthcare professionals. In general, however, each state permits and licenses the following: medical doctors (MD); osteopaths (DO); nurses (RN and LPN); nurse practitioners (ARNP), including nurse anesthetists and nurse midwives; psychologists (PhD), therapists, mental health counselors, and social workers; pharmacists; occupational, speech, and physical therapists; dentists; chiropractors; podiatrists; physician and nursing assistants; and various specialty technologists and assistants, such as radiology and laboratory technicians. Several states have passed legislation to license alternative practitioners such as naturopaths. Others have also established statutory qualifications for alternative practitioners such as hypnotists, massage therapists, and acupuncturists. Each of these specialties has varied areas of practice that often intersect and sometimes overlap. When these intersecting or overlapping responsibilities are pursuant to established protocols, questions of practice scope, authority, responsibility, and accountability are relatively straightforward.

When those relationships are not well defined or there exists conflicting or competing standards regarding scope of practice, these intersections are much more complex and difficult to reconcile. The U.S. Constitution reserves to the states the power to regulate health, safety, and welfare, which includes the licensing of healthcare providers. As a result, there is a broad diversity of licensing and scope of practice rules across states that must be considered in any integrated practice environment.

Generally, healthcare practitioners can be authorized to practice independently, be required to collaborate, be required to be supervised, or be expected to practice under a combination of these provisions. There is no single practice arrangement accepted in all jurisdictions; there are, however, some generally accepted principles. If supervision is required, the required supervision is usually one of two types. Direct supervision usually requires the supervisor to be physically on the premises and readily available. Indirect supervision typically requires the supervisor to be physically on the premises or readily available by electronic communication and/or able to be on the premises in a specified period of time and from a limited distance. Direct supervision usually applies to those practitioners that serve more of a supportive role and that have more limited training such as physician assistants. Indirect supervision is more prevalent where independent licensed practitioners, such as nurses and nurse practitioners, are involved. Regardless of the arrangement, however, a system of shared responsibility and accountability is necessary to ensure safe and appropriate care. Several states have established a mechanism for the joint rulemaking between the boards whose practitioners are involved in collaborative or integrated practices. These are intended to promote frank and open discussions regarding practice expectations, scope limitations, and enforcement criteria related to existing or proposed regulation.

The complexity of relationships among healthcare practitioners, when combined with the need to ensure collaboration and coordination between these practitioners, has caused many commentators and industry organizations to question the traditional structure of healthcare regulation (Eisenberg et al., 1998; Eisenberg et al., in press).

- The 1998 Pew Commission Taskforce on Health Care Workforce Regulation's report included several recommendations regarding scope of practice. One in particular recommended the creation of a national advisory body to develop standards for uniform scopes of practice and continuing competency standards for healthcare professions (O'Neil, 1998).
- The 2001 Institute of Medicine (IOM) report *Crossing the Quality Chasm: A New Health System for the 21st Century* asserted that "scope of practice acts and other workforce regulations need to allow for innovation in the use of all types of clinicians to meet patient needs in the most effective and efficient way possible" (p. 19).

- In 1999, NCCAM was established within the NIH (Omnibus Appropriations Act, 1999) to address the growing interest in and need for research in CAM practices.
- In 2000, the Clinton administration established the White House Commission on Complementary and Alternative Medicine Policy, which reported its findings in March 2002 (National Institutes of Health, 2002), to look at the growing integration of nontraditional practices in medical care.

The 2003 IOM report *Health Professions Education: A Bridge to Quality* acknowledged that "efforts to change scope of practice acts are often the focus of turf battles among professions fought out in State legislatures; the result is distrust and hostility among professions that are supposed to be collaborating to provide coordinated care" (p. 107). The Federation of State Medical Boards formed a Special Committee on Scope of Practice. In response to these reports, the federation developed guidelines, which it recommended that state regulators and legislators review when considering scope of practice initiatives. The federation concluded that patient safety and accountability should be the most important factors in establishing expectations and limitations associated with scope of practice changes and that it is the state's responsibility to establish and enforce standards for healthcare delivery by physicians and other healthcare professionals to protect the public from unqualified practitioners (Federal and State Medical Boards, 2003). In evaluating safety and risk prevention strategies, all practitioners should consider these guidelines and the views expressed in the report to assess the factors that will be considered by state regulators in assessing scope of practice issues. These include the following.

1. *Referral to a physician.* The symptoms, conditions, diseases, and complications that healthcare practitioners should recognize are beyond their training and expertise and should be referred to a physician or other more qualified expert.
2. *Minimum education, training, and examination.* Are the practitioners qualified, capable, and competent as a result of appropriate and relevant education, training, examination, and experience? Are there accreditation processes and requirements? Is there an objective and independent accrediting body or an established and recognized accrediting organization?
3. *Licensure, certification, registration, and regulation.* Are there minimum standards for entry into practice, renewal, demonstration of continuing competency, prescribed procedures for enforcement of established practice standards, and discipline of problem practitioners? Are the particular practitioners in an integrated, complementary, or alternative practice all appropriately licensed, and is there any history of disciplinary or other adverse regulatory actions that may bear on their individual competence?
4. *Complaints and disciplinary action.* Complaint investigations and disciplinary processes are the responsibility of individual regulatory boards. Provisions for communication among boards on cases involving multiple practitioners vary greatly among the states. Are there specific rules, regulations, or disciplinary guidelines that have been adopted regarding a particular type of practitioner?
5. *Disclosure and public awareness.* Consumers generally assume that the practitioner performing a service is properly trained, competent, and practicing appropriately.

Consumers also tend to trust that services being offered are safe and that the practitioners are qualified to provide them. Whether the practitioner performing a service is a physician or other healthcare practitioner, consumers should be informed about the education and credentials of the practitioner and the name of the supervising practitioner, if there is one. Consumers should also be informed as to whether or not the practitioner is under the jurisdiction of a regulatory board.

6. *Liability.* Liability statutes and case law vary significantly from state to state. Integrated practices and practitioners should review state liability laws and evaluate how they apply to the multiple practitioners that may be involved in patient care. For example, supervising practitioners may be liable for the acts of those under their supervision if they fail to provide adequate and reasonable supervision. Also, supervised practitioners may also be held independently liable. In addition, independent practitioners should be individually liable for their own diagnoses and treatment recommendations and for failure to refer patients when appropriate.

In a recent pilot study, Cohen, Hrbek, Davis, Schacter, and Eisenberg (2005) suggested that hospitals across the United States are implementing vastly different practices and policies concerning CAM providers and therapies as regards credentialing, malpractice liability, and use of dietary supplements. The current environment creates significant impediments to the delivery of consistent clinical care and the implementation of multisite evaluations of the safety, efficacy, and cost-effectiveness (or lack thereof) of CAM therapies (or integrative models) as applied to the management of common medical conditions. Specific obstacles include the following: (1) inconsistency of state laws regarding provider licensure of acupuncturists, massage therapists, chiropractors, naturopaths, and mind-body therapists, and corresponding divergence of hospital practices concerning credentialing, limitations on practice authority and provider mix in the integrative team; and (2) divergence of approaches to liability management strategies, including minimum malpractice liability insurance, informed consent practices and documentation, and provider hiring status.

They further surmised that hospitals are not likely to increase standardization of integrative care teams in the absence of data concerning what combinations of providers or therapies are most effective (and safe) for any given condition. Furthermore, potential liability exposure, which is difficult to predict given changing case law and changing levels of evidence for specific therapies, and variations in local institutional policies and politics are likely to continue playing a significant role in the emergence of models of integrative care.

ROLE OF FACILITY AND PEER REVIEW IN DETERMINING SCOPE OF PRACTICE

An argument can be made that a provider's scope of practice is most effectively determined by way of the healthcare facility's credentialing process and the rights of the facility to grant, limit, or retract privileges through credentialing and peer review activity. When laws regulating the medical profession are attacked, substantive due process requires that the exercise of the state's police power not be unreasonable or unduly oppressive and that the regulatory means employed by the legislature have a real and substantive relation to the objects sought to be obtained (Katz v. State Bd. of Medical & Osteopathic Examiners, 1988). The U.S. Supreme Court has held that "there is no right to practice medicine which is not subordinate to the police power of the States" (Access to Medical Treatment Act, 2003). However, who in the state is better qualified to regulate its healthcare professionals' scope of practice other than the healthcare providers themselves and the facility that also may share in the liability of that provider?

Vociferous assertions that the state was abusing its policing powers with regard to intimate aspects of healthcare, coupled with the belief that so-called establishment hubris was interfering with the rights of competent individuals to access novel modes of therapy, gave rise to the Access to Medical Treatment Act of 2003. This bill, considered repeatedly by Congress since 1997 but not enacted, represents a statutory response to the paternalistic philosophy exemplified by *United States v. Rutherford* (1979). In *Rutherford,* the U.S. Supreme Court held the unanimous view that substantial evidence of a drug's safety and effectiveness and distribution is under the sole jurisdiction of the Food and Drug Administration. Furthermore, there was no exemption under the act for so-called new drugs that are used by the terminally ill, thus precluding terminally ill cancer patients from obtaining drugs for their illness that may be determined as useful in other countries. To the contrary, the act grants individuals

the right to be treated by a health care practitioner with any medical treatment (including a treatment that is not approved, certified, or licensed by the Secretary of Health and Human Services) that such individual desires or the legal representative of such individual desires, if the practitioner personally examines and agrees to treat the individual and the administration of the treatment is within the provider's authorized scope of practice. (§ 2618 IS; H.R. 2792, 2006)

Traditionally, providers are not entitled to membership or staff privileges at a healthcare facility as a matter of right. Although a license to practice a profession is a valuable right deserving of protection by the law, staff membership is not afforded the same considerations as a constitutional or inherent right (Wallington v. Zinn, 1961). Private hospitals have an absolute right to exclude licensed physicians from their medical staffs, and decisions regarding the granting or denial of medical staff privileges are not subject to judicial review (Pepple v. Parkview Memorial Hospital, Inc., 1987). Public hospitals have similar authority. (Hayman v. Galveston, 1927).

Therefore healthcare facilities, through the decisions and actions of their member credentialing and peer review committees, may select the membership of their staffs and determine the scope of practice of each individual healthcare provider. State peer review statutes have already provided considerable, albeit qualified, legal protections that allow hospitals to extend, deny, or revoke any individual physician's medical staff privileges or scope of practice. This right of staff membership has most often been used to exclude practitioners. However, the proliferation of forward looking programs that incorporate integrative protocols and employ a wider variety of disciplines can also create a climate for broader peer review and wider acceptance of an integrated scope of practice.

The study by Cohen et al. (2005) offered a number of recommendations both on macro and micro levels that addressed the issues of standardization of integrative teams, scope of practice, and peer review. The latter included, among others, recommendations to enhance opportunities for licensees to participate in clinical residency in integrative care centers, with the intent of receiving supervision by senior clinicians from both the conventional and CAM communities; create performance standards and assessment of clinical skills for conventional and complementary care providers who work in integrative care settings; and, individually and collectively, encourage relevant professional organizations and agencies to consider creative ways of using integrative care centers to help further consistent clinical care and research.

As part of its strategic planning efforts for the years 2005–2009, NCCAM has prepared five background reports on the major areas of CAM. These brief overviews of biologically based practices; energy medicine; manipulative and body-based practices; whole medical systems; and mind-body medicine are "intended to provide a sense of the overarching research challenges and opportunities in particular CAM approaches" (NCCAM, 2004, p. 2).

RISK MANAGEMENT STRATEGIES

As stated previously, the primary risk management and patient protection tool related to any complementary, alternative, or integrated practice arrangement and treatment protocol is an assessment of the risks of that treatment and the prevailing professional standards related to its delivery (Nahin & Strauss, 2001). Because the determination of recognized standards at a trial or disciplinary proceeding almost always requires expert testimony, the primary places to begin the search for applicable standards are professional literature and research; professional societies' position papers or practice guidelines; any specific state statutes or rules that relate to licensure, scope of practice, and discipline of the involved practitioners; or the requirements of any designating, certifying, or accreditation bodies. It is axiomatic that if the treatment at issue follows a specific state law or regulation, recognized professional guidelines or standards, or promulgated criteria from an objective and independent certifying organization, then it is much easier to defend that treatment from criticism or rebuke. It is also clear that the existence of only a few, conflicting, or no guidelines creates a much more uncertain and potentially risky situation for the patient and practitioner. It is indisputable that any actions that are contrary to any existing laws, regulations, or binding professional guidelines would likely be considered either per se negligence, presumptive evidence of negligence or a licensure violation, or even a criminal act subject to prosecution. Consultation with an attorney with expertise in health law is strongly recommended. In some jurisdictions it may be possible to seek an advisory opinion from the relevant regulatory agency regarding a particular practice method or modality. In others, there may be local or national professional organizations that will provide guidance to their members.

Regardless of the method chosen to determine an appropriate treatment plan or practice arrangement, it is imperative that health practitioners document the basis for clinical and therapeutic recommendations. Inaccurate, incomplete, or missing documentation in the medical record can and usually will be used to demonstrate a failure to exercise due care and can support an array of civil, administrative, quasi-criminal, or criminal sanctions (Cohen, 1998, 1999, 2000, 2001; Studdert et al., 1998). Conversely, good documentation and maintenance of a library of supporting materials can help defend against any allegations of improper, unsafe, or unauthorized practices (Scott, 2000). In those where the clinical environment requires the granting of privileges to perform certain procedures, then review and preauthorization of your proposed protocol and supporting materials by the appropriate facility board or committee should be considered. At a minimum, consultation with colleagues in the same field and relevant overlapping fields should be made, along with a detailed note regarding these consultations and conclusions.

Even if the practitioner has reviewed the literature, identified the appropriate standards, documented the chart, and obtain preauthorization, no course of treatment, whether conventional, integrated, complementary, or otherwise, should be undertaken without a full and complete disclosure of the recommended treatment; the persons that will be performing, providing, or assisting with the treatment; the material risks and benefits of that treatment; and the reasonable alternative treatments that are available. The choice, ultimately, is the patient's, not the practitioner's, and a competent adult is allowed to accept or reject any course of treatment, as long as that treatment is recommended and given within recognized parameters and, if experimental, fully disclosed as such and given pursuant to approved protocols. Any treatment provided without informed consent is a technical battery and a basis for civil, administrative, or criminal actions. Conversely, in most states, the existence of a signed written consent is presumptive evidence of consent and protection against a claim for an injury if the risk of that injury was disclosed and accepted. A patient cannot consent to negligence, so a signed consent will not protect against improper acts. It will, however, protect against injuries that have been known to occur as a complication of the proposed treatment without negligence (Ernst & Cohen, 2001).

REIMBURSEMENT ISSUES

In addition to basic issues of scope of practice and malpractice, another issue of legal importance that is rarely mentioned is reimbursement. Clearly the easiest manner in which to practice CAM is with private payment from clients. Government programs, such as Medicare or Medicaid, rarely, if ever, fund alternative therapies. Payments for newer treatments are often denied due to their so-called experimental nature. One such example in Medicare is acupuncture, although it has been 10 years since the NIH determined that acupuncture is beneficial in medical treatment (National Institutes of Health, 1997), and despite the fact that continuous reports from the NIH indicate a wide range of uses. Given this scenario, legal inconsistencies arise when a physician who is paid by Medicare for an office visit provides the patient acupuncture on that visit—even though the physician may be credentialed in acupuncture and finds it to be the most appropriate intervention of choice.

Another concern is related to the teamwork inherent in CAM treatments. The holistic framework needed for communication to best meet the patient's needs makes use of a variety of treating specialists. However, team conferences and group treatments are poorly reimbursed by most insurers, and never by Medicare or Medicaid. Coordination during such meetings is vital, and group treatments are beneficial in integrating treatment goals.

As previously mentioned in this chapter, documentation to address issues of legality in reimbursement is of utmost importance. Treating professionals must be able to document observations, rationale, and outcomes of interventions that are specific to the individual profession and the patient's needs. An important challenge is for professionals working as part of CAM teams to be able to design research and determine successful outcomes based on mind-body interventions. Additionally, cutting-edge programs that provide integrative care must hold the highest standards for clinical and evidence-based protocols. The health professionals that work together in these endeavors must be proactive in peer review and credentialing for such facilities. This will serve to help justify the need for such treatments. It will also provide a fertile ground for appropriately broadening the definition of scope of practice and reimbursement needed to provide a more comprehensive medical system in the United States.

TOOL KIT FOR CHANGE

Role and Perspective of the Healthcare Professional

1. Licensing and scope of practice rules across states must be considered in any integrated practice environment.
2. Accurate and complete documentation for the basis of clinical and therapeutic recommendations is essential for all disciplines in an integrative practice. A good library of supporting materials and peer consultation are also helpful in risk management of integrative practices. Documentation of peer consultation is also recommended.
3. A signed consent for treatment by a patient is essential. Consents should indicate disclosure of the recommended treatment; the persons that will be performing, providing, or assisting with the treatment; the material risks and benefits of that treatment; and the reasonable alternative treatments that are available.

Role and Perspective of the Patient/Participant

1. Patients should actively request information about the training of their healthcare providers, whether traditional or nontraditional.
2. Patients should be familiar with licensing laws and regulating boards for various healthcare professionals in their state.
3. Patients should be active participants in gathering information about prospective integrative treatment protocols.

Interconnection: The Global Perspective

1. Greater opportunities for clinical residency in integrative care centers are warranted.
2. Relevant professional organizations and agencies need to consider creative ways to further consistent clinical care, research and development of performance standards, and competency using integrative care centers and training models.
3. Traditional and nontraditional healthcare professionals in cutting-edge programs and facilities need to be proactive in peer review of one another and support interdisciplinary and transdisciplinary treatments that are clinically efficacious and/or evidence based to expand the boundaries of scope of practice appropriately.

REFERENCES

Access to Medical Treatment Act, H.R. 2085 (2003).

Astin, J. (1998). Why patients use alternative medicine: Results of a national study. *Journal of the American Medical Association, 279*, 1548–1553.

Cohen, M. (1998). *Complementary and alternative medicine: Legal Boundaries and regulatory perspectives.* Baltimore: Johns Hopkins University Press.

Cohen, M. (1999). Malpractice considerations affecting the clinical integration of complementary and alternative medicine. *Current Practice of Medicine, 2,* 87–89.

Cohen, M. (2000). *Beyond complementary medicine: Legal and ethical perspectives on health care and human evolution.* Ann Arbor: University of Michigan Press.

Cohen, M. (2001). Legal and ethical issues in complementary and alternative medicine. In E. Ernst, M. Pittler, C. Stevenson, A. White, & D. Eisenberg (Eds.), *The desktop guide to complementary and alternative medicine: An evidence based approach* (pp. 404–411). London: Mosby.

Cohen, M., Hrbek, A., Davis, R., Schacter, S., & Eisenberg, D. (2005). Emerging credentialing practices, malpractice liability policies, and guidelines governing complementary and alternative medical practices and dietary supplement recommendations: A descriptive study of 19 integrative health care centers in the United States. *Archives of Internal Medicine, 165,* 289–295.

Eisenberg, D., Davis, R., Ettner, S., Appel, S., Wilkey, S., & Van Rompay, M. (1998). 1990–1997: Results of a follow-up national survey. *Journal of the American Medical Association, 280,* 1569–1575.

Eisenberg, D., Cohen, M., Hrbek, A., Grayzel, J., Van Rompay, M., & Cooper, R. (2002). Credentialing, complementary and alternative medical providers. *Annals of Internal Medicine, 137*(12): 965–973.

Ernst, E., & Cohen, M. (2001). Informed consent in complementary and alternative medicine. *Archives of Internal Medicine, 161,* 2288–2292.

Federal and State Medical Boards. (2003). *Model guidelines for the use of complementary and alternative therapies in medical practice.* Retrieved June 5, 2007, from http://www. fsmb.org/pdf/2002_grpol_complementary_alternative_therapies.pdf

Hayman v. Galveston, 273 U.S. 414 (1927).

Institute of Medicine. (2001). *Crossing the quality chasm: A new health system for the 21st century.* Washington, DC: Author.

Institute of Medicine. (2003). *Health professions education: A bridge to quality.* Washington, DC: Author.

Katz v. State Bd. of Medical & Osteopathic Examiners, 432 N.W.2d 274 (S.D. 1988).

Nahin, R., & Strauss, S. (2001). Research into complementary and alternative medicine: Problems and potential. *British Medical Journal, 322,* 161–164.

National Center for Complementary and Alternative Medicine. (2002). *What is complementary and alternative medicine?* Washington, DC: Author.

National Center for Complementary and Alternative Medicine. (2004). *Strategic plan 2005–2009.* Washington, DC: Author.

National Institutes of Health. (1997). Acupuncture. *NIH Consensus Statement, 15*(5), 1–34.

National Institutes of Health. (2002). White house commission on complementary and alternative medicine policy final report. (NIH Publication No. 03–5411). Washington, DC: U.S. Department of Health and Human Services.

Omnibus Appropriation Act, P.L. 105–277 (1999).

O'Neil, E. (1998). *Recreating health professional practice for a new century.* Washington, DC: Pew Commission.

Pepple v. Parkview Memorial Hospital, Inc., 511 N.E.2d 467 (Ind. Ct. App. 1987).

Scott, R. (2000). *Legal aspects of documenting patient care.* Gaithersburg, MD: Aspen.

Studdert, D., Eisenberg, D., Miller, F., Curto, D., Kaptchuk, T., & Brennan, T. (1998). Medical malpractice implications of alternative medicine. *Journal of the American Medical Association, 280,* 1610–1615.

United States v. Rutherford, 442 U.S. 544 (1979).

Wallington v. Zinn, 118 S.E.2d 526 (W. Va. 1961).

Wetzel, M., Eisenberg, D., & Kaptchuk, T. (1998). Courses involving complementary and alternative medicine at U.S. medical schools. *Journal of the American Medical Association, 280,* 784–787.

Chapter Thirteen

DOLLARS AND SENSE: MAKING IT HAPPEN (PART I)

Marie A. DiCowden, PhD, Russ Newman, PhD, JD, and Bree Johnston, MD, MPH

OVERVIEW

The U.S. healthcare system produces the greatest portion of the cutting-edge scientific knowledge and research initiatives developed in the world. It also provides the majority of highly honed technical resources and professional skills. The U.S. healthcare system is endowed with the capacity to produce near-miracles every day through groundbreaking biomedical technology and innovative life-extending procedures. However, large portions of the American population cannot access the jewels of this healthcare system. Almost 47 million Americans have no health insurance, and many more are intermittently uninsured or underinsured. Families USA (2005) and the Institute of Medicine (2006 & 2002) report that at the current rate, 53 million people in the United States will have no health insurance coverage for at least a full year by 2010. The report goes on to describe the individuals who are uninsured: "Contrary to popular belief, the overwhelming majority of uninsured people are workers or members of a family in which at least one member works. Researchers have estimated that four in five individuals without health insurance are employed or in a family with an employed adult" (p. 12). At any point in time, 60 million people are without insurance coverage or have inadequate coverage (Schoen, Doty, Collins, & Holmgren, 2005).

The United States is the only industrialized nation without a universal system of healthcare for its citizens, and U.S. healthcare outcomes suffer as a result. The World Health Organization ranks the U.S. healthcare system 37th in the world overall. The U.S. system is also ranked ninth in life expectancy and seventh in infant mortality for its citizens. Furthermore, there are also significant health disparities depending on race and income and, as noted in another chapter 8 in this book, ethnicity, class, and gender (Schuster, McGlynn, & Brook, 1998).

The financial underpinnings of the healthcare system in this country are a complex jumble of public and private financing, special programs designed to try to close gaps in coverage, perverse incentives, and high administrative overhead. The United States spends more than any other country on healthcare—about $2 trillion annually. This amount is 15.3 percent of the gross domestic product (GDP), or $6,000 per person. This cost is approximately double what most other countries pay per capita or as a percentage of their GDPs (Woolhandler & Himmelstein, 2004).

On balance, what can be said about the healthcare system in America is that it is incredibly expensive and produces miracles for many, yet overall, its outcomes are poor. Additionally, millions of Americans are delayed access to needed medical care or denied that care altogether.

CURRENT FINANCING MECHANISMS

Before a discussion about funding any healthcare reform, including integrative care, a brief review of the funding mechanisms of the current healthcare system is needed. Despite the perception that the U.S. health system is private, government expenditures account for 44.9 percent of healthcare costs, including Medicare, Medicaid, the Veterans Administration, and the military healthcare system. If tax subsidies for businesses that provide health insurance to their employees are included, that percentage rises to more than two-thirds; private sources represent 55.1 percent of expenditures, of which about one-quarter are out-of-pocket expenses (Woolhandler & Himmelstein, 2004).

Medicare

Medicare was introduced in 1965 as one of Lyndon Johnson's Great Society Programs. Today, Medicare is the major insurer for the elderly and chronically disabled population. Medicare has four major programs: Medicare Part A, Medicare Part B, Medicare Advantage, and Medicare Part D. Because Medicare does not provide comprehensive coverage, most Medicare beneficiaries supplement their coverage with private so-called Medigap policies. These supplemental policies are designed to cover deductibles and copayments. Providers cannot waive this deductible or copay, under penalty of law, merely because the patient cannot afford it. The patient must provide a statement or proof of inability to pay the nonfunded amounts, or the provider must document that a good faith effort was made to secure payment.

Medicare Part A is paid for through payroll taxes and is available to any elderly or chronically disabled person who has paid into the system for a sufficient amount of time (defined as being employed for 13 quarters). Medicare Part A funds hospital care, hospice, some home healthcare services, and a limited amount of inpatient rehabilitation and nursing home care. Eligibility for Medicare Part B also requires prior employment for 13 quarters and is paid via payroll taxes and a premium paid by beneficiaries. Part B funds most outpatient care. A person with both Medicare A and B still faces large out-of-pocket expenses and deductibles. Consequently, the majority of enrollees also require Medigap policies. These policies range in coverage and price but are designed to pay for the major portions of Medicare deductibles and copayments that are approved, but not fully covered, by Medicare Part B. If an individual does not have a Medigap policy, payment is required from the individual directly and is mandated by federal policy.

The Medicare Modernization Act was passed into law in 2003. As a result, the Medicare Part D drug benefit was implemented in 2006. This program is administered through private insurers and is exceedingly complex and incomplete in its coverage, with a donut hole gap after several thousand dollars in insurance. The Medicare Modernization Act of 2003 also contained a number of other provisions, including demonstration projects of Medicare privatization, which will begin in the next few years in designated geographic areas.

Medicare Advantage programs (formerly Medicare Plus Choice) are capitated health programs (health maintenance organizations (HMOs) or preferred provider organizations (PPOs)) that patients can choose that integrate benefits from Parts A, B, and D. A specific payment is made prospectively to the insurer by the government. The specific insurer then provides designated benefits to the individual to cover, in theory, all costs incurred for healthcare services needed.

Medicare has been a remarkably successful program on many levels, but it also has substantial limitations. Medicare is consistently ranked higher than private insurance policies on quality and satisfaction by beneficiaries. Its administrative costs—about three percent—are substantially lower than the 15–30 percent administrative costs of private insurers. Most importantly, Medicare has improved the lives and financial stability of elders in the United States (National Economic Council/Domestic Policy Council, 2000).

Medicare continues to reimburse high-technology, procedure-oriented specialties much more generously than primary, preventive, and team-oriented care. Some providers will not accept Medicare due to its reimbursement structure, so access to care under Medicare is not guaranteed for all specialties in all regions (American Medical Association, 2006). As care of patients with chronic illnesses, such as dementia, diabetes, and congestive heart failure, accounts for an ever-increasing portion of healthcare expenditures, innovations in this government-funded program will be necessary to optimize health outcomes under Medicare in a cost-effective manner.

Medicaid

Medicaid, also introduced in the 1960s, is the primary insurance program for low-income Americans. Medicaid is an income-based health insurance program that covers low-income populations, the disabled, and the elderly. Although Medicaid has improved healthcare immeasurably for low-income individuals, there are many localities where few or no professionals accept Medicaid, and thus access to care continues to remain a problem for many Medicaid recipients (California Healthcare Foundation, 2006; Pew Center on the States, 2006). Medicaid is administered through a federal-state partnership. The federal government sets minimum program requirements that states can supplement, if they so choose. Medicaid also pays for about half of nursing home care in the United States. Because Medicaid accounts for about 21 percent of state budgets, state governments face tremendous pressures to limit Medicaid expenditures, and a number of states are experimenting with new approaches that would limit Medicaid spending, many of which will reduce access and limit services to Medicaid recipients (Pew Center on the States, 2006).

Elders or chronically disabled persons who are poor can receive both Medicare and Medicaid. These so-called dual eligibles receive crossover coverage that pays for acute care, long-term care, and supportive in-home services. For many frail patients, Medicare/Medicaid, or "Medi-Medi," is the most comprehensive plan available; however, Medicare/Medicaid crossover funding is not accepted by all providers.

The Veterans Administration and Military Systems of Care

The Veterans Affairs (VA) Healthcare System is the largest healthcare system in the country, providing follow-up through a continuum of care. It provides services for about five million veterans. Twenty years ago, the VA system of care was considered by many to be a plodding dinosaur of a healthcare system that delivered mediocre care at best. Over the past 10 years, the VA has undergone a major transformation and is now considered to be one of the highest-quality healthcare systems in the country. Innovative elements of VA care include a state-of-the-art electronic medical record system, a capitation system that adjusts risk sufficiently for even the sickest veterans to be covered adequately, and a coordinated service delivery system that is more cohesive than traditional fee-for-service care (Asch et al., 2004; Longman, 2005).

Other Government-Funded Programs

States and counties also provide services for patients that are not covered by other state and federal programs. The State Children's Health Insurance

Program (SCHIP) covers many near-poor children that do not qualify for Medicaid but whose families are still considered to be from disadvantaged economic circumstances. Counties have various programs that care for the indigent and underserved. Workers' compensation programs, generally regulated by the states, are designed to pay for people who are hurt or made ill by their jobs. Employers must make payments to the state government on a regular basis to assist in funding this mechanism. However, in some cases, employers can elect to be self-insured to take care of employees hurt on the job. But by any measure, these programs are under heavy fiscal and programmatic pressures in the current antitax, antigovernment environment.

Private Insurance

In 2004, the majority of Americans (63%) purchased private health insurance through their employers or through the employer of somebody in their family. Only five percent of people purchased health insurance individually (Aaron, 2005).

Employers may purchase coverage with a health insurance company (for-profit and not-for-profit private) or self-fund. Almost half of those covered by private employer-based insurance have PPOs, which tend to be cheaper than traditional fee-for-service plans. Twenty-three percent of those covered by employer-based health insurance are enrolled in HMOs. Twenty-two percent are covered by point-of-service/indemnity plans that allow free choice of providers, although choosing contracted providers is usually rewarded in the form of more extensive benefit coverage. Only seven percent still have the traditional fee-for-service plans that used to be the norm.

Self-Pay

In 2003, 16 percent of healthcare expenditures were paid for out of pocket by the consumer (Krugman & Wells, 2006). Additionally, because complementary and alternative medicine (CAM) is generally not covered by insurance, with the exception of some healthcare insurance policies that now cover acupuncture, naturopathy, massage, and chiropractic, most funding for integrative medicine was paid out of pocket. Two landmark studies by David Eisenberg, Davis, Ettner, Appel, Wilkey, Rompay, et al. (1998) reveal the growing trend of increased dollars paid directly by patients for such care. In 1993, $13.7 billion was spent on CAM. In 1997, a conservative estimate of $27 billion—an increase of 100 percent in five years—was paid for CAM services out of pocket. Surveys indicate that 42 percent of all Americans use CAM, with 75 percent of these individuals not informing their traditional physicians about the use of such care. Visits to CAM practitioners increased by 47 percent between 1993 and 1998, with Americans logging 629 million visits to CAM providers in 1998.

In Washington State, which has required that private insurance cover licensed CAM providers since 1996, only 14 percent of enrollees made CAM claims in 2002 (Lafferty, Tyree, Bellas, Watts, Lind, Sherman et al., 2006). Other studies also suggest that CAM therapies account for a small proportion of insurance claims overall, about one to three percent (Eisenberg et al., 2006; Lafferty et al., 2004; Lind, Lafferty, Grembowski, & Diehr, 2006).

THE IMPACT ON EQUITY OF CARE AND PAYMENT

Today, the U.S. healthcare system is a contradiction in terms. Well-insured people enjoy some of the best healthcare in the world and have access to expensive, high-technology services that are lifesaving for many. Unfortunately, as a whole, however, many of our health outcomes are shocking. The Institute of Medicine (IOM) estimates that 18,000 adults die each year due to lack of health insurance coverage. For any given illness, a person without health insurance is about 25 percent more likely to die than a person with the same condition with insurance (Institute of Medicine, 2002).

Even people with health insurance coverage are at significant financial risk due to underinsurance. A 2005 Harvard study (Himmelstein, Warren, Thorne, & Woolhandler, 2005) found that about half of bankruptcies in the United States are related to medical costs. Perhaps even more alarming, about two-thirds of those who declared bankruptcy due to medical costs were insured at the time of the onset of their bankrupting illness.

In addition, the complexity of the system entails a high cost of administration. Part of the astronomical cost of healthcare is due to the fact that 25 percent of every healthcare dollar is spent on administration, including 15 percent on insurance paperwork (Kahn, Kronick, Kreger, & Gans, 2004). Additionally, physicians, patients, nurses, and others often feel frustrated and beleaguered by the enormous amount of time spent on navigating the complex system to receive reimbursement for needed medical services that were provided.

PITFALLS AND CHALLENGES IN THE CURRENT REIMBURSEMENT SYSTEM

Free Market—Not

The current healthcare funding mechanism is a unique and cumbersome system. It is basically resistant to the demands of the free market. In most cases, because the patient is paying very little of the bill, and because healthcare is not a standard economic commodity, the traditional supply and demand model is ineffective. Fee-for-service, the payment mechanism for traditional health insurance, is paid by a third party—a nameless bureaucracy removed from the patient-provider relationship. From the provider side, healthcare professionals are in a special position because they can actually generate more demand at their own discretion through recommendations for testing, medication, return visits, and opinions and treatment from other healthcare providers. The public must trust that integrity, professionalism, and concern for the welfare of the patient are the primary motivators of the healthcare provider. However, because of the present system focus on healthcare as a business, a dangerous potential for misuse presents itself. If the system breaks down, the opportunity for healthcare providers and patients to collude to obtain higher reimbursement for the provider, and in some cases, lower out-of-pocket costs for the patients, is a concern. Fee-for-service, then, motivates providers to supply services, even though services may be coded at a higher reimbursement level or provided on a more frequent basis.

From the insurance company perspective, the profit motive is central. A required end product of health insurance for most private companies offering policies in the current system—and potentially detrimental to good health—is profits. The end product of health insurance, for most private companies offering policies in the current system, is not necessarily good health but, primarily, profits. Consequently, insurers can often distort the market by determining where patients can go to receive healthcare services. With the supply side held captive, HMOs and other managed care systems can collude to undercut the free market benefits of supply/demand and quality control. Healthcare can then be steered or denied altogether by cutting dollars flowing to healthcare treatment and/or reimbursement. The mechanisms of capitation and/or prospective payment favored by managed care plans and health maintenance organizations are also administered by a third party. Capitation can then place healthcare providers in an ethical bind. They may be motivated to minimize covered services or upcode carved-out services—a mechanism where the provider submits a charge for a service that has a higher value than the one actually performed. Overutilization or fraudulent upcoding by a network provider then becomes a problem inherent in the system The focus of the health insurance business can then be turned to the more traditional concerns of business: quarterly profits rather than patient care.

The federal government, as previously discussed, is a major purchaser of healthcare services. This fact further distorts the free market as well. Private insurance and workers' compensation carriers are geared to cover acute care needs. Because of this, private carriers and workers' compensation funders can deny payments for treatment, especially for chronic conditions, and cost-shift these to the public sector, forcing patients to use their Medicare or Medicaid coverage. This places the burden of healthcare costs squarely on taxpayers. It also allows private insurers to ration coverage for medically necessary care—but it ensures a more positive bottom line for insurance companies.

CHALLENGES IN HEALTHCARE REFORM

There is broad recognition that the U.S. healthcare system is in crisis related to rising costs, access problems, and deficiencies in the quality of care provided. It is not surprising that in our ideologically polarized country, different policy makers and stakeholder groups propose markedly polarized solutions that would take the direction of healthcare in the United States in very different directions.

Cost

Whether a short- or long-term perspective is taken, there is no denying that healthcare costs continue to spiral upward. In the first three years of this millennium, percentage increases in healthcare costs for premiums have risen in the double digits (Colliver, 2003). But even averaging healthcare costs over a 40-year period, costs have still risen on at average of seven percent annually (Aaron, 2005).

Increasing costs of administering the complex and cumbersome healthcare system that has evolved piecemeal over time is one contributing factor. However, the rapid expansion of information and technology in the medical field that has led to the miracle discoveries over the last 40 years has also been a factor. Increased technology produces more and more services and generates more research to improve the existing technology and services. Healthcare then begins to operate on the costly edge of cutting-edge medicine, which drives the costs for all services to their highest points.

Aging and Diversity of Population

Add to the cost issue the fact that the majority of the American population is aging at a rate unprecedented in this country, the cost figures for healthcare become even more daunting. In 1900, people 65 and older numbered 3.1 million. By 2000, this group encompassed 35.0 million, 11 times as large. And according to the *Report on Special Populations* from the Department of Health and Human Services (2005), this is only going to continue:

> According to U.S. Census Bureau projections, a substantial increase in the number of older people will occur when the Baby Boom generation (people born between 1946 and 1964) begins to turn 65 in 2011. The older population is projected to double from 36 million in 2003 to 72 million in 2030, and to increase from 12 percent to 20 percent of the population in the same time frame. By 2050, the older population is projected to number 86.7 million.
>
> The oldest-old population (those aged 85 and older) is also projected to double from 4.7 million in 2003 to 9.6 million in 2030—and to double again to 20.9 million in 2050. The latter increase will reflect the movement of Baby Boomers into the oldest-old category. . . . As the older population grows larger, it will also grow more diverse.

The increasing age of the American population will require that more services be provided for chronic health conditions, for example, cardiovascular problems, diabetes, stroke, and dementia, all health challenges that the current system is ill equipped to handle. The increasing diversity of the population will also challenge the healthcare system to be responsive to needs of aging, currently marginalized individuals.

Belief System

Currently, 35 percent of all healthcare costs are incurred for the first month and the last six months of life (Jones, 2002). A recent report indicates that medical care at the end of life consumes 10 to 12 percent of the total healthcare budget and 27 percent of the Medicare budget (Emmanuelle, 2006). A review of existing data also suggests that hospice and advance directives can save between 25 and 40 percent of healthcare costs during the last month of life, with savings decreasing to 10–17 percent over the last 6 months of life, and decreasing further to 0–10 percent over the last 12 months of life (Emmanuelle, 2006). There is an internal conflict of values that is emerging, and must be confronted, in healthcare as technology provides more and more advances to prolong life—advances that also result in more costly services.

Studies are emerging that indicate that healthcare consumption can decrease parallel with an increase in quality of life for older patients (Iruthayanathen, Zou, & Childs, 2005). Changing the belief system in healthcare to reorient from acute medical interventions to focus on improving quality of life and promoting good health as a necessary part of healthcare is a fundamental shift that is antithetical to the current philosophies of healthcare funding. Reorienting this philosophy is a major challenge in any kind of healthcare reform debate.

FUNDING OUR WAY

Mind, Body, and Behavior

The unprecedented public focus, however, that is now being placed on the effects of lifestyle, behavior, and stress on health and illness holds the potential for shifting the underlying philosophy in healthcare. Such a focus is unprecedented ("New Science," 2004). The so-called mind-body connection—the intersection of psychological and physical health—is, for the first time, receiving mainstream media coverage. Also for the first time, real dollars are starting to flow into funding approaches that affect quality of life—prevention, health promotion, and disease management. These areas are where behavior and behavior change provide the foundation for ensuring health and preventing illness. Policy makers are even looking to these areas for solutions to the country's broken healthcare system. Just recently, the Robert Wood Johnson Foundation (Hearne, Elliot, Juliano, & Segel, 2005) concluded that "the United States needs to develop a proactive approach for health, focusing on prevention of illness and injury. . . . This type of approach would save lives and money and improve our overall health." Integrating mind with body, behavior with health, and the psychological with the physical holds a credible promise of achieving the long sought after, elusive goal of improved healthcare, while simultaneously controlling, if not reducing, healthcare costs.

Health and Behavior Codes

In 2002, Medicare accepted and began implementation of health and behavior Current Procedural Terminology codes for medical treatment. These codes are used by physicians and psychologists to bill for psychologically and behaviorally based interventions to treat an individual with a physical health *(not mental health)* diagnosis. This was a major step forward in acknowledging the mind-body-behavior connection by a major purchaser of services in the healthcare delivery system. Of course, acceptance of these codes did not automatically mean widespread use of the codes, yet increased use since their creation has been quite apparent (Centers for Medicare and Medicaid, 2007). The number of health and behavior claims submitted to Medicare increased almost 400 percent, from 64,000 claims in 2002, the first year they were available, to over one-quarter of a million claims in 2003. While reimbursement for this category of treatment also increased, it is anticipated that overall healthcare cost savings due to mind-body-behavior interventions will be substantial. It is important that demonstration projects and studies be designed to examine this issue more closely.

Use of the codes in the private insurance market has been much slower to catch on since each company makes its own determination about accepting the codes. To date, however, virtually every large, private insurer is accepting the health and behavior codes, and there is consistent effort to increase that number. The impact of behavior on health and illness, which is now being taken seriously by the public, payers, and policy makers, provides an opportunity for the country's healthcare system to address cost and quality problems.

Integrated Care

At the federal level, a recently funded demonstration project in Pennsylvania is highly noteworthy. Through the efforts of the Practice Directorate of the American Psychological Association and the Pennsylvania Psychological Association, Congressional seed money was provided to integrate mental health screening and treatment with primary medical care for older adults. This effort holds promise as a prototype for other projects and studies that need to be developed to advance the understanding of cost savings, delivery of quality care, and improved functioning and quality of life of the patient derived from integrating mind-body-behavior care. Given Congress's increased interest in supporting demonstrations based on the integration of behavior and health, such an approach has good merit. Other possible demonstration projects on tap to use congressionally appropriated money to showcase integrated services include psychological interventions combined with medical interventions in the treatment of Medicare cardiac patients and the treatment of childhood obesity in school-based health centers (American Psychological Association, 2001, 2005; Holloway, 2005).

In the private sector, there is also a growing recognition of the connection between health and behavior. Structures that had previously been built to keep behavioral health and physical health separate are now being dismantled. The creation of the health and behavior codes has contributed to this, but insurers are also beginning to eliminate behavioral health carve-outs to integrate medical and behavioral services. For example, Blue Cross and Blue Shield of Massachusetts eliminated its Magellan behavioral health carve-out contract for almost half a million subscribers who work for state-based companies with the intention of providing more integrated behavioral and physical healthcare (Kowalczyk, 2005). A company spokesperson pegged its move to the desire to have the ability to look at both medical and behavioral health claims when developing disease management programs to improve members' healthcare.

Even the managed behavioral healthcare carve-outs are themselves developing more integrative disease management capabilities. This change appears motivated by several factors, including an expected synergistic effect between mental health and medical conditions, increasing respect for the impact disease management programs can have on health outcomes and medical costs, and more pressure on insurers to slow premium increases.

Prevention: Beyond Integrated Disease Management

But the role of behavior goes far beyond disease management. Behavior is integrally linked with the promotion of health and the prevention of disease. The growing public understanding of such a concept is new. Much more prominent today than in the past 30 years is the realization that the six leading causes of death are related to behavior—heart disease, cancer, liver disease, lung disease, car crashes, and suicides. Some 60–90 percent of visits to a medical doctor, depending on which study is referenced, are considered to be for stress-related complaints. Forty-three percent of all adults suffer adverse health effects from stress. People are beginning to understand, perhaps for the first time, that things such as having a good support system or maintaining an optimistic outlook on life can lead to better health, a longer life, and lower costs of healthcare (Anderson & Anderson, 2003).

THE CURRENT STATE OF HEALTHCARE REFORM

No good comprehensive health reform plan, or even an organized vision of one, seems able to emerge in response to recent years of turmoil in the country's health system. A number of approaches, however, are being debated in an attempt to shed new light on the current system issues that darken the horizon.

Consumerism and Health Savings Accounts

Among the few visible so-called reform trends that can be found is the movement toward consumer-driven healthcare. In the absence of any organized healthcare reform effort by Congress, consumerism appears to be gaining traction in the healthcare marketplace. This concept means different things to different people, but it usually means empowering consumers to make decisions about their healthcare, rather than deferring to a third party. This concept intends to better enable individual consumers, as opposed to employers or other third-party payers, to be better purchasers of their health services, not just the beneficiaries of services purchased for them by a third party. In theory, consumer-driven healthcare intends to produce an informed consumer of healthcare who will make smart purchasing choices based on quality and cost. In its nascent form, it typically consists of a high-deductible insurance plan, with the potential for a combined employer and employee–funded health reimbursement account or health savings account (HSA), used by the employee to pay for services within that deductible.

One policy application of this framework has been promoted by the Bush administration. Under these plans, a person buys a relatively low cost health insurance policy that has a deductible in the $2,000–5,000 range (a high-deductible plan, or HDHP). In addition, he opens a tax-sheltered health savings account of $2,000–5,000 that can be used toward the deductible. The employer and employee would contribute tax-free dollars that can accumulate from year to year. Money in the account can be used to pay for plan deductibles, coinsurance, or copayments, which the employee historically has paid with after-tax dollars. Money in the HSA can also be used to cover nonplan expenses recognized by the IRS as qualified medical expenses. The employee is responsible for all expenses up to the deductible. In theory, this structure positions the employee to control decision making about how to spend his healthcare dollars and, importantly, choose the desired healthcare services.

Proponents see consumer-driven healthcare as a way to bring the power of informed consumer decision making to healthcare to remedy the distorted purchasing decisions and uncontrollable inflation in a system where someone other than the patient is paying the bill. Some think consumer-driven healthcare offers a way of replacing managed care's efforts to limit the supply side of healthcare with incentives that influence and control the demand side of healthcare

Opponents of consumer-driven healthcare point to significant problems with HSAs. They are of no help to low-income or uninsured individuals. They do not necessarily curb healthcare costs because HSAs are built on fatally flawed assumptions about consumer behavior regarding healthcare. For example, people diagnosed with a life-threatening disease would not look to price as their first concern. People do not shop for emergency care.

Opponents also believe that HSAs will cause further fragmentation in the health insurance market. The healthiest individuals will gravitate to HSAs, while sicker people will remain in traditional insurance plans, causing premiums to rise and employers to stop offering plans. In the end, critics say, HSAs drive people out of the group insurance market and into an individual insurance market that is ill equipped to handle the shift.

Even supporters of consumer-driven healthcare agree that the individual insurance market needs alteration if it is to be part of any effective healthcare system transformation. But they are also quick to point out that HDHPs with HSAs are far from the whole story with consumer-driven healthcare. Supporters say that consumer-driven healthcare is about changing incentives that influence all participants in the healthcare system. Its ultimate focus is behavior change leading to wellness, prevention, early intervention, and better disease management.

But adoption of this approach has not been what was hoped for. According to Mercer Health and Benefits Consulting, the number of consumer-driven plans grew by only two percent among small employers in 2005—the very population that was supposed to be most advantaged by the plans (Appleby, 2005). The Mercer study found that the plans are more popular among jumbo employers with 20,000 or more workers, where 22 percent offer some form of consumer-driven health plan, up from 12 percent in 2004. But even in those companies, enrollment in the plans averaged only eight percent of workers.

A survey by the Employee Benefits Research Institute (2005) and the Commonwealth Fund found lower consumer satisfaction and higher out-of-pocket costs with consumer-driven plans than with more comprehensive health plans. Importantly, the study found that individuals with consumer-driven health plans were more likely to avoid, skip, or delay healthcare because of costs than those in comprehensive plans. The study also found that few health plans of any type provide the cost and quality information sufficient to enable informed decisions, and it found very low levels of trust by consumers in the information provided by these health plans.

Information Technology

Another area where hope springs eternal for reforming healthcare is the adoption of information technology to create a more effective, more efficient, and better integrated healthcare system. Despite the promise, one health commentator sums it up this way:

> If the state of U.S. medical technology is one of our great national treasures, then the state of U.S. health information technology is one of our great national disgraces. We spend $1.6 trillion a year on health care—far more than we do on personal financial services—and yet we have a 21st century financial information infrastructure and a 19th century health information technology infrastructure. Thousands of small organizations chew around the edges of the problem, spending hundreds of millions of dollars per year on proprietary clinical IT products that barely work and do not talk to each other. Health care organizations do not relish the problem, most vilify it. Many are spending vast sums on proprietary products that do not coalesce into a system-wide solution, and the investment community has poured nearly a half-trillion dollars into failed health information technology ventures that once claimed to be the solution. Nonetheless, no single health care organization or health information technology venture has attained anything close to the critical mass necessary to effect such a fix. This is the textbook definition of a market failure. (Kleinke, 2005, pp. 1246–1262)

Quality-Based Reform

An information-driven health system appears to be faring no better than a consumer-driven health system as a vehicle for reform. Nor have attempts to administratively limit services or realign incentives done much to cure the woes of the current healthcare system. And until recently, little has been done in an attempt to improve health as a means of improving the healthcare system. Efforts are emerging, however, to refocus on quality and, it is argued, move the system away from the historical obsession with costs. Tools such as pay-for-performance, evidence-based practice, and outcome measures are being touted as a potential remedy for the system's problems. Pay-for-performance is most frequently described as an effort, initiated by payers, to realign incentives in healthcare services delivery so as to provide incentives for improving the quality of care. The major focus of the 100 or so current employer-initiated pay-for-performance programs is to attempt to determine how well health professionals care for their patients and reward the ones whose outcomes are best, usually with bonus pay at the end of the year. Centers for Medicare and Medicaid Services has also been experimenting with pay-for-performance programs, and the Medicare law recently enacted by Congress includes language requiring some limited type of pay-for-performance component in Medicare beginning in July 2007.

At present, however, what constitutes a pay-for-performance program is far from standardized, or even clear. There is considerable confusion as to whether incentives should be provided in response to performance-based measures or clinical outcome measures. Some programs include measures of preventive services such as cancer screening, mammography, and immunizations. Some include measures of care for such chronic diseases as asthma, diabetes, and cardiovascular disease; others do not. Many programs also use client satisfaction measures. Some incorporate utilization measures such as percentage of generic drugs prescribed or medically unnecessary tests ordered. Some actually reward physicians for using various forms of information technology. Some attempt to incent performance and good quality, while others incent quality improvement.

Universal Coverage

There is also a movement in some quarters toward universal access and a single-payer system. At the state level, some legislatures have proposed and/or enacted universal health coverage for residents of their states. The National Conference of State Legislatures (2006) reports that "while the legislative trend in the states is to fill in the gaps public and private systems leave behind, some states are still considering a single-payer, universal health insurance system that would cover every citizen within their borders" (http://www.ncsl.org/programs/health/uvinhc2006.htm).

By and large, the single-payer system approaches differ philosophically from the past assumptions that have funded private/public healthcare in this country. Rather than a business approach, single-payer proposals view healthcare as an integral part of a strong social infrastructure and a basic right of every citizen. As the Physicians' Working Group for Single-Payer National Health Insurance (2003) states, "The United States alone treats health care as a commodity distributed according to the ability to pay, rather than as a social service to be distributed according to medical need" (http://www.pnhp.org/single_payer_resources/proposal_of_the_physicians_working_group_for_singlepayer_national_health_insurance.php).

In 2003, Maine became the first state to pass legislation aimed at providing every citizen with access by 2009. In 2005, Illinois passed the All Kids Health Insurance program. This program provides that all children under 18 who are not covered through parents' health policies or another government-funded plan are eligible for sliding scale payments for hospital and routine physician visits, vision and dental benefits, and prescription drug coverage. Both programs are designed to fill in gaps for the uninsured so that there is universal access to services, though the systems are not based on a single-payer model. As of 2006, eight states are considering universal healthcare bills, and seven more states have commissioned studies to look at the possibility of such a system. Missouri, Hawaii, Connecticut, and California have all had bills proposed in 2006 that would provide universal access to healthcare for all residents of the state and be funded by a single-payer system. However, these bills died at various points in the legislative process (http://www.ncsl.org/programs/health/universalhealth2006.htm).

The California proposal (SB 840) for a universal access, single-payer healthcare system was actually passed by the assembly but was vetoed by the governor in September 2006. Some aspects of that proposal are well worth noting. For example, eligibility under the plan was determined by residence in the state of California, not by employment or income. The plan involved no new spending on healthcare. The system was to be paid for by federal, state, and county monies already being spent on healthcare and by affordable insurance premiums that replaced all premiums, deductibles, out-of-pocket payments, and copays now paid by employers and consumers.

A study by the Lewin Group, a Virginia-based consulting firm, predicted that the legislation would save California $343.6 billion in healthcare costs over the next 10 years, mainly by cutting administration and using bulk purchases of drugs and medical equipment. By consolidating the administrative functions of many insurance companies into one agency, it was estimated that savings would reach $20 billion the first year alone. Furthermore, the combined purchasing power of all California residents was to be consolidated to provide more effective negotiating power with pharmaceutical companies to save another $5.2 billion (Lawrence, 2005).

Additionally, California residents would be free to choose their own healthcare providers. Benefits coverage included all care prescribed by a patient's healthcare provider that met accepted standards of care and practice. Specifically, coverage included hospital, medical, surgical, and mental health; dental and vision care; prescription drugs and medical equipment such as hearing aids; emergency care, including ambulances; skilled nursing care after hospitalization; substance abuse recovery programs; health education and translation services, including services for those with hearing and vision impairments; transportation needed to access covered services; diagnostic testing; and hospice care.

If such a plan were to be enacted in California or any state, a major challenge would be the retooling of the insurance industry, which is a huge industry. Although the proposed California legislation addresses this issue to some degree, the economic impact of such a transition would need to be comprehensively modeled and planned to avoid making a substantial negative economic impact on the economy.

NEXT STEPS

A number of surveys indicate that the vast majority of Americans support both universal health coverage and major reform in our health system (Pew Report 2005, Harris Poll 2005, Washington Post/ABC News Poll, 2003). How that support can be translated effectively into the financial and political arenas is another matter. The U.S. healthcare system is unique in its combination of vast technological advances, skyrocketing costs of healthcare, and multiple mechanisms of reimbursement. Models of healthcare that exist in other industrialized countries tend to have more built-in mechanisms for cost control. It is these models that are often used to elucidate issues of financial and political reform in the United States. These issues necessarily include hard discussions about the low benefit–high cost values of some medical procedures and the rationing of healthcare services (Aaron, 2005).

These discussions are important to have. The changing demographics and healthcare economic profile of this county mandate such discussions. However, given the basic value and belief systems of Americans, which range from mind-body to end-of-life issues, any discussion of healthcare reform—and the hard decisions that entails—may be more effective if financing reform is buttressed with healthcare delivery system reform. This means a greater emphasis on wellness than illness; a greater emphasis on the impact of the mind and behaviors on physical health; a greater emphasis on the importance of community connectedness to overall health; and a greater emphasis on the end product of healthcare as good health.

The Institute of Medicine (2004) suggested that the following criteria be used to judge any health reform effort:

- healthcare coverage should be universal
- healthcare coverage should be continuous
- healthcare coverage should be affordable to individuals and families
- the health insurance strategy should be affordable and sustainable for society
- health insurance should enhance health and well-being by promoting access to high-quality care that is effective, efficient, safe, timely, patient-centered, and equitable.

Substantive healthcare reform will be a challenging undertaking that will expose the deep philosophical differences that Americans hold on whether healthcare is a right or a market good and the role of society, government, and individuals in providing healthcare. It is imperative that any considered system of reform move beyond medical care to healthcare. If that can be accomplished, the future of healthcare in the United States may be able to move beyond health rationing to health realization.

TOOL KIT FOR CHANGE

Role and Perspective of the Healthcare Professional

1. Overall, the product of good healthcare should be good health, not profits.
2. Thirty-five percent of all healthcare costs are incurred in the first month and the last six months of life.
3. Studies indicate that reorienting from acute medical interventions to a focus on improving quality of life can decrease healthcare consumption during the life span.

Role and Perspective of the Patient/Participant

1. Surveys indicate that the vast majority of Americans support both universal health coverage and major reform in our health system.
2. Americans are focusing on how the mind and body work together to create health or illness.
3. The current healthcare system is not responsive to free market principles and consumer demands. It is paid for primarily by third parties, where healthcare decisions can be rendered independently of the patient through denial of services or denial of access to particular practitioners.
4. The primary motive of insurance companies is profit.

Interconnection: The Global Perspective

1. Healthcare coverage should be universal and enhance health and well-being.
2. The goal must be to provide access to high-quality care that is effective, efficient, safe, timely, patient-centered, and equitable.
3. Any considered system of healthcare reform must move beyond medical care to healthcare. Only then can the United States move beyond health rationing to health realization.
4. Studies indicate that through integrating administration of healthcare, vast financial savings can result, which can be channeled into services.

REFERENCES

Aaron, H. (2005, October 20). *Putting the lid on health care costs: An industry perspective.* Retrieved December 18, 2006, from http://www.brookings.edu/comm/events/20051020health.pdf

American Medical Association. (2006). *New AMA survey shows Medicare cuts will harm seniors' access to physician care.* Retrieved December 13, 2006, from http://www.ama-assn.org/ama/pub/category/16117.html.

American Psychological Association. (2005). *Positive aging act.* Retrieved December 12, 2006, from http://www.apa.org/ppo/aging/PAA05.pdf.

American Psychological Association. (2001). *APA uses actuarial model to plan cardiac demonstration project.* Retrieved December, 12, 2006, from http://www.apa.org/monitor/jan01/actuarial.html.

Anderson, N. B., & Anderson, P. E. (2003). *Emotional longevity: What REALLY determines how long you live.* New York: Viking Penguin.

Appleby, J. (2005, November 4). High health care deductibles not a hit. *USA Today.*

Asch, S. M., McGlynn, E. A., Hogan, M. M., Hayward, R. A., Shekelle, P., Rubenstein, L., et al. (2004). Comparison of quality of care for patients in the Veterans Health Administration and patients in a national sample. *Annals of Internal Medicine, 141,* 938–945.

California Healthcare Foundation. (2006, January). *Medi-Cal facts and figures: A look at California's medical program*: *Medi-Cal budget and cost drivers.* Retrieved November 28, 2006, from http://www.chcf.org/documents/policy/MediCalBudgetAndCost Drivers2006.pdf.

Centers for Medicare and Medicaid. (2007, February 2). *Physician fee schedule: Overview.* Retrieved December 6, 2006, from http://www.cms.hhs.gov/Physician FeeSched/01_ overview.asp

Colliver, V. (2003, December 8). Health Care Costs Continue Double Digit Increase. *San Francisco Chronicle.* Retrieved December 3, 2006 from http://www.commondreams. org/headlines03/1208-03.htm.

Eisenberg, D. M., Davis, R. B., Ettner, S. L., Appel, S., Wilkey, S., Van Rompay, M., et al. (1998). Trends in alternative medicine use in the United States, 1990–1997: Results of a follow-up national survey. *Journal of the American Medical Association, 18,* 1569–1575.

Emanuel, E. J. (2006). Cost savings at the end of life: What do the data show? Center for Outcomes and Policy Research, Division of Cancer Epidemiology and Control, Dana-Farber Cancer Institute. Boston, MA: Harvard Medical School.

Employee Benefits Research Institute. (2005). *Early experience with high deductible and consumer-driven health plans: Findings from the ebri/commonwealth fund consumerism in health care survey.* Retrieved November 28, 2006, from http://www.ebri.org/ publications/ib/index.cfm?fa=ibDisp&content_id=3606.

Families USA. (2005). Paying a premium: The increased cost of care for the uninsured. Retrieved December 13, 2006, from http://www.familiesusa.org/resources/ publications/reports/paying-a-premium-findings.html.

Health & Human Service, NIH Report on Aging. (2005). Dramatic changes in U.S. aging highlighted in new census, Impact of baby boomers anticipated. Retrieved December 3, 2006, from http://www.nih.gov/news/pr/mar2006/nia-09.htm.

Hearne, S., Elliot, K., Juliano, G., & Segel, L. M. (2005). *Shortchanging America's health—A state by state look at how federal public health dollars are spent.* Retrieved November 28, 2006, from http://healthyamericans.org/reports/budget05/ StateHealthSpending05.pdf.

Himmelstein, D. U., Warren, E., Thorne, D., & Woolhandler, S. (2005, February 2). MarketWatch: Illness and injury as contributors to bankruptcy. *Health Affairs,* doi:10.1377/ hlthaff.w5.63. Retrieved November 29, 2006, from http://content.healthaffairs.org/ cgi/content/full/hlthaff.w5.63/DC1.

Holloway, Jennifer (2005). Health funding for prevention on the rise. Retrieved Dec 12, 2006 from http://www.apa.org/monitor/feb05/funding.html. p. 66.

Institute of Medicine. (2002, May 21). *Care without coverage: Too little, too late.* Retrieved February 2, 2005, from http://www.iom.edu/CMS/3809/4660/4333.aspx.

Institute of Medicine. (2004). *Insuring America's health: Principles and recommendations.* Retrieved December 7, 2006, from http://www.iom.edu/CMS/3809/4660/17632.aspx.

Institute of Medicine. (2006). Examining the health disparities research plan of the national institutes of health: Unfinished business. Retrieved December 7, 2006, http://www. iom.edu/CMS/3740/22356/33275.aspx.

Iruthayanathen, M., Zou, Y-H., & Childs, G. (2005). Deydroepiandorsterone restoration of growth hormone gene expression in aging female rats in vivo and in vitro: Evidence for actions via estrogen receptors. *Journal of Endocrinology, 146,* 5176–5187.

Jones, C. (2002). *Why have health expenditures as a share of GDP risen so much?* Retrieved December 3, 2006, from http://www.nber.org/~confer/2002/efgf02/jones.pdf

Kahn, J., Kronick, R., Kreger, M., & Gans, D. (2004). The cost of health insurance administration in California: Estimates for insurers, physicians and hospitals. *Health Affairs, 24,* 1629–1639.

Kleinke, J. (2005). Dot-gov: Market failure and government intervention. *Health Affairs, 24,* 1246–1262.

Kowalczyk, L. (2005, February 11). Blue Cross to take back oversight of some Magellan Health patients. *Boston Globe.*

Krugman, P., & Wells, R. (2006, March 23). The health crisis and what to do about it. *The New York Review of Books, 53,* article 18802. Retrieved November 26, 2006, from http://www.nybooks.com/articles/18802

Lafferty, W., Bellas, A., Corage Baden, A., Tyree, P. T., Standish, L. J., & Patterson, R. (2004). The use of complementary and alternative medical providers by insured cancer patients in Washington State. *Cancer, 100,* 1522–1530.

Lafferty, W., Tyree, P. T., Bellas, A. S., Watts, C. A., Lind, B. K., Sherman, K. J., et al. (2006). Insurance coverage and subsequent utilization of complementary and alternative medicine providers. *American Journal of Managed Care, 12,* 397–404.

Lawrence, S. (2005, January 19). Lew group analysis of Senator Kuehl's single payer plan. *San Francisco Chronicle.*

Lind, B. K., Lafferty, W. E., Grembowski, D. E., & Diehr, P. K. (2006). Complementary and alternative provider use by insured patients with diabetes in Washington State. *Journal of Alternative and Complementary Medicine, 12,* 71–77.

Longman, P. (2005, January/February). The best care anywhere. *Washington Monthly.*

National Conference of State Legislatures. (2006). Universal health care: 2005 legislation. Retrieved December 12, 2006, from http://www.ncsl.org/programs/health/universalhealth.htm.

National Conference of State Legislatures. (2006). 2006 bills on universal health care coverage legislatures fill in the gaps. Retrieved December 12, 2006, from http://www.ncsl.org/programs/health/uvinhc2006.htm.

National Economic Council/Domestic Policy Council. (2000, February 29). *America's seniors and Medicare: Challenges for today and tomorrow.* Washington, DC: White House.

The new science of mind and body. (2004, September 27). *Newsweek.*

Pew Center on the States. (2006). *Special report on Medicaid.* Retrieved December 18, 2006, from http://www.pewcenteronthestates.org/report_A2.html.

Physicians Working for a Single-Payer National Health Insurance. (2003). Proposal of the physicians' working group for single-payer national health insurance executive summary. Retrieved December 7, 2006, from http://www.pnhp.org/single_payer_resources/proposal_of_the_physicians_working_group_for_singlepayer_national_health_insurance.php.

Schoen, C., Doty, M., Collins, S., & Holmgren, A. (2005, June 14). Insured but not protected: How many adults are underinsured? *Health Affairs,* doi:10.1377/hlthaff. w5.289. Retrieved June 14, 2005, from http://content.healthaffairs.org/cgi/content/abstract/hlthaff.w5.289

Schuster, M., McGlynn, E., & Brook, R. (1998). How good is the quality of health care in the United States? *Milbank Quarterly, 76*, 517–563.

U.S. Census Bureau. (2006). 65+ in the United States. Special Report on Aging.

Woolhandler, S., & Himmelstein, D. (2004). The high costs of for-profit care. *Canadian Medical Association Journal, 170*, 1814–1815.

Chapter Fourteen

THE POLITICS OF HEALTHCARE: MAKING IT HAPPEN (PART II)

Marie A. DiCowden, PhD

IT'S BROKEN, BUT HOW DO WE FIX IT?

Our nation continues to suffer from debilitating and costly preventable health conditions. Seven of the top 10 leading causes of death are related to behavior (National Committee on Vital and Health Statistics, 2002). A recent survey on stress (American Psychological Association, 2006) found that Americans most concerned about their stress levels were more likely to smoke and use so-called comfort foods and less likely to exercise than people not concerned about their stress levels. Those individuals that used food to cope with stress were more likely to report hypertension and high cholesterol and be overweight or obese. Forty-three percent of all adults, according to one study (Miller, Smith, & Rothstein, 1993), were found to suffer adverse health effects from stress.

At the same time, costs for treating health problems are spiraling out of control. Double-digit increases in premiums for health insurance have been the norm in recent years (Colliver, 2003). Currently, almost 47 million people in this country are uninsured, and up to 60 million are without health insurance or have inadequate coverage at some point during the year (Schoen, Doty, Collins, & Holmgren, 2005). Most of the uninsured find their way to emergency rooms, which are their only resource when they must seek treatment. This situation has now led to a crisis in emergency rooms. The Institute of Medicine (2006a) has reported that emergency rooms are on the verge of collapse: "Ambulances are turned away from emergency departments once every minute on average and patients in many areas may wait hours or even days for a hospital bed" (p. 23).

The debate around healthcare reform has primarily centered on how to limit costs and limit supply in the face of the seemingly endless demand for services in the medical system. Peripherally, issues of health and prevention of illness have also been discussed. However, arguments focusing primarily on limiting expenditures are still predominant. Discussions in favor of promoting health have not led, in any significant way, to reorganization of the delivery system to reflect health promotion and prevention (Schoen et al., 2005). It is a discussion that has much in common with the blind men discussing what the elephant actually looks like. To those worried about cost control, the elephant is like a wall. To those promoting health as a means of cost control, the elephant is exactly like a rope. One group seems to be talking about rationing healthcare, the other about expanding it. To those who focus primarily on the funding and cost aspects, there is a heightened sense of fear that promoting health services will only escalate costs. And when you add this fear to the discussions, then the elephant clearly looks more and more like a wall. Consequently, political backers of reform on both sides end up at loggerheads.

The Citizens' Health Care Working Group was formed to query the American people at a grassroots level and address the issue of healthcare from a bipartisan perspective. The participants in 98 community forums around the country indicated that a clear majority want a mandated, basic benefit for everyone and are "not comfortable with bare-bones benefit packages"—even if this means paying higher taxes. Yet the full reform needs are daunting, and "it will involve difficult decisions about how health care is organized, delivered and financed" (Citizens' Health Care Working Group, 2006).

The parameters are clear. The elephant is really more than its individual parts. We cannot talk about meaningful healthcare reform in the political arena unless we discuss all aspects simultaneously—what health services are delivered, how they are delivered, and how they are paid for. A fragmented delivery system no longer works and is no longer viable financially. "Integrated community health networks to improve quality of care, efficiency and provide basic benefits are essential" (Citizens' Health Care Working Group, 2006), but who determines what kind of benefits Americans receive, and how should they be paid for?

THE PLAYERS: WHO HAS THE INFLUENCE?

Elected officials, whether they be legislative or executive, are responsible for guiding the system. Addressing conflicting social and economic demands to move the policies of this country ahead are what they are given a mandate to do. However, over the last decade, the conflicting issues in healthcare have fallen victim to partisan politics: "national health insurance, Medicare, prescription drug coverage, and stem cell research served as wedge issues during presidential and major congressional campaigns from 1991 through 2004" (Heaney, 2006, p. 893).

But who influences the politicians on these wedge issues? Heaney's (2006) landmark study of influence on the brokering of public health issues reports that there is no single architect or interest group that stands as the broker of influence on health policy. While the American Medical Association may have played that role in the past, it no longer enjoys that status today. Instead, there is a focus on "multiple, coequal elites as the driving force in the policy process" (McFarland, 2004). The elite interest groups who are "regarded as devoted partisans" wield the most influence within political parties and, in turn, with elected politicians (Heaney, 2006, p. 899).

In a 2003 survey, the Pharmaceutical Research and Manufacturers of America was considered to be the most influential group in determining health policy. Second in influence was the American Medical Association, followed by the American Association for Retired Persons, then the American Hospital Association (Heaney, 2004).

The insurance industry, which is one of the greatest contributors to economic growth in this country over the last several years (Bureau of Economic Analysis, 2005), was ranked among the top 25 most influential organizations, along with general business interests, unions, and other major health trade associations (Heaney, 2004). The analysis of how these groups collaborated for trade-offs in other areas to influence the passage of the Medicare prescription drug legislation in 2003 should be required reading for any preparation for passing healthcare reform (Heaney, 2006).

However, political dynamics in the legislative process aside, the recent elections have brought a revitalized awareness to politicians of the role of the American public in determining the eventual outcome of the governing and legislative processes. While the meaning of the midterm elections are not yet completely clear, Pew Research (Kohut, 2006) indicates that something very different took place during the 2006 elections. The election was determined by "the shifting sentiments of independents and moderates" and the "views of the least ideological voters decided this election for the Democrats." The composition of the voters also shifted. The electorate that made the difference tended to be younger voters, women, and seculars who joined the ranks of the more liberally leaning Democrats. While there is no clear consensus that the American voters are moving significantly to the Left, there is a clear message that they are dissatisfied with performance failures—the war in Iraq, corruption, and the aftermath of Katrina.

While healthcare has remained fourth on the agenda in reported voter concerns (Americans for Health Care, 2005), there is evidence that it is an issue that is increasing in salience for Americans. A recent survey (Americans for Health Care, 2005) indicated that people are more concerned about politicians not taking action on healthcare than they are about higher taxes due to healthcare reform or government being overly involved in healthcare. Sixty-six percent of those surveyed feel that healthcare was discussed far too little in the last campaign. Seventy-four percent believe it should be considered a "high, very high, or the single highest priority" when Congress reconvenes. The American people want healthcare reform, not partisan attacks. Voters have loudly repudiated partisanship and poor performance of elected officials in the last election on both international and national issues. Continued avoidance of healthcare reform may well be interpreted in the 2008 election as a performance failure as well.

Americans see the provision of healthcare as a core value. But if the politicians do not understand what Americans view as important about healthcare, if they continue to avoid reform, or simply pass reform that is not reflective of the will of the people, they may well pay the price—losing their job of representing the people. Fears about the changes needed to implement healthcare reform remain for both the electorate and their representatives. Leadership, such as can evolve out of the Citizens' Health Care Working Group to study and determine what Americans need to address both healthcare reform and the fears about reform, is crucial.

WHAT DO AMERICANS VALUE?

For healthcare reform to be viable in the political arena, legislators and the executive branch must understand what the American people want and provide leadership to overcome the fear of change. It is essential that the models of healthcare delivery and financing considered be flexible, innovative, and allow change to evolve in incremental ways (Newman, 2006). Healthcare must be accessible, of sufficient quality, and affordable. Consequently, basic services, organization of the delivery system, and the capacity to fund it must all be addressed simultaneously.

Quality Care

Americans want humane treatment that promotes quality care of the whole person, both in the community and at the end of life (Citizens' Health Care Working Group, 2006). Americans recognize that health includes both the body and the mind. There is an increasing public focus being placed on the effects of lifestyle, behavior, and stress on health and illness. The "mind-body connection," as it is often referred to by the public, is, for the first time, receiving mainstream media coverage. There is a generally acknowledged connection between psychological and physical health (American Psychological Association, 1995). A *Newsweek* cover story in October 2005 highlighted the link between stress, psychological health, and cardiovascular health. A January 2006 *New York Times* series, "The Stealth Epidemic," put a spotlight on diabetes and clearly fingered the culprit for this epidemic as behavior—faulty diet and inactivity.

There is extensive research, an existing knowledge base, and technologies that exist about how to change behavior in ways that benefit people's health. The early research of Neal Miller demonstrated instrumental learning of visceral responses and led to biofeedback treatment for hypertension, cardiac arrhythmias, gastrointestinal symptoms, and headaches (Miller, 2007). The understanding of the influence of behavior, lifestyle, and personality on health issues such as diabetes, asthma, and cardiovascular disease has also led to better management protocols for those diseases. The knowledge of brain-behavior relationships through neuropsychology and rehabilitation psychology has contributed greatly to such things as the management of attention deficit disorder, hyperactivity, and autism (Newman, 2005).

Forty years ago, a young research and clinical cardiologist named Herbert Benson began investigating a connection between stress and hypertension and discovered that monkeys could be trained to regulate their blood pressure levels with brainpower alone. This eventually led to the publication of *The Relaxation Response* (Benson, 1975), which offered a useful application of the mind-body connection.

Corporate America has also taken note of the growing role of lifestyle and behavior in health. Wellness programs are springing up in the workplace as companies look to promote employee health and positively influence their financial bottom line. Perhaps as a testament to how influential lifestyle and behavior have become, even some corporate marketing departments are taking note. One large, well-known food company, for example, recently presented elements of its new marketing strategy to a gathering of health industry and consumer advocates. It described three categories of products being sold to consumers: "good-for-you foods," such as oatmeal and orange juice, with known health benefits; "better-for-you foods," which have undergone processes to squeeze out as much of the saturated fats and sugar as possible; and "fun-for-you foods," which are those foods likely to contain little else besides fat and sugar (Newman, 2005). The real point to be made here is that the company is redistributing its marketing dollars away from the historical consumer favorite fun-for-you foods and toward the better-for-you and good-for-you foods. This change, of course, is designed to reflect consumers' changing behaviors, priorities, and purchasing patterns.

What is important here for healthcare reform is that the public is beginning to recognize and value the promotion of health and also recognize that paying attention to psychological health is necessary for promoting overall good health. Despite the growing public awareness of this, there has been a lack of reform at the national level. Even recognition of the importance of achieving parity of mental and physical health benefits, which has bipartisan congressional support, has not resulted in a good federal parity law. But educated policy makers at the state level have been more progressive. In 2006, mental health parity laws were enacted by Washington, Oregon, Iowa, and South Carolina, bringing the total number of states with some form of parity to 41 (Newman, 2005). The American people, at some level, want services that treat the whole person.

Accessible and Affordable Care

One of the greatest contributors to spiraling costs in healthcare is the fragmentation of the healthcare system. The U.S. healthcare system is highly inefficient in both the delivery and funding of services. International comparisons indicate that we spend twice as much on healthcare per capita than France and 2.5 times per capita more than Britain. Yet life expectancy is lower in the United States, and infant mortality is higher (Krugman & Wells, 2006).

Increasing the efficiency of healthcare delivery by organizing more highly integrated centers and networks would have the combined effect of decreasing costs as well as providing more humane, higher-quality services (Citizens' Health Care Working Group, 2006). These centers need to be accessible in the local community. Complaints from Americans about the current healthcare system include a paucity of primary care practitioners, difficulty in gaining access to specialty care, and problems navigating a complex system to obtain needed services, especially for people with chronic illnesses.

The bipartisan Citizens' Health Care Working Group (2006) emphasized the importance of "fix[ing] the delivery system first." Although funding remains a critical issue, without changes in the delivery system that occur simultaneously, there is not true healthcare reform, only healthcare rationing. The Citizens' Health Care Working Group enumerated several salient points about reorganization of healthcare delivery that could translate into affordable care:

- focus on locally based clinics where evidence-based, integrative care is accessible
- emphasize wellness and prevention at the community level
- use multiple medical and health personnel, including qualified extenders, to provide services
- employ best practices in health-based services by including mental health with physical health, health education, nutrition, and wellness checks
- develop core benefits to be delivered in an integrated, community-based center through use of the growing body of information from evidence-based practices.

Accountability

But changing policy is only half the battle—implementation of the new policy is the other half. Accountability at all levels is a critical factor in implementation. For healthcare reform, this means accountability of the system in providing access to quality care, coordinated and efficient administration, and feasible funding and reimbursement levels. It is important to define access to quality care as the ability of Americans to receive care that integrates the best available research with clinical practice. The result of an effort to rely on an overly narrow approach that defines quality only in terms of so-called empirically validated treatments is quite different from a truly evidence-based practice approach that integrates the best available research with clinical expertise in the context of patient characteristics, values, culture, and preferences (American Psychological Association, 2005). During meetings with citizen groups held by the bipartisan Citizens' Health Care Working Group (2006) during its data-gathering stage, participants emphasized the importance of keeping access to healthcare simple as well as available and responsive to the local communities. Given the current disparities in healthcare that are an issue in the system today, responsiveness to local community culture is of critical importance (Agency for Healthcare Research and Quality, 2003).

A locally responsive system with an integrated administration and an affordable reimbursement mechanism that provides quality, integrated healthcare is the voiced goal of the American people (Citizens' Health Care Working Group, 2006). Supported by existing research in mind-body therapies, it is possible that high-benefit, low-cost protocols that are evidence based and provided in a team approach can meet this goal.

READINESS FOR CHANGE

Knowing what is important in the belief system and values of American voters when it comes to healthcare reform is important for politicians to weigh. The recent midterm elections have indicated that there is a shift in voter profiles and an emphasis on holding politicians accountable for poor performance or failure to take right action. At the same time, politicians engaged in the political process must assess the readiness for change. There is still an existing fear of vulnerability that the American electorate acknowledges when it comes to healthcare reform (Americans for Health Care, 2005).

When it comes to change, people move through a series of stages from precontemplation, to contemplation, to preparation, to action and maintenance. Prochaska and DiClemente (1984) have identified the underlying process that it takes to move from one stage to the next. Change as an end goal is unlikely to occur until an individual is ready to take the actions necessary to bring about change. This involves incremental steps in consciousness-raising, emotional arousal, reflecting on the consequences of change, self-reevaluation, commitment and confidence in the ability to change, countering the pros and cons of change, developing helping relationships that provide support for change, and experiencing the rewards that maintain change.

When Lyndon Johnson's plan for Medicare and Medicaid was passed in 1965 as the capstone of the Great Society, Congress and the country were ready to accept the change. But the movement toward that change had been contemplated some 20 years before. In 1945, President Truman had actually begun advocating for national health insurance for all Americans. His first proposal was sent to Congress in November 1945. In 1948, he stated before Congress, "The greatest gap in our social security structure is the lack of adequate provision for the Nation's health....I have often and strongly urged that this condition demands a national health program. The heart of the program must be a national system of payment for medical care based on well-tried insurance principles. This great Nation cannot afford to allow its citizens to suffer needlessly from the lack of proper medical care. Our ultimate aim must be a comprehensive insurance system to protect all our people equally against insecurity and ill health" (President Truman, 1948). In 1949, Truman submitted another proposal for national healthcare to Congress, but like the prior proposed bills, it did not pass into law (Corning, 1969/1969).

Truman's ideas were revived again in 1951 in the form of a scaled back version of healthcare that would provide healthcare benefits for those who were aged 65 years and older. However, the concept languished during the Eisenhower years. In 1960, John Kennedy campaigned on a platform that promised healthcare benefits for the disabled and retirees. He had already introduced such legislation in the Senate. While he won the presidency, his bill failed to pass the Senate by four votes that year. A new version in 1962 also failed to pass the Senate by two votes. In 1965, despite strong opposition from the Republican Party and the American Medical Association, President Lyndon Johnson, pushing the populist sentiment, was able to get the legislation passed. The message, the timing, and the person to carry the message was right. That same year, the Kerr-Mills bill, which eventually became Medicaid, was also passed (Dewitt, 2001). As Prochaska and DiClemente (1984) would analyze it, the matter had been contemplated. For 20 years, the issues had been evaluated, the consequences considered, the pros and cons countered. The time had now come for action, and the emotional fervor reached a peak, where the scale tipped and the legislation we know today as Medicare was enacted.

In later years, Nixon and Carter also introduced legislation that had some variation on the theme of national health insurance. However, this issue was not a major part of either president's agenda. In 1992, Bill Clinton, as did his predecessor President John F. Kennedy, made national health reform a major part of his election campaign. After he took office, the passage of national health reform legislation was the centerpiece of his domestic agenda. He very quickly named Hillary as head of his Health Care Task Force to pursue this legislation. Clinton spent much of 1993 and 1994 working tirelessly for the passage of a bill he believed to be modest in nature and encompassing compromises for all sectors. But despite initial intense public interest, national health legislation remained on the table and died in the 103rd Congress.

What are the reasons for its failure? Laham (1996), in his political analysis *A Lost Cause,* cites four reasons: (1) intense opposition from the healthcare industry, including the combined interest groups of doctors, hospitals, private insurance companies, and pharmaceutical and nursing home industries; (2) fading public support due to the complexity of the plan and a successful public relations campaign waged by opponents of the bill; (3) lack of support from the business community, which felt that the plan would be too costly for them; and (4) deep divisions within the Democratic Party as to what type of national health plan was actually needed. Clearly, while change had been contemplated for some time, and there was extensive preparation in the political arena, the public lacked confidence in the ability to change; the pros and cons had not been fully aired within the Democratic Party, and there was very little collaboration among groups that allowed for a win-win situation to provide a sense of support for the change.

Leadership

Evaluating where both politicians and the American voters are in relation to the stages of change, and the process that is needed to move from one stage to the next, is a reciprocal process. Currently, 12 years after the failure of the Clinton Health Security Act, the public is ready for the debate. The issue has long been contemplated, and there is a greater psychological preparedness to address the change (Americans for Health Care, 2005). There is a split in the healthcare industry. No one interest group now drives healthcare policy (Heaney, 2006). Helping relationships to provide support for change are now derived from new aggregates of collaborative groups. The positions of doctors, hospitals, and business have changed and are no longer allied, for the most part, with the insurance industry. Providers and patients are more often "losers" in the current configuration of the healthcare system and, consequently, more allied with one another. The public appears primed to air the pros and cons and develop new alliances to support change.

Leadership is needed to move the process of healthcare reform ahead in the political arena. Leadership can emerge both from within the ranks of the politicians and/or from within the community as a whole. However, the need for leadership raises a fundamental question of whether leading such change is simply a variation of traditional leadership, or whether it is a qualitatively different kind of leadership (Newman, 2006). Traditional leadership has often been described as tactical. Tactical leadership works best when the objective is very clear—win a game, or defeat the enemy. The people involved in the effort are being led in the execution of a plan. The tactical leader clarifies the goal, persuades others that the goal is important, explains the strategies and tactics necessary to advance the goal, and coordinates the activities of those involved. Traditional leadership is also typically leadership by virtue of a position at the top of a functional structure. But, in their book about leadership, Chrislip and Larson (1994) argue that this traditional leadership does not work well when collaboration among people or groups or communities is required. In their research on successful collaboration, they found another form of leadership with distinctly different roles and tasks—they termed it *collaborative leadership*.

The typical tactical or positional leader works with a homogeneous group. A collaborative leader, on the other hand, must work with a mix of people, a range of stakeholders or different communities over which the leader holds no formal power or authority. Leadership must be exercised in a peer-to-peer context. The strategies for getting results in situations requiring collaboration are usually less clear because of the complexity of the problem and the fact that different stakeholders typically have different interests in the outcome—at least at the start—of a collaborative process. Additionally, collaborative leaders are more focused on promoting and safeguarding the collaborative process.

In a nutshell, according to Chrislip and Larson (1994), collaborative leaders challenge the way things are being done by bringing new approaches to complex public issues when nothing else is working. They convince others that something can be done by working together. They inspire collaborative action that leads to shared vision. They empower people by engaging them on issues of shared concern and helping them achieve results by working together constructively. Their credibility comes from the congruence of their beliefs with their actions. If they espouse collaboration, they collaborate themselves. They recognize that their ability to get things done must come from respect since they have no formal authority. They keep people at the table through difficult and frustrating times by reminding them of the common purpose and of the difficulties of achieving results with other approaches. They "encourage the heart" by helping to create and celebrate successes along the way to sustain hope and participation.

Heaney (2006) extends this model of collaborative leadership to brokerage of influence among groups. While he cites a "hollow core" of leadership among interest groups in healthcare—that is, there is now no monolithic power broker in healthcare playing the center role of the American Medical

Association in the 1950s—he does indicate that coalitions of collaborative groups are drawn to the core. These collaborative groups move in and out of leadership and the wielding of influence, depending on the issue and the representative individuals involved in the collaboration:

> The neopluralist context of contemporary health politics prevents a single interest group from holding public policy hostage, but well-positioned brokers collectively can influence the outcomes of debates on specific issues. As a result, prominent health policy debates are demonstrably affected by the emergence or absence of skilled interest group brokers in a policy domain once thought to lack this kind of leadership. (p. 829)

Heaney (2006) suggests that there are three types of communication that promote collaborative leadership among interest groups and allow them to influence otherwise disconnected organizations. These are informal communications among leaders and members, formal collaborative communications and the formation of coalitions, and specific bridge building across boundaries normally difficult to cross. A specific example of the latter type of leadership and brokerage revolves around the issue of stem cell research:

> Stem cell research is an example of an issue on which interest group advocates have played an enormously effective part in building bridges across party boundaries. The Coalition for the Advancement of Medical Research (CAMR) was founded in 2001 by opponents of President Bush's policy on stem cell research. The coalition had ninety-three member organizations by 2005, spanning advocates for patients, disease research, universities, and medical professionals. Although stem cell research is largely a Democratic issue, CAMR was able to build support among Republican-leaning interest groups and politicians because of the leadership of groups like the Juvenile Diabetes Research Foundation International (JDRF). As a result, it won support early from prominent Republican senators, especially Arlen Specter and Orrin Hatch, and later from Majority Leader Bill Frist.

In the public domain, it has also joined such diverse supporters as Michael J. Fox and Nancy Reagan.

New collaborative leaders are needed within the political arena, within interest groups, and within the community of Americans at large if we are to counter the pros and cons of healthcare reform and move it to the next level of action. The complexity of such leadership challenges does not offer a specific road map. Where leading change is involved and requires a commitment to a vision to do something that has never been done before, some believe that there is no way to absolutely know how to get there. Robert Quinn (2004), who has written extensively on leading change, describes the process as "building the bridge as we walk on it," which clearly depicts the uncertainty we face. He alternately describes the process of what it is like to lead change as "walking naked into the land of uncertainty" or "learning how to walk through hell effectively" (p. 9). Clearly leading change is not for the faint of heart. In spite of any uncertainty or even adversity we may face, we must move ahead and build that bridge to healthcare reform using the tools at our disposal. It has been, and continues to be, a slow and arduous process. However, there is a point in time when the scales tip.

The Tipping Point

Malcolm Gladwell (2000), in *The Tipping Point*, advances the belief that new ideas are like viral epidemics—contagious and capable of spreading at one dramatic moment. Little causes can have big effects. Little things can make a big difference. Incremental changes or almost imperceptible changes at the margins accumulate. Ultimately, significant change happens, not gradually, but at one dramatic moment, when everything can change all at once—the tipping point. Take, for example, Rosa Parks. A single act of conscience by this one African American woman who, in 1955, refused to give up her seat on a bus became the tipping point for a wave of events that changed the nation (Newman, 2006). So what is the epidemic of change for which we seek a tipping point? Simply put, it is a solution to our broken healthcare system that provides quality, affordable care for the whole person, and that is accountable to the values of dignity and social justice. This is the conclusion of the Citizens' Health Care Working Group after listening in countless meetings to the American people speak.

The bigger question for today is, How do we spread the word that healthcare reform is feasible? How do we persuade policy makers that the solution to at least some of their biggest problems is right at our fingertips? How do we move employers and other payers to appreciate the cost to them of unhealthy behaviors and lifestyles so that they are eager to pay for efforts to create healthy ones? And how do we create the social epidemic, as Gladwell (2000) would call it, that flows from the single tipping point and leads people to literally demand thoughtful healthcare reform? How do we create the epidemic that leads people away from feeling entitled to good healthcare and leaves them feeling entitled to good health?

The Paul Revere Initiative

Perhaps Gladwell (2000) himself can offer some wisdom on that point. Among his many metaphors, he describes Paul Revere's ride as the most famous historical example of a word-of-mouth epidemic—a piece of extraordinary news that traveled a long distance in a very short period of time and that mobilized an entire region to arms. At first blush, it seems straightforward why this would occur. Revere was carrying news that no one could ignore—the British were coming. But, on further inspection, there appears to be more to it than just a compelling message.

Gladwell (2000) reminds us that at the same time Revere began his ride north and west of Boston, a fellow revolutionary named William Dawes carried the same urgent message to Lexington via a different route. Yet few people from the towns Dawes rode through materialized for the battle the next day. Why did Revere succeed where Dawes failed? Gladwell concludes that Revere's news "tipped," while Dawes's did not, because of differences between the two men, not the messages. Revere, according to Gladwell, was a "connector"—someone who provided the link for collections of people who would not otherwise come together. It was his ability as a connector that enabled his message to succeed, while Dawes's failed. In Gladwell's (2000) words:

> When Revere set out for Lexington that night, he would have known just how to spread the news as far and wide as possible. When he saw people on the roads, he was so naturally and irrepressibly social he would have stopped and told them. When he came upon a town, he would have known exactly whose door to knock on, who the local militia leader was, who the key players in the town were. He had met most of them before. And they knew and respected him as well. (p. 58)

Gladwell (2000) also tells us that Paul Revere was a "maven," or someone considered to be very knowledgeable and, therefore, credible. What he never tells us, however, is that Revere was actually arrested by the British that night and later released without a horse to continue his now famous midnight ride. No matter the actual events of that April night in 1775, it is the lesson that is important here. A good message alone cannot succeed without the right people to carry it; a social epidemic depends as much on the people who support it as the idea they spread. Modern leadership for healthcare reform demands that the Paul Reveres among us step forward. Convening the right people to carry the message that tips, and cultivating the support necessary for the message to spread, is what collaborative leadership is all about. The challenge is to continue to find more ways to spread the word, to continue to work to trigger the tipping point that starts an epidemic of good health and healthcare reform in this country (Newman, 2006).

Our nation is increasingly preoccupied by virtual epidemics of health conditions, such as obesity and diabetes, in which behavior plays a significant role in both causes and effective treatments. Second, our country is desperately looking for strategies to control healthcare costs without sacrificing quality of care or quality of life. Third, consumers are spending billions of dollars—much of it out of pocket—on mind-body remedies. Fourth, this is a time in our health system's history where evidence-based practice is defining health beyond the traditional treatment provided by MDs, and integrative services are being actively sought by the American people.

It is important in addressing these issues to act nationally and locally. To initiate healthcare reform, it is important to survey the local community landscape to see where and how strategic networks can be expanded to further the spread of the message of what Americans want in healthcare reform. Publicize and talk about the Citizens' Health Care Working Group findings. Speak with people both inside and outside your normal collaborative groups. Call it a community networking initiative, a community leadership initiative, or call it the Paul Revere initiative (Newman, 2006). No matter what we call it, it will ultimately be the cumulative effect of the message, the collective persistent efforts to carry that message and collaborate with communities beyond our own, that enables us to succeed and impact the political arena. If we can do these things, a dramatic change in healthcare may just be the country's next health epidemic.

TOOL KIT FOR CHANGE

Role and Perspective of the Healthcare Professional

1. Healthcare professionals need to band together to shift the healthcare delivery paradigm to a more social value than a marketplace value.
2. Healthcare professionals must look beyond the medical system and champion a larger definition of the healthcare system for true healthcare reform to take place.
3. Healthcare professionals can step forward into leadership roles and bring about this change within their practices, their professional organizations, and in their communities on a larger level.

Role and Perspective of the Patient/Participant

1. The Citizens' Health Care Working Group assessment indicates that Americans consider healthcare services as a social responsibility, not as market-produced goods.
2. Patients can demand parity of mental and physical health services to reflect the growing patient awareness of the mind-body connection.
3. Patients can be active as citizens in contacting their public representatives about healthcare delivery and payment problems. Most importantly, patients can activate their belief system by refusing to vote for leaders who avoid the difficult issues of healthcare or want to maintain healthcare delivery as a business.

Interconnection: The Global Perspective

1. Americans see the provision of healthcare as a core value.
2. Americans want humane treatment that promotes quality care of the whole person, both in the community and at the end of life.
3. Americans want an increased focus on locally based clinics where evidence-based, integrative care is accessible and wellness and prevention are emphasized.
4. Americans can begin a Paul Revere initiative, where ordinary Americans and American leaders speak out and spread the word that reform of both the healthcare delivery system and financing is necessary and feasible.

REFERENCES

Agency for Healthcare Research and Quality. (2003). *National healthcare disparities report.* Retrieved November 26, 2006, from http://www.qualitytools.ahrq.gov/disparitiesreport/2003/download/download_report.aspx

American Psychological Association. (1995). *Public perceptions of the value of psychological services.* Washington, DC: Author.

American Psychological Association. (2005, August). *Policy statement on evidence-based practice in psychology.* Washington, DC: Author.

American Psychological Association. (2006). *Stress survey.* Washington, DC: Author.

Americans for Health Care. (2005). *Findings from a national survey on health care: Lakeside Partners.* Retrieved November 26, 2006, from http://www.americansforhealthcare.org/survey_voters.cfm

Benson, H. (1975). *The relaxation response.* New York: William Morrow & Co.

Bureau of Economic Analysis. (2005). *Gross domestic product by industry.* Retrieved November 26, 2006, http://www.bea.gov/newsreleases/industry/gdpindustry/gdpindnewsrelease.htm.

Chrislip, D., & Larson, C. (1994). *Collaborative leadership: How citizens and civic leaders can make a difference.* San Francisco: Jossey-Bass.

Citizens' Health Care Working Group. (2006). *Health care that works for all americans. Final recommendations.* Retrieved November 26, 2006, from http://www.citizenshealthcare.gov/recommendations/finalrecommendations_print.pdf.

Colliver, V. (2003, December 8). Health care costs continue double digit increase. *San Francisco Chronicle.* Retrieved December 3, 2003, from http://www.commondreams.org/headlines03/1208-03.htm.

Corning, P. (1969). *The evolution of Medicare...from idea to law.* U.S. Social Security Administration, Office of Research and Statistics. Washington, D.C.: U.S. Government Printing Office.

Dewitt, L. (2001). *Oral history collection: Robert M. Ball—Interview #3.* Retrieved November 26, 2006, from http://www.ssa.gov/history/orals/ball3.html

Gladwell, M. (2000). *The tipping point: How little things can make a big difference.* Boston: Little, Brown.

Health Care That Works for All Americans. (2006, September 29). *Citizens' Health Care Working Group. Report to the president.* Retrieved November 26, 2006, from http://www.citizenshealthcare.gov

Heaney, M. (2004). Outside the issue niche: The multi-dimensionality of interest group identity. *American Politics Research, 32,* 611–651.

Heaney, M. (2006). Brokering health policy: Coalitions, parties and interest group influence. *Journal of Health Policy, Politics, and Law, 31,* 887–944.

Institute of Medicine. (2006a, June). *Emergency medical services at the crossroads.* Washington, DC: National Academies Press.

Institute of Medicine. (2006b, June). *The future of emergency care: Key findings and recommendations.* Future of Emergency Care Series. Retrieved November 26, 2006, from www.iom.edu/CMS/3809/16107/17962.aspx.

Kohut, A. (2006). *The real message of the midterms.* Retrieved November 26, 2006, from http://pewresearch.org/pubs/91/the-real-message-of-the-midterms.

Krugman, P., & Wells, R. (2006, March 23). The health crisis and what to do about it. *The New York Review of Books, 53,* article 18802. Retrieved November 26, 2006, from http://www.nybooks.com/articles/18802

Laham, N. (1996). *A lost cause: Bill Clinton's campaign for a national health insurance.* Westport, CT: Praeger.

McFarland, A. (2004). *Neopluralism: The evolution of political process theory.* Lawrence: University of Kansas Press.

Miller, Neal E. (2007). Preliminary guide to the Neal E. Miller papers, manuscript group 1770. Retrieved June 4, 2007, from http://mssa.library.yale.edu/findaids/stream.php?xmlfile=mssa.ms.1770.xml.

Miller, L., Smith, A., & Rothstein, L. (1993). *The stress solution: An active plan to manage the stress in your life.* New York: Pocket Books.

National Committee on Vital and Health Statistics. (2002). *National Vital Statistics System.* Atlanta, GA: Centers for Disease Control.

Newman, R. (2005, March 2). *Staying the course in uncertain times.* Paper presented at the American Psychological Association State Leadership Conference, Washington, DC.

Newman, R. (2006, March 4). *Psychology and communities: Advancing health, building resilience and changing behavior.* Paper presented at the American Psychological Association State Leadership Conference, Washington, DC.

Prochaska, J., & DiClemente, C. (1984). *The transtheoretical approach: Crossing traditional boundaries of change.* Homewood, IL: Dorsey Press.

Quinn, R. (2004). *Building the bridge as you walk on it: A guide for leading change.* San Francisco: Jossey-Bass.

Schoen, C., Doty, M., Collins, S., & Holmgren, A. (2005). Insured but not protected: How many adults are underinsured? *Health Affairs,* doi:10.1377/hlthaff.w5.289. Retrieved June 14, 2005, from http://content.healthaffairs.org/cgi/reprint/hlthaff.w5.289v1.

Truman, President Harry (January 7, 1948). Annual Message to the Congress on the State of the Union, Retrieved June 4, 2007 from http://everything2.com/index.pl?node_id=1676849.

AFTERWORD

Margaret Heldring, PhD

Humanizing Healthcare is a volume that speaks with multiple voices about the challenges of delivering quality, cost effective healthcare to the American people. Authors from a variety of healthcare disciplines present recurring themes. First is the generally accepted assumption that the United States has the most technologically advanced and expensive medical care in the world. Second is the evidence-based awareness that health status and healthcare outcomes are not at the same high level as U.S. technological achievement, nor are they acceptably cost effective for the money that is spent. In fact, other industrialized countries that spend less on healthcare achieve far better results. The burden of these disappointments falls disproportionately on racial and ethnic minorities, and this disparity is an increasing focus of public policy.

A case can be made that the focus of the healthcare system in the United States is *not* really healthcare, but medical care. Medical care is essential for specialty care, trauma, and acute interventions. However, the major challenge in healthcare that the United States faces today is not acute care but chronic care. Heart problems, cancer, strokes, chronic respiratory disease, Alzheimer's disease, and diabetes are all among the top ten causes of death in the United States, and all involve ongoing healthcare management. The stress, coping behaviors and social support systems needed to cope with these chronic diseases and achieve the best outcomes fall more within a definition of healthcare rather than strictly medical care. But for too long the United States has suffered from myopia and, up close, has confused medical care with healthcare. And focusing on medical care alone is no longer efficacious or cost effective in this country.

This volume presents a series of wide-ranging chapters about integrative healthcare. The definition of integrative care goes beyond what is normally denoted by this term. Authors in this volume make the case that true integrative healthcare combines physical, emotional, and social care. It encompasses the work of traditional physicians, psychologists, and mental health professionals along with complementary and alternative practices that are evidence based. The focus of Humanizing Healthcare is to present a perspective of the importance of *medical care* embedded in a more humane *healthcare* system. It seeks to more fully recognize the health, and medical needs, of the whole person. It places the person squarely within his or her social circumstances and attempts to move healthcare upstream—to the roots of the illnesses and injuries that require medical care. It also seeks to bring an awareness that health needs can be met cost effectively and efficaciously. In so doing, a more humane *healthcare* system in the United States can integrate with and help to solve some of the problems of our current medical care system.

While reflecting a myriad of perspectives, this collection of chapters attempts to elucidate some of the most important aspects of healthcare from a variety of clinical providers, public health reviewers, and policy makers. The concept of healthcare—and integrative healthcare—is often diversely defined, even within the group of advocates of an integrative healthcare system. But by following the outline of the chapters in this book, some common ground and conclusions emerge.

In Humanizing Healthcare, integrative healthcare is defined with a more encompassing view. Chapters 1 and 2 show the development of this enlarged definition as a natural progression of the history of integrative medicine and healthcare. This enlarged definition also reflects what the Citizens' Health Care Working Group, an example of one of many advocacy groups in the United States, found that most Americans want—and are willing to pay for—from the United States healthcare system. This common ground is a place for discussion to begin among healthcare providers, government policy makers, and funders. Working models for providing this kind of quality healthcare along with frontline medical care in an efficacious and cost-effective manner exist and are presented here. These models bear closer study and development of demonstration projects to assess their suitability for duplication and application in various areas.

Chapters 3 through 10 address the application of this enlarged definition of integrative healthcare on various populations. Although discussions among practitioners who work on integrative teams in real life vary widely, basic respect of each other and the patient can lead to greater understanding and effectiveness in care. People treated in the context of their families and community, as well as in an environment that takes human sensitivities into account, can marshal their own healing abilities in a more effective, culturally meaningful manner. An expanded definition of healthcare is an approach that works in the rehabilitation of trauma and chronic disease. It also provides support for development of children, especially those with special needs, and with marginalized populations where health disparities in the current medical system abound.

Chapters 10 and 11 address training and research in integrative healthcare. Training and disseminating integrative knowledge is a challenge. But it does occur currently in areas where a broader healthcare, rather than strictly medical care, perspective is found. The International Classification of Functioning (ICF), developed by the World Health Organization, also provides a means to develop research on these integrative health training and treatment models. The ICF is currently being used to assess healthcare delivery and improvement of function in other developed countries. A more expanded definition of healthcare sets the stage for implementation of the ICF in this country and can allow a move from a focus strictly on illness to a focus on health and improved function.

Given these emerging approaches in healthcare, the legal ability to minimize risks and protect patients is also emerging. Chapter 12 presents some of the current laws, court cases, and systems approaches to integrative healthcare teams. Providers, patients, and policy makers are recognizing that integrative healthcare is warranted and that the delivery and accountability for such services can be appropriately managed in the public arena.

Embedding medical care in an expanded definition of healthcare does not have to increase expenditures. Chapter 13 reviews the history of medical care funding in the United States and the current research and issues that surround the practicability of reorienting funding from strictly medical care to healthcare. Chapter 14 also reflects the debate, and process, in the political arena that is needed to bring about this change.

The American people are asking for policy makers to show leadership to address the current problems of medical care and establish a true healthcare system. This does not mean throwing the baby out with the bath water. Technologically advanced medical care will continue to be an important contribution to the health and welfare of the American people. But, as the Citizens' Health Care Working Group points out in their September 29, 2006 report, Americans want a more humane health system that recognizes the individual's quality of health and life.

There are many steps to be taken on the journey to a new healthcare system. But this volume sets the tone for moving in that direction. The many voices of various healthcare practitioners, patients with differing needs, funding sources and policy makers, and Americans of all ages—who bear the cost of caring for the young and old—clamor to be heard on this journey. Humanizing Healthcare provides an initial map to the terrain. It is useful as a text for practitioners of medicine and nursing, psychology, social work, and counseling, as well as physical, occupational, and speech therapies. It is also useful for training complementary and alternative practitioners and bringing them together with current needs and practice issues. At the same time, it provides a background text for professionals in the legal and public health policy arena. Additionally, the individual citizen, concerned with what is happening in our healthcare system and the direction our country is taking, can also gain a broader perspective on not only healthcare needs, but on what needs to be done. Finding a new direction in healthcare requires disparate perspectives, disparate voices. The writers in Humanizing Healthcare can help to make these voices heard and, in the process, help to chart the way.

ABOUT THE GENERAL EDITOR

Ilene Ava Serlin, PhD, ADTR, is a recognized leader and has been practicing whole person health care for over 35 years. She is a clinical psychologist and registered dance/movement therapist at Union Street Health Associates in San Francisco and Marin County. She is a fellow of the American Psychological Association (APA), past-president of the APA's Division of Humanistic Psychology, and served on APA's Presidential and Division 42 (Independent Practice) Health Care Task Force. She is the founder of the Arts Medicine program at the Institute of Health and Healing at California Pacific Medical Center and of the movement support group at the Integrative Health Care for Women with Breast Cancer at the University of California, and is on the advisory committee for Sutter Hospital's Integrative Health and Healing Services in Santa Rosa. Her videotape called *Dance Movement Therapy for Women with Breast Cancer* was awarded the Marian Chace Award by the American Dance Therapy Association.

Dr. Serlin has taught at Saybrook Graduate School, UCLA, Lesley University, and abroad. She is on the Editorial Board of *PsycCritiques PsycCRITIQUES—Contemporary Psychology: APA Review of Books*, the *American Journal of Dance Therapy*, and *The Journal of Humanistic Psychology* and is a reviewer for APA's *Professional Psychology: Research and Practice* and *Division 32's The Humanistic Psychologist*. Her writings include the following:

Serlin, I. A. (2000). Symposium: Support groups for women with breast cancer. *The Arts in Psychotherapy, 27*(2), 123–138.

Serlin, I. A. (2004a). Religious and spiritual issues in couples therapy. In M. Harway (Ed.), *Handbook of couples therapy* (pp. 352–369). New York: John Wiley & Sons.

Serlin, I. A. (2004b). Spiritual diversity in clinical practice. In J. Chin (Ed.), *The psychology of prejudice and discrimination* (pp. 27–49). Westport, CT: Praeger.

Serlin, I. A. (2005). Year of the whole person. *Psychotherapy Bulletin: Division 29 (APA)*, *40*(1), 34–39.

Serlin, I. A. (2006). Expressive therapies. In M. Micozzi (Ed.), *Complementary and integrative medicine in cancer and prevention: Foundations and evidence-based interventions* (pp. 81–91).

Her Web site is www.ileneserlin.com.

ABOUT THE VOLUME EDITORS

VOL. I

Marie A. DiCowden, PhD, is a nationally known healthcare psychologist and behavioral medicine specialist. Dr. DiCowden joined the University of Miami/Jackson Memorial Hospital staff in the Department of Orthopedics and Rehabilitation in 1981. She maintains her adjunct faculty position at the medical school in addition to faculty affiliations with Nova University and Saybrook Graduate School. In 1988 Dr. DiCowden founded The Biscayne Institutes of Health and Living, Inc. and The Biscayne Foundation in Miami, Florida. This program was an extension of her work on the medical campus and evolved into the HealthCare Community model. This innovative program provides frontline, integrative care for disabled children and adults in addition to integrative health programs for mind and body for the community at large. She serves as the executive director of this program. Dr. DiCowden is a Fellow of the American Psychological Association and a member of the National Academy of Practice. She writes and lectures extensively, both nationally and internationally, on issues of disability, healthcare, and healthcare policy.

VOL. II

Kirwan Rockefeller, PhD, is the director of arts and humanities continuing education at the University of California, Irvine. His expertise includes psychology, visual and performing arts, humanities, and body-mind modalities. He has taught organizational behavior and social psychology at the doctoral level and has consulted with top national and entertainment organizations on the accurate depiction of social and mental health issues, including the Entertainment Industries Council, ABC, CBS, NBC, FOX, Paramount Pictures, Universal Studios, Warner Bros., Centers for Disease Control and Prevention, National Institute on Drug Abuse, The Robert Wood Johnson Foundation, and Ogilvy Public Relations Worldwide. He is the author of *Visualize Confidence: How to Use Guided Imagery to Overcome Self-Doubt.* He has presented at the Susan Samueli Center for Integrative Medicine and is a member of the American Psychological Association and the California Psychological Association.

Stephen S. Brown, MA, is a freelance editor in San Francisco, California. He holds a master's degree in philosophy from San Francisco State University, where he studied with Jacob Needleman and taught philosophy and religion. His interests include contemporary spiritual thought, aesthetics, particularly the philosophy of music, and the philosophy of technology and culture.

VOL. III

Jill Sonke-Henderson, BA, is cofounder and codirector of the Center for the Arts in Healthcare Research and Education (CAHRE) at the University of Florida (UF) and is on the faculty of the School of Theatre and Dance at the University of Florida. She has been an artist in residence in the Shands Arts in Medicine program since 1994, where she founded the Dance for Life program. She has been developing and teaching arts in healthcare coursework and conducting research at UF for over a decade, and is a frequent lecturer throughout the United States and abroad. Jill serves on the board of directors and as a consultant for the Society for the Arts in Healthcare, and is the recipient of a New Forms Florida Award, an Individual Artist Fellowship Award from the State of Florida, and a 2001 Excellence in Teaching Award from the National Institute for Staff and Organizational Development (NISOD).

Ilene Ava Serlin, PhD, ADTR, is a nationally known clinical psychologist and registered dance/movement therapist in private practice in San Francisco and Marin County. She is a Fellow of the American Psychological Association, is past president of the Division of Humanistic Psychology, and served on APA's Presidential Task Force on Whole Person Psychology. She is the founder of the Arts Medicine program at the Institute of Health and Healing at California Pacific Medical Center, and has taught at Saybrook Graduate School, University of California at Los Angeles, Lesley University, and abroad. She is on the editorial board of *PsycCritiques, American Journal of Dance Therapy,* and *The Journal of Humanistic Psychology.*

Rusti Brandman, PhD, is codirector of the Center for the Arts in Healthcare Research and Education (CAHRE) and is coordinator of dance at the University of Florida. Credits include directorships of professional dance companies, international appearances in Holland, receipt of awards from the Florida Fine Arts Council, the National Dance Association, and the American College Dance Festival Association, and service as a national officer for ACDFA. She was a founder of CAHRE and has served as an artist in residence at Shands Hospital at UF and at AGH. She has presented internationally on the arts in healthcare for the American Holistic Medical Association, the Society for the Arts in Healthcare, the International Institute on the Arts in Healing, the Congress on Research in Dance, and the Hawaii International Conference on the Arts and Humanities. She has received five Scholarship Enhancement grants for her arts in health research, producing the Dancing in Hospitals video.

John Graham-Pole, MD, graduated from London University in 1966, and has been on the faculties of London and Case Western Reserve Universities. He is now professor of pediatrics, adjunct professor of clinical and health psychology, medical director of Shands Arts in Medicine, University of Florida, and medical director of Pediatric Hospice of North Central Florida. He has authored or edited five books and made a CD of original poetry and music. He has published about 250 book chapters, articles, and poems in peer-reviewed journals. He has given several hundred presentations across the world on holistic medicine, palliative care, humor, and the healing arts.

ABOUT THE CONTRIBUTORS

Martha E. Banks, PhD, is a research neuropsychologist for ABackans DCP, Inc., a former professor of Black Studies at the College of Wooster, and a retired clinical psychologist. She is editor of *Women with Visible and Invisible Disabilities: Multiple Intersections, Multiple Issues, Multiple Therapies* and coauthor of the *Ackerman–Banks Neuropsychological Rehabilitation Battery.*

William Benda MD, FACEP, FAAEM, received his professional training at Duke University, University of Miami School of Medicine, Harbor-UCLA Medical Center, and the Program in Integrative Medicine at the University of Arizona. His research and clinical work has focused on patients with breast cancer, animal-assisted therapy, and physician health and well-being. He was principal investigator on two National Center for Complementary and Alternative Medicine–funded investigations of therapeutic horseback riding in the treatment of children with cerebral palsy and is currently extending this research to the field of pediatric autism. Dr. Benda is a cofounder of the National Integrative Medicine Council, a nonprofit organization for which he has served as director of medical and public affairs. He is an editor, contributor, and medical advisory board member for a number of conventional and alternative medicine journals and has lectured extensively on a variety of topics in the integrative arena.

Lydia P. Buki, PhD, conducts research and teaches in the Department of Educational Psychology at the University of Illinois at Urbana-Champaign.

As a counseling psychologist, she brings multicultural, developmental, and social justice frameworks to her work with medically underserved Latina populations. Her research examines psychosocial factors that influence health disparities in cancer outcomes.

Mark L. De Santis, PsyD, is currently the director of neuropsychology and biofeedback at the Biscayne Institutes of Health and Living in Miami, Florida. Additionally, he is an adjunct faculty member at both Nova Southeastern University and Art Institute University. He has published numerous articles that have appeared in professional journals. His emphasis of study is on pediatrics with special needs.

Marie A. DiCowden, PhD, is a nationally known healthcare psychologist and behavioral medicine specialist. Dr. DiCowden joined the University of Miami/Jackson Memorial Hospital staff in the Department of Orthopedics and Rehabilitation in 1981. She maintains her adjunct faculty position at the medical school in addition to faculty affiliations with Nova University and Saybrook Graduate School. In 1988 Dr. DiCowden founded the Biscayne Institutes of Health and Living, Inc. and the Biscayne Foundation in Miami, Florida. This program was an extension of her work on the medical campus and evolved into the HealthCare Community model. This innovative program provides frontline, integrative care for disabled children and adults in addition to integrative health programs for mind and body for the community at large. She serves as the executive director of this program. Dr. DiCowden is a fellow of the American Psychological Association and a member of the National Academy of Practice. She writes and lectures extensively, both nationally and internationally, on issues of disability, healthcare, and healthcare policy.

Mark G. DiCowden, JD, is a graduate from St. Thomas University School of Law in Miami, Florida. Prior to entering the legal profession, he worked for over 10 years as the administrator and chief of operations of the Biscayne Institutes of Health and Living, Inc. Mark has been a member of the State of Florida Department of Health's Brain and Spinal Cord Injury Advisory Council and is currently active in the Agency for Health Care Administration's Managed Care Ombudsman Committee. He also serves as a director for the Biscayne Foundation and is involved in other civic programs such as the Kiwanis Club of Aventura.

Tristan Haddad DiCowden, MS, is an assistant principal and classroom instructor at the Biscayne Academy, Biscayne Institutes of Health and Living, in Miami, Florida. Mrs. DiCowden holds her master of science degree in pre-K primary education and is working toward her PhD in curriculum and instruction. Mrs. DiCowden has been teaching for nine years and has been a coach for the Special Olympics for 10 years.

Diane Batshaw Eisman, MD, is a family medicine physician and practices with her husband, Eugene Eisman, MD, who is a cardiologist. She is a voluntary clinical faculty member of the University of Miami School of Medicine. Dr. Diane has been named as one of the *South Florida Women of Valor* by *Miami* magazine and has been a member of the Dade County Judge's Standing Committee on Domestic Violence. She is coauthor with her husband of *Your Child and Cholesterol* and has been a contributing editor and writer for the national monthly publication *Deepak's Chopra's Infinite Possibilities.* She has served on the editorial board of *Miami Medicine* and written scripts for *Healthy Women 2000,* a weekly television series that aired on the Discovery Channel, hosted by U.S. Assistant Surgeon General Dr. Susan Blumenthal. In 1999 Dr. Diane wrote the video documentary *Breast Cancer, Know the Facts,* which was nominated for Time Inc.'s International Health and Medical Film Freddie award and was awarded second place honors.

Eugene Eisman, MD, is an internist/cardiologist who practices with his wife, Dr. Diane Eisman, a family medicine physician in Miami. He is a voluntary clinical faculty member of the University of Miami School of Medicine. He is coauthor with his wife of *Your Child and Cholesterol.* Dr. Eugene has been contributing editor and writer for the national monthly publication *Deepak's Chopra's Infinite Possibilities.* He has also served on the editorial board of *Miami Medicine* and played an integral role in the design of the magazine, winning three first place Florida Medical Association editorial awards. Dr. Eugene has served as chief of the Department of Internal Medicine at the North Miami Medical Center, was an army physician in Vietnam, and served as chief of professional services. He also practices Eastern martial arts. He holds a third-degree black belt in Tae Kwon Do and practices Kum Do (Korean sword fighting).

James Ferguson, PA-C, has worked in northwestern Alaska for the last 13 years. Jim currently works in Gambell on St. Lawrence Island as a clinical PA and community health aide practitioner (CHA/P) trainer. Jim did his medical training at Wake Forest University's School of Medicine PA Program from 1988 to 1990.

Susan J. Frey, PhD, ND, RN, founder of Avalon Health Associates, combines her knowledge of healthcare with architectural design. Frey integrates principles, research, and application of naturopathy to the built environment. Her book, articles, and professional speaking span issues of healing, cultural influences, sustainability, neuroscience, and holism in public education and healthcare.

Jeanette Gallagher, ND, is a naturopathic physician trained in Arizona who recently returned to the New Orleans area prior to Katrina. She has been working in all areas of healthcare, from corporate to personal care, for the last 30 years. Currently, Gallagher is working in Louisiana to instill changes in the current healthcare system.

Miguel E. Gallardo, PsyD, is an assistant professor at Pepperdine University Graduate School of Education and Psychology and a licensed clinical psychologist. His areas of clinical and research interest include Chicano/Latino mental health and psychology, culture and disability, cultural responsiveness in therapy, and multicultural organizational development.

Robert L. Glueckauf, PhD, is professor in the Department of Medical Humanities and Social Sciences at the Florida State University College of Medicine. He has authored over 75 empirical and theoretical articles, books, and chapters in the fields of telehealth and rehabilitation. His primary interests lie in the development and evaluation of alternative healthcare delivery systems (i.e., telehealth) for individuals with chronic illnesses and their family caregivers.

Alan L. Goldberg, PhD, JD, Tucson psychologist and attorney, is a member of APA Divisions 41, 40, and 22. He has been active in APA divisional activities as well as state and local professional organizations. He is the Arizona Psychological Association's chair of Health and Disability Issues Committee. With expertise in social justice, advocacy, psychology, and law, Dr. Goldberg has made pivotal contributions in the drafting of insurance and criminal laws (consumer access, timely pay, antideath penalty legislation for juveniles and for individuals with mental retardation). He maintains a private practice concentrating on forensic issues, and he adjudicates Social Security disability cases.

Margaret Heldring, PhD, is a clinical psychologist whose career spans independent practice to public policy. She has served as a clinical assistant professor in family medicine at the University of Washington and senior health advisors to former U.S. Senators Bill Bradley and Paul Wellstone. In 2000, she founded and is president of a national health policy nonprofit organization, America's Health Together (AHT). Funded by the Robert Wood Johnson Foundation, AHT led a groundbreaking partnership after 9/11 to investigate the mental health effects of that disaster and to build capacity in primary healthcare to respond to natural and manmade disasters. AHT is currently working to strengthen philanthropic activity in mental health, both domestically and globally.

Gerry E. Hendershot, PhD, is a consultant on disability statistics. Formerly, he held various research and supervisory positions in federal government statistical agencies. Prior to his government service, Dr. Hendershot was on the sociology faculties of Brown University, Vanderbilt University, the University of the Philippines, and the College of Wooster. He has published about 50 articles and coedited four books.

Bree Johnston, MD, MPH, is an associate professor of medicine at University of California, San Francisco and the San Francisco Veterans' Administration Medical Center. She is the copresident of the California Physician's Alliance and a board member of Physicians for a National Health Program.

Don Lollar, EdD, is a senior research scientist, National Center on Birth Defects and Developmental Disabilities, at the Centers for Disease Control and Prevention (CDC) in Atlanta, Georgia. Prior to coming to the CDC, Dr. Lollar practiced rehabilitation psychology for 25 years, providing assessment and therapy services to children, adults, and families across the life span. His advanced degrees are from Indiana University, and his most recent writings include articles for the *Annual Review of Public Health, Public Health Reports,* and the *Journal of Developmental and Behavioral Pediatrics.*

Frank Maye, DOM, ND, is the director of alternative medicine at Biscayne Institutes of Health and Living, Inc. in Miami, Florida. His private practice is at the forefront of the integrative medical movement. Dr. Maye received his masters in Chinese philosophy and Oriental medicine from the Community School for Traditional Chinese Healthcare in Miami, Florida, and his doctorate in naturopathic medicine from the American Naturopathic Medical Institute. His research and clinical work focus on autism, neurology, and autoimmune disease. Dr. Maye is the cofounder and medical director for the Lancaster Research Institute, a nonprofit organization designed to provide research articles and data from around the world to both patients and professionals. He also maintains a private practice in South Miami, Florida. Dr. Maye is a board member of the International University Center for the Study of Spirituality. He has lectured extensively and appeared in local and national media. He is the author of a monthly newsletter in *Acupuncture Today.*

Scott E. Miller, MA, is currently attending the clinical psychology doctorate program at Nova Southeastern University in the neuropsychology concentration supervised by Dr. Charles Golden. Scott is employed at the Biscayne Institutes for Health and Living, Inc. as a member of the Behavioral Medicine and Neuropsychology Department. Scott has presented original research at the National Academy of Neuropsychology and at the American Psychological Association.

Russ Newman, PhD, JD, is a clinical psychologist and lawyer who currently serves as executive director for professional practice for the American Psychological Association (APA). He is responsible for spearheading and promoting the association's multifaceted agenda on behalf of practicing psychologists and individuals in need of psychological care. For the last two decades, Dr. Newman has been engaged in legislative advocacy and policy development related to health and mental healthcare in this country. He received his PhD in clinical psychology from Kent State University in 1979 and his JD from Capital University Law School in 1987.

Barry Nierenberg, PhD, is assistant professor, University of Miami Miller School of Medicine, within the Department of Family Medicine, where he currently directs behavioral medicine. He is a diplomate of the American Board of Professional Psychology and has been practicing psychology for the past 25 years. He has focused on issues affecting families and health.

Dean Ornish, M.D., is the founder and president of the non-profit Preventive Medicine Research Institute in Sausalito, California, where he holds the Safeway Chair. He is Clinical Professor of Medicine at the University of California, San Francisco. Dr. Ornish received his medical training in internal medicine from the Baylor College of Medicine, Harvard Medical School, and the Massachusetts General Hospital. He received a BA in Humanities summa cum laude from the University of Texas in Austin, where he gave the baccalaureate address.

For the past 30 years, Dr. Ornish has directed clinical research demonstrating, for the first time, that comprehensive lifestyle changes may begin to reverse even severe coronary heart disease, without drugs or surgery. Recently, Medicare agreed to provide coverage for this program, the first time that Medicare has covered a program of comprehensive lifestyle changes. He recently directed the first randomized controlled trial demonstrating that comprehensive lifestyle changes may stop or reverse the progression of prostate cancer. His current research is focusing on whether comprehensive lifestyle changes may affect gene expression.

He is the author of five best-selling books, including New York Times' best-sellers *Dr. Dean Ornish's Program for Reversing Heart Disease, Eat More,*

Weigh Less, and *Love & Survival.* He writes a monthly column for both *Newsweek* and *Reader's Digest* magazines.

The research that he and his colleagues conducted has been published in the *Journal of the American Medical Association, The Lancet, Circulation, The New England Journal of Medicine, the American Journal of Cardiology,* and elsewhere. A one-hour documentary of their work was broadcast on *NOVA,* the PBS science series, and was featured on Bill Moyers' PBS series, *Healing & The Mind.* Their work has been featured in all major media, including cover stories in *Newsweek, Time,* and *U.S. News & World Report.*

Dr. Ornish is a member of the boards of directors of the U.S. United Nations High Commission on Refugees, the Quincy Jones Foundation, and the San Francisco Food Bank, and a member of the Google Health Advisory Council. He was appointed to The White House Commission on Complementary and Alternative Medicine Policy and elected to the California Academy of Medicine. He is Chair of the PepsiCo Blue Ribbon Advisory Board and the Safeway Advisory Council on Health and Nutrition and consults directly with the CEO's of McDonald's and Del Monte Foods to make more healthful foods and to provide health education to their customers in this country and worldwide.

He has received several awards, including the 1994 Outstanding Young Alumnus Award from the University of Texas, Austin, the University of California, Berkeley, "National Public Health Hero" award, the Jan J. Kellermann Memorial Award for distinguished contribution in the field of cardiovascular disease prevention from the International Academy of Cardiology, a Presidential Citation from the American Psychological Association, the Beckmann Medal from the German Society for Prevention and Rehabilitation of Cardiovascular Diseases, the "Pioneer in Integrative Medicine" award from California Pacific Medical Center, the "Excellence in Integrative Medicine" award from the Heal Breast Cancer Foundation, the Golden Plate Award from the American Academy of Achievement, a U.S. Army Surgeon General Medal, and the Bravewell Collaborative Pioneer of Integrative Medicine award. Dr. Ornish has been a physician consultant to The White House and to several bipartisan members of the U.S. Congress. He is listed in *Who's Who in Healthcare and Medicine, Who's Who in America,* and *Who's Who in the World.*

Dr. Ornish was recognized as "one of the most interesting people of 1996" by *People* magazine, featured in the "TIME 100" issue on integrative medicine, and chosen by *LIFE* magazine as "one of the 50 most influential members of his generation."

Alan P. Pearson, OD, PhD, received his doctorate of optometry in 1992 from the Pacific University College of Optometry and a master of education with emphasis on visual processes in education in 1993 from that same institution.

He received his doctorate in psychology in 2005 from Saybrook Graduate School and Research Institute. He is the chief clinical officer for Developmental Vision Associates, PLLC, Bellevue, Washington. His research interests lie in collaborative systems for interdisciplinary service delivery models.

Marc Pilisuk, PhD, is a retired professor of psychology from the University of California at Davis and is currently a faculty member of the Saybrook Graduate School and Research Institute. He has conducted extensive research, including heading various research projects for Kaiser Permanente. He is the author of numerous articles and books.

Annette Ridenour is founder and president of Aesthetics, Inc., a multidisciplinary design firm creating healing environments since 1980. Annette is a nationally recognized specialist in interior design, wayfinding, art, and music for healthcare and is a highly sought after consultant and lecturer. She is currently authoring books on wayfinding and evidence-based art programs.

Wayne Ruga, PhD, founder and president of the CARITAS Project, is an internationally recognized healthcare architect. Now in the fourth decade of his practice, his distinguished work has produced many changes in the current system, with bold, pioneering, strategic, practical, and tangible demonstrations of how the environment can be used more effectively to improve health.

Ilene A. Serlin, PhD, ADTR, is a clinical psychologist and registered dance/movement therapist. She is the founder and director of Union Street Health Associates and the Arts Medicine Program at California Pacific Medical Center. She is a fellow of the American Psychological Association, past president and council representative of the Division of Humanistic Psychology of the American Psychological Association, on the editorial boards of *The Arts in Psychotherapy,* the *Journal of Dance Therapy,* and the *Journal of Humanistic Psychology,* and has taught and published widely in the United States and abroad. Dr. Serlin's approach draws on her extensive background of training and experience in dance and the arts, Gestalt and depth psychotherapy, and behavioral medicine. She has been dancing for 40 years and trained in Labanotation with Irmgard Bartenieff. She studied and taught with Laura Perls at the New York Gestalt Institute, did her predoctoral internship at the Children's Clinic of the C. G. Jung Institute of Los Angeles, and taught at the University of California, Los Angeles, Lesley University, Saybrook Graduate School, and the California School of Professional Psychology.

Steven E. Stark, JD, LHCRM, is a 1985 graduate of the University of Miami School of Law. He has an undergraduate bachelor's degree in business administration and holds licensure (inactive) as a Florida certified public accountant. From 1985 to October 2004, he was an attorney (shareholder) in a private law firm in Miami. He practiced primarily in the area of torts and insurance defense, with specialization in medical malpractice defense and health law. He holds specialty certification from the Florida Bar Board of Legal Specialization and Education in health law and appellate law. He is also a Florida licensed healthcare risk manager. Since 2004, he has held the position of executive director of the Office of Patient Protection and Risk Prevention at the University of Miami Miller School of Medicine.

Barbara W. K. Yee, PhD, is professor at the University of Hawaii, a fellow of the American Psychological Association and Gerontological Society of America, and appointed to the National Institutes of Health Advisory Committee on Women's Health Research. She has examined how acculturation, gender, and health literacy influence chronic disease health beliefs and lifestyle practices among southeast Asians and Pacific Islanders in the United States.

ABOUT THE ADVISERS

Laura Barbanel, EdD, ABPP, served as professor and program head of the graduate program in the School Psychology at Brooklyn College of the City University of New York for many years. She also served as deputy dean for graduate studies for the School of Education at Brooklyn College. Dr. Barbanel is currently in private practice in Brooklyn, New York. She works with adults and children, couples, and families.

Dr. Barbanel is a fellow of the American Psychological Association (APA) and a diplomate of the American Board of Professional Psychology. She has served in a number of elected and appointed positions in the APA, on its board of directors, and currently on the Committee for the Advancement of Practice. She is president-elect of Division 42, the division of independent practice. In this capacity, she has established a Task Force on Health Care for the Whole Person, which focuses on the collaboration of psychologists with physicians in the delivery of healthcare.

William Benda, MD, FACEP, FAAEM, received his professional training at Duke University, University of Miami School of Medicine, Harbor-UCLA Medical Center, and the Program in Integrative Medicine at the University of Arizona. His research and clinical work has focused on patients with breast cancer, animal-assisted therapy, and physician health and well-being. He was principal investigator on two National Center for Complementary and Alternative Medicine–funded investigations of therapeutic horseback riding in the treatment of children with cerebral palsy and is currently extending this research to the field of pediatric autism. Benda is a co-founder of the National Integrative Medicine Council, a nonprofit organization for which he has served as director of medical and public affairs. He is an editor, contributor, and medical advisory board member for a number of conventional and alternative medicine journals and has lectured extensively on a variety of topics in the integrative arena.

Lillian Comas-Diaz, PhD, is the executive director of the Transcultural Mental Health Institute, a clinical professor at the George Washington University Department of Psychiatry and Behavioral Sciences, and a private practitioner in Washington, DC. The former director of the American Psychological Association's Office of Ethnic Minority Affairs, Comas-Diaz was also the director of the Yale University Department of Psychiatry Hispanic Clinic. She is the senior editor of two textbooks: *Clinical Guidelines in Cross-Cultural Mental Health* and *Women of Color: Integrating Ethnic and Gender Identities in Psychotherapy.* Additionally, Comas-Diaz is the founding editor in chief of the American Psychological Association Division 45 official journal, *Cultural Diversity and Ethnic Minority Psychology.* She is a member of numerous editorial boards and currently is an associate editor of *American Psychologist.*

Rita Dudley-Grant, PhD, MPH, ABPP, is a psychologist currently serving as clinical director of Virgin Islands Behavioral Services, a system of residential services for emotionally disturbed and behaviorally disordered adolescents. She has published and presented extensively on child and adolescent mental health and substance abuse both locally and nationally. A practicing Nichiren SGI Buddhist for the past 26 years, she has presented on Buddhism and psychology as well as spirituality at meetings of the American Psychological Association since 1998. Dudley-Grant is co-editor of *Psychology and Buddhism: From Individual to Global Community.*

Jeffrey E. Evans, PhD, is clinical associate professor in the Department of Physical Medicine and Rehabilitation, Division of Rehabilitation Psychology and Neuropsychology, University of Michigan where he treats patients with brain injuries and other conditions. He also holds an appointment in the Residential College at U of M where he has taught courses on the psychology of creativity, psychology of consciousness, and brain and mind since the 1970s. His dissertation, "The Dancer from the Dance: Meaning and Creating in Modern Dance Choreography" (1980), is a life historical exploration of creative style. Recent research includes executive mental processes involved in task switching.

Joseph S. Geller, JD, has been active in policy-making, government relations, and community service for many years. He was elected mayor of the City of North Bay Village, Florida, in 2004 and was reelected in 2006. He previously served North Bay Village as an interim city attorney in 2003. He was chair of the Dade County Democratic Party from 1989 to December 2000. He also served as a member of the Democratic National Committee. He was an attorney for the Gore campaign during the recount litigation and represented former Attorney General Janet Reno in regard to the gubernatorial primary in 2002 and the John Kerry campaign in 2004. Geller is a partner in the Hollywood, Florida, law firm of Geller, Geller, Fisher & Garfinkel, LLP. The partners specialize in governmental relations, real estate, land use, civil litigation, municipal law, administrative and appellate practice, and corporate practice. Geller is admitted to practice in the Supreme Court of the State of Florida, the United States District Court, Southern District of Florida, and the United States Court of Appeals for the Eleventh Circuit.

Marjorie S. Greenberg, MA, is chief of the Classifications and Public Health Data Standards staff at the National Center for Health Statistics (NCHS), Centers for Disease Control and Prevention, Department of Health and Human Services (DHHS). Greenberg, who has been with NCHS since 1982, also serves as executive secretary to the National Committee on Vital and Health Statistics, which is the external advisory committee to DHHS on health information policy, and as head of the World Health Organization Collaborating Center for the Family of International Classifications for North America. Her areas of interest and expertise include health data standardization, uniform health data sets, health classifications, data policy development, and evaluation policy. She received her bachelor's degree from Wellesley College and a master's degree from Harvard University.

Stanislav Grof, MD, is a psychiatrist with more than fifty years of experience in research of nonordinary states of consciousness. He has served as principal investigator in a psychedelic research program at the Psychiatric Research Institute in Prague, Czechoslovakia; chief of psychiatric research at the Maryland Psychiatric Research Center; assistant professor of psychiatry at the Johns Hopkins University; and scholar-in-residence at the Esalen Institute. He is professor of psychology at the California Institute of Integral Studies and Pacifica Graduate Institute, conducts professional training programs in holotropic breathwork and transpersonal psychology, and gives lectures and seminars worldwide. He is one of the founders and chief theoreticians of transpersonal psychology. He has contributed 18 books and more than 130 papers to the professional literature. Among his books are *Psychology* *of the Future, The Ultimate Journey, When the Impossible Happens, The Cosmic Game,* and *The Stormy Search for the Self* (with Chr istina Grof). His Web site is www.holotropic.com.

Gay Powell Hanna, PhD, MFA, is the executive director of the Society for the Arts in Healthcare. Through faculty positions at Florida State University and the University of South Florida (USF) from 1987 to 2002, Hanna directed VSA arts of Florida, an affiliate of the John F. Kennedy Center for the Performing Arts, providing arts education programs for people with disabilities including people with chronic illness. In 2001, she established the Florida Center for Creative Aging at the Florida Policy Exchange Center on Aging at USF to address quality of life issues. A contributing author to numerous articles and books, including the *Fundamentals of Arts Management,* 4th edition, published by the Arts Extension Service of University of Massachusetts Amherst, Hanna is noted for her expertise in accessibility and universal design. In addition, she is a practicing artist who maintains an active studio with work in private and corporate collections through the southeastern United States.

Margaret Heldring, PhD, is a clinical psychologist whose career spans independent practice to public policy. She has served as a clinical assistant professor in family medicine at the University of Washington and senior health advisors to former U.S. Senators Bill Bradley and Paul Wellstone. In 2000, she founded and is president of a national health policy nonprofit organization, America's Health Together (AHT). Funded by the Robert Wood Johnson Foundation, AHT led a groundbreaking partnership after 9/11 to investigate the mental health effects of that disaster and to build capacity in primary healthcare to respond to natural and manmade disasters. AHT is currently working to strengthen philanthropic activity in mental health, both domestically and globally.

James G. Kahn, MD, MPH, is a professor of health policy and epidemiology at the University of California, San Francisco, in the Institute for Health Policy Studies. Kahn is an expert in policy modeling in healthcare, cost-effectiveness analysis, and evidence-based medicine. His work focuses on the use of cost-effectiveness analysis to inform decision-making in public health and medicine. Kahn and colleagues recently published a study in *Health Affairs* entitled "The Cost of Health Insurance Administration in California: Insurer, Physician, and Hospital Estimates." This is the first study to quantify U.S. healthcare administration costs by setting (i.e., insurer, hospital, and physician groups) and within setting by functional department (e.g., billing). It found that insurance-related administration represents at least 21 percent of physician and hospital care funded through private insurance. The research led to the following in

Harper's Index: "Estimated amount the U.S. would save each year on paperwork if it adopted single-payer healthcare: $161,000,000,000" (http://harpers.org/HarpersIndex2006-02.html). Kahn was the leader of a team of Physicians for a National Health Program physicians who submitted a single-payer proposal for the California Health Care Options project.

Gwendolyn Puryear Keita, PhD, is the executive director of the Public Interest Directorate of the American Psychological Association, where she had previously served as director of the Women's Programs Office for 18 years. She has written extensively and made numerous presentations on women's issues, particularly in the areas of women's health and women and depression, and on topics related to work, stress, and health. She has convened three conferences on psychosocial and behavioral factors in women's health and is coauthor of *Health Care and Women: Psychological, Social and Behavioral Influences.* Keita was instrumental in developing the new field of occupational health psychology, has convened six international conferences on occupational stress and health, and coauthored several books and journal articles on the subject, including *Work and Well-Being: An Agenda for the 1990s* (1992), *Job Stress in a Changing Workforce: Investigating Gender, Diversity, and Family Issues* (1994), and *Job Stress Interventions* (1995). Keita has presented before Congress on depression, violence, and other issues.

Kenneth Kushner, PhD, received his PhD in psychology from the University of Michigan in 1977. He is a professor in the Department of Family Medicine of the University of Wisconsin. He has practiced Zen for over 25 years and is a Zen Master in the Chozen-ji lineage. He is founder of the Chozen-ji Betsuin/International Zen Dojo of Wisconsin and the author of *One Arrow, One Life: Zen, Archery and Enlightenment.*

William Mauk, MBA, has a long history in public service and in the private healthcare and administrative consulting arena. Graduating from the University of California, Los Angeles, with an MBA degree in finance, Mauk has worked with the Agency for International Development. He was appointed by President Carter to serve as deputy comptroller of that agency in 1977 and in 1979 by President Carter as deputy administrator of the Small Business Administration. Beginning in the 1980s, he was senior vice president of administration for the John Alden Life Insurance Company. From 1995 to 2002, he was chief executive officer for the Health Maintenance Organization, Neighborhood Health Partnership. Since that time he has been active as a business and political consultant. He is currently CEO of VIVA Democracy, providing Internet software consultation for political campaigns.

Susan McDaniel, PhD, is professor of psychiatry and family medicine, associate chair of family medicine, and director of family programs and the Wynne Center for Family Research in Psychiatry at the University of Rochester School of Medicine and Dentistry. Her special areas of interest are behavioral health in primary care and family dynamics and genetic conditions. She is a frequent speaker at meetings of both health and mental health professionals. McDaniel is co-editor of the journal *Families, Systems & Health.* She coauthored or edited the following books: *Systems Consultation* (1986), *Family-Oriented Primary Care* (1990 and 2005), *Medical Family Therapy* (1992), *Integrating Family Therapy* (1995), *Counseling Families with Chronic Illness* (1995), *The Shared Experience of Illness* (1997), *Casebook for Integrating Family Therapy* (2001), *Primary Care Psychology* (2004), *The Biopsychosocial Approach* (2004), and *Individuals, Families, and the New Era of Genetics (2007).* Her books have been translated into seven languages.

Marc Micozzi, MD, is a physician-anthropologist who has worked to create science-based tools for the health professions to be better informed and productively engaged in the new fields of complementary and alternative (CAM) and integrative medicine. He was the founding editor-in-chief of the first U.S. journal in CAM, *Journal of Complementary and Alternative Medicine: Research on Paradigm, Practice and Policy* (1994). He organized and edited the first U.S. textbook, *Fundamentals of Complementary & Alternative Medicine* (1996), now in its third edition. In addition, he has served as series editor for Medical Guides to Complementary and Alternative Medicine with 18 titles in print on a broad range of therapies and therapeutic systems within the scope of CAM. In 1999, he edited *Current Complementary Therapies,* focusing on contemporary innovations and controversies, and *Physician's Guide to Complementary and Alternative Medicine.* In 2002, he became founding director of the Policy Institute for Integrative Medicine in Washington, DC.

Geoffrey M. Reed, PhD, is a clinical and health psychologist who, from 1995 to 2006, was assistant executive director for professional development at the American Psychological Association. He has worked with the World Health Organization (WHO) on the development and implementation of the International Classification of Functioning, Disability, and Health (ICF) since 1995. He continues to lead the development of a multidisciplinary procedural manual and guide for standardized application of the ICF with the official involvement of national professional associations representing psychology, speech-language pathology, occupational therapy, recreational therapy, physical therapy, and social work. He is senior consultant for WHO projects with the International Union of Psychological Sciences and is an international consultant on healthcare issues. He is a member of the WHO International Advisory Group for the revision of the Chapter V: Mental and Behavioural Disorders of the International Classification of Diseases and Related Health Problems. He lives in Madrid, Spain.

Elaine Sims, AB, MA, is the director of the University of Michigan Hospitals and Healthcare Centers Gifts of Art program. She has worked in arts in healthcare since 1990. Her areas of expertise include the visual and performing arts, healing gardens, caring for the caregiver initiatives, as well as the full spectrum of arts in healthcare offerings including art cart programs, bedside music, artists-in-residence, medical school arts curriculum, and running a full medical center orchestra. Sims is serving her third term on the board of the Society for the Arts in Healthcare (SAHCS). She is also a consultant for the SAHCS consulting service. Sims is a member of the Ann Arbor Commission for Art in Public Places. She also serves on the University of Michigan Health System Environment of Care Committee and the Interior Design Standards Committee. She particularly enjoys collaborating with university and community partners in exploring and promoting the world of arts in healthcare.

Louise Sundararajan, PhD, received her doctorate in history of religions from Harvard University and her EdD in counseling psychology from Boston University. Currently a forensic psychologist, she was president of the International Society for the Study of Human Ideas on Ultimate Reality and Meaning. A member of American Psychological Association and the International Society for Research on Emotions, she has authored over forty articles in refereed journals and books, on topics ranging from Chinese poetics to alexithymia.

Tobi Zausner, PhD, who has an interdisciplinary PhD in art and psychology, is also an art historian and an award-winning visual artist with works in major museums and private collections around the world. Zausner writes and lectures widely on the psychology of art and teaches at the C. G. Jung Foundation in New York. She is an officer on the board of ACTS (Arts, Crafts, and Theatre Safety), a nonprofit organization investigating health hazards in the arts, and was chair of art history in the Society for Chaos Theory in Psychology and the Life Sciences. Zausner is writing a book on physical illness and the creative process of visual artists titled *When Walls Become Doorways: Creativity and the Transforming Illness.*

CUMULATIVE INDEX